HIP
REPLACEMENT

HIP REPLACEMENT

Current Trends and Controversies

edited by

Raj K. Sinha

University of Pittsburgh Medical Center
Pittsburgh, Pennsylvania

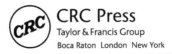

CRC Press
Taylor & Francis Group
Boca Raton London New York

CRC Press is an imprint of the
Taylor & Francis Group, an **informa** business

CRC Press
Taylor & Francis Group
6000 Broken Sound Parkway NW, Suite 300
Boca Raton, FL 33487-2742

© 2002 by Taylor & Francis Group, LLC
CRC Press is an imprint of Taylor & Francis Group, an Informa business

First issued in paperback 2019

No claim to original U.S. Government works

ISBN 13: 978-0-367-44699-4 (pbk)
ISBN 13: 978-0-8247-0789-7 (hbk)

Visit the Taylor & Francis Web site at
http://www.taylorandfrancis.com

and the CRC Press Web site at
http://www.crcpress.com

Preface

Total Hip Replacement: Current Trends and Controversies was undertaken to address several shortcomings that I perceive in the cast of currently available orthopaedics textbooks. I have had the good fortune to be invited to contribute chapters to many textbooks, as well as the overwhelming task of being editor of a 250-page, 19-chapter section of a 1000-page text. From these invaluable experiences, I have been struck by the multidisciplinary nature of orthopaedic medicine, from research to clinical practice. No other subspecialty calls equally upon surgeons, internists, trainers, physical therapists, molecular biologists, cell biologists, geneticists, biomaterials scientists, and biomechanical engineers as orthopaedics does. Yet, despite working closely with members of related disciplines, we are all guilty of being unfamiliar with the true nature and tenets of one another's work.

Open any of the currently popular orthopaedic texts. You will find chapters written by biomechanical engineers that are lauded by other engineers yet leave the clinical practitioner perplexed as to how these principles apply to performing a hip replacement using the available implants and instruments. In the same volume, you will find chapters written by well-known surgeons who discuss at great length the clinical results of fracture fixation devices and methods that violate the biomechanical principles discussed elsewhere in the same text. Basic science sections will catalog hundreds of experimental papers, differentiating the fine nuances of one animal model versus another, or the limitations of one cell culture system versus another, but make cursory mention of human application. The result is that clinicians deride the basic science sections as being impractical and boring, while scientists deride the clinical sections as being superficial and nonfactual.

To address this shortcoming, I arranged for several chapters of *Total Hip Replacement: Current Trends and Controversies* to be written by scientists and surgeons who work closely together. My hope was that multidisciplinary research teams would be put in the position of truly determining where they agree and disagree on experimental approaches and relevance to clinical orthopaedics. The result would be a chapter that was equally satisfactory to the clinical and basic science faculty. Each of these chapters contains a background section that details the current scientific understanding of a particular topic followed by an explanation of how that knowledge has been applied clinically, and with what results. This structure is particularly true for the chapters on alternate bearings, biologic fixation, and osteolysis. In these chapters the contributors have succeeded in assembling information of significant value for scientists and surgeons alike.

Another common pitfall for authors writing primarily clinical chapters is the compulsion to exhaustively catalog the previous hundred years of literature in order to provide background information. Typically, authors then will explain their preferred method, never referring to how the literature they have just outlined helped them choose their techniques. Rather than ask authors to provide complete lists of the pertinent literature, I asked them to describe their historic experience with a particular technique, and explain how they have evolved to the current technique employed. I think the chapters by Drs. Cameron, Bourne, Gross, and Masri et al. accomplish this objective quite well. In addition, since most readers will recognize these authors' names, they can import their ideas into their own operating rooms with confidence.

A third common area of obvious improvement in our literature is the discussion of new and emerging technologies. In most texts, the future of a particular field receives scant attention, often just a paragraph or two at the end of a long chapter. I wanted readers of this book to become familiar with some new techniques that I believe will have wide-ranging impact on the future of hip surgery. Specifically, the chapter on surgical navigation and computer assistance, by DiGioia and associates, nicely explains these technologies, their current limitations, and possible future impact. The reader will become versed with unfamiliar terms and concepts that in the future will become commonplace. Similarly, although the chapter on hip arthroscopy would seem out of place in a book on hip replacement, I included it to familiarize surgeons with techniques and concepts that are being applied more commonly to arthroplasty. I believe that hip arthroscopy will have a future role in the implantation of hip components, the evaluation of failing components, and the treatment of failed components. Possible applications may include minimally invasive implantation of components or targeted delivery of drugs or growth factors. Thus, this chapter should also be perceived as an indicator of things to come in arthroplasty.

Finally, I also wanted to put my personal bias somewhere in the text. I chose the chapters on cemented stems and revision stems—my residents, fellows, and partners know that I have very strong feelings about both these topics. Specifically, since I use cement in less than 3% of the hip replacements I perform, I provide the cynical view of cement, one that is wholly contrarian to the NIH consensus panel. The literature generally conveys the message that cement is reliable, durable, and forgiving. I disagree. I have underscored the importance of the technical details of cement implantation, and the various design and insertion details, all of which must be reproduced every time to achieve an adequate cement mantle. Despite my bias, I think the chapter presents a well-balanced view of our current state of understanding of cement utilization. Similarly, I have been an enthusiast of modular stems for revision arthroplasty. In Chapter 8, I compare modular stems with monoblock stems, and I think this chapter also presents a balanced view.

No text that desires to be timely can be comprehensive in all aspects of arthroplasty. I specifically chose to stay away from the complications of hip replacement, which could easily comprise an entire book of the same length as this. Instead, I asked Dr. Saluja to describe how to avoid these complications through proper preoperative planning. In addition, since the planning of this text began, minimally invasive surgery has appeared as an emerging trend. We could not examine this technology here; it will be the subject of future chapters in future texts.

In closing, I would like to thank the many people without whom this project never would have reached fruition: all the chapter authors who have allowed us to borrow their intellectual property; at Marcel Dekker, Inc., Geoffrey Greenwood, who originally approached me and gave me tremendous leeway in how I put together this book, and Ted Allen and Dana Bigelow, who kept pushing me forward toward completion; at the University of Pittsburgh, my administrative assistants Lou Duerring and Catherine Zerbach, who kept track of all my communications with authors and publishers, and who tracked the authors' progress; my wife Kavita, who amazes me in her effortless adjustments to the inconsistencies of a surgeon's schedule, and my son Abhishek, who is more understanding of my commitment to my patients than any 12-year-old should ever have to be.

Raj K. Sinha

Contents

Contributors

Harlan C. Amstutz, M.D. Professor Emeritus, University of California–Los Angeles, and Medical Director, Joint Replacement Institute at Orthopaedic Hospital, Los Angeles, California

William L. Bargar Sutter Orthopedic Center, Sacramento, California

Paul E. Beaulé, M.D., F.R.C.S.C. Assistant Clinical Professor, University of California–Los Angeles, and Joint Replacement Institute at Orthopaedic Hospital, Los Angeles, California

Robert B. Bourne, M.D. University of Western Ontario, London, Ontario, Canada

Hugh U. Cameron, M.B., Ch.B., F.R.C.S.(C) University of Toronto, Toronto, Ontario, Canada

Steven M. Dellose, M.D. Department of Orthopedic Surgery, University of Pittsburgh Medical Center, Pittsburgh, Pennsylvania

Rohit R. Dhir St. Luke's Hospital Medical Center, Milwaukee, Wisconsin

Anthony M. DiGioia III, M.D. Center for Medical Robotics and Computer Assisted Surgery, The Western Pennsylvania Hospital and Carnegie Mellon University, Pittsburgh, Pennsylvania

Clive P. Duncan, M.D., F.R.C.S.(C)   Professor and Chairman, Department of Orthopaedics, University of British Columbia, Vancouver, British Columbia, Canada

David J. Dunlop, M.B., Ch.B., F.R.C.S.(Tr&Orth)   Clinical and Research Fellow, Division of Reconstructive Orthopaedics, Department of Orthopaedics, University of British Columbia, Vancouver, British Columbia, Canada

Donald S. Garbuz, M.D., F.R.C.S.(C)   Assistant Professor, Division of Reconstructive Orthopaedics, Department of Orthopaedics, University of British Columbia, Vancouver, British Columbia, Canada

Nelson V. Greidanus, M.D., F.R.C.S.(C)   Assistant Professor, Division of Reconstructive Orthopaedics, Department of Orthopaedics, University of British Columbia, Vancouver, British Columbia, Canada

Allan E. Gross, M.D., F.R.C.S.(C)   Professor of Surgery, University of Toronto, and Division of Orthopaedic Surgery, Mount Sinai Hospital, Toronto, Ontario, Canada

Noreen J. Hickok, Ph.D.   Cell & Tissue Engineering Program, Department of Orthopaedic Surgery, Thomas Jefferson University, Philadelphia, Pennsylvania

Gun-Il Im, M.D.*   Department of Orthopaedic Surgery, Massachusetts General Hospital and Harvard Medical School, Boston, Massachusetts

Branislav Jaramaz, Ph.D.   Center for Medical Robotics and Computer Assisted Surgery, The Western Pennsylvania Hospital and Carnegie Mellon University, Pittsburgh, Pennsylvania

Andrew H. Kim, M.D.   Department of Orthopedic Surgery, University of Pittsburgh Medical Center, Pittsburgh, Pennsylvania

Steven M. Kurtz, Ph.D.   Principal Engineer, Exponent Inc.; Director, Implant Research Center, Drexel University; and Department of Orthopaedic Surgery, Thomas Jefferson University, Philadelphia, Pennsylvania

---

Current affiliation: Department of Orthopaedic Surgery, Hallym University Hospital, Chunchon, South Korea.

Michele Marcolongo, Ph.D. Department of Materials Science, School of Biomedical Engineering, Science and Health Systems, Drexel University, Philadelphia, Pennsylvania

Bassam A. Masri, M.D., F.R.C.S.(C) Associate Professor and Head, Division of Reconstructive Orthopaedics, Department of Orthopaedics, University of British Columbia, Vancouver, British Columbia, Canada

James Moody, M.S. Center for Medical Robotics and Computer Assisted Surgery, The Western Pennsylvania Hospital and Carnegie Mellon University, Pittsburgh, Pennsylvania

Orhun K. Muratoglu, Ph.D. Department of Orthopaedic Surgery, Harvard Medical School; Department of Chemical Engineering, Massachusetts Institute of Technology; and Orthopaedic Biomechanics and Biomaterials Laboratory, Massachusetts General Hospital, Boston, Massachusetts

James T. Ninomiya, M.D., M.S. Department of Orthopaedic Surgery, Medical College of Wisconsin, Milwaukee, Wisconsin

Frederic Picard, M.D. Center for Medical Robotics and Computer Assisted Surgery, The Western Pennsylvania Hospital and Carnegie Mellon University, Pittsburgh, Pennsylvania

Anton Plakseychuk, M.D. Center for Medical Robotics and Computer Assisted Surgery, The Western Pennsylvania Hospital and Carnegie Mellon University, Pittsburgh, Pennsylvania

James J. Purtill, M.D. Department of Orthopaedic Surgery, Thomas Jefferson University, Philadelphia, Pennsylvania

Harry E. Rubash, M.D. Department of Orthopaedic Surgery, Massachusetts General Hospital and Harvard Medical School, Boston, Massachusetts

Rajit Saluja Department of Orthopedic Surgery, St. Luke's Hospital Medical Center, Milwaukee, Wisconsin

Rajiv K. Sethi, M.D. Department of Orthopaedic Surgery, Massachusetts General Hospital and Harvard Medical School, Boston, Massachusetts

Arun S. Shanbhag, Ph.D.   Department of Orthopaedic Surgery, Massachusetts General Hospital and Harvard Medical School, Boston, Massachusetts

Raj K. Sinha, M.D.   Department of Orthopedic Surgery, University of Pittsburgh Medical Center, Pittsburgh, Pennsylvania

Rocky S. Tuan, Ph.D.   Cartilage Biology and Orthopaedics Branch, National Institute of Arthritis and Musculoskeletal and Skin Diseases, National Institutes of Health, Bethesda, Maryland

HIP
REPLACEMENT

1

Alternate Bearing Surfaces in Hip Replacement

Orhun K. Muratoglu
*Harvard Medical School, Massachusetts Institute of Technology,
and Massachusetts General Hospital, Boston, Massachusetts*

Steven M. Kurtz
*Exponent, Inc., Drexel University, and Thomas Jefferson University,
Philadelphia, Pennsylvania*

I. INTRODUCTION

During total hip arthroplasty, both the femoral and acetabular bearing surfaces are surgically replaced with metallic, polymeric, and/or ceramic components. Throughout the twentieth century, many different combinations of these materials have been explored as candidate bearing surfaces for total hip arthroplasty. Metal-on-metal total hip replacements were first implanted by Wiles in the 1930s (1) and later developed in the 1950s and 1960s by pioneering surgeons like McKee and Ring (2). In 1958, Charnley introduced a "low-friction arthroplasty" based on the principle of a metallic femoral component articulating against a polymeric acetabular component, and in 1970, Boutin developed the first ceramic-on-ceramic total hip replacement (Table 1). Charnley's hard-on-soft bearing concept eventually dominated the other hard-on-hard bearing alternatives.

Today the most widely accepted *bearing couple* (i.e., combination of bearing materials for the hip joint) consists of a femoral head fabricated from cobalt chromium molybdenum (cobalt chrome or CoCr) alloy articulating against a polymeric component fabricated from ultrahigh molecular-weight polyethylene (UHMWPE). The use of the CoCr/UHMWPE bearing couple has provided consistent results in total hip arthroplasties around the

1

Table 1 First-Generation Prostheses and Orthopedic Bearing Configurations

Date	Prosthesis	Bearing Materials	Fixation Method	Reference
1923–1938	Smith-Petersen mold arthroplasty	Glass, Viscaloid, Pyrex, Bakelite, CoCr	None	21
1938	Wiles metal-metal	SS/SS	Screws	1
1950	Judet hemiprosthesis	PMMA femoral head	Steel stem	22
1956–1960	McKee	CoCr/CoCr	Screw-type implant design	2
1958–1962	Charnley low-friction arthroplasty	CoCr/PTFE	Acrylic cement	15, 26, 170
1962	Charnley low-friction arthroplasty	CoCr/UHMWPE	Acrylic cement	26, 170
1962–1966	McKee-Farrar	CoCr/CoCr	Acrylic cement	2
1964–1968	Ring	CoCr/CoCr	Uncemented, screw-type implant design	171
1970	Boutin	Al_2O_3/Al_2O_3	Uncemented design	92
1971	Oonishi	CoCr/UHMWPE (1000 kGy)	Acrylic cement	76
1977	Shikata	Al_2O_3/UHMWPE	Acrylic cement	80
1978	Grobbelaar	CoCr/UHMWPE (100 kGy)	Acrylic cement	82

KEY: SS = stainless steel; PMMA = polymethylmethacrylate; CoCr = cobalt-chromium-molybdenum; PTFE = polytetrafluoroethylene; UHMWPE = ultrahigh-molecular-weight polyethylene.

world for the past four decades. In 1998, an estimated 1.4 million UHMWPE components were implanted worldwide, with approximately half of these bearings being implanted in the hip. Based on discussions with major orthopaedic manufacturers, at most 200,000 metal-on-metal or ceramic-on-ceramic components have been implanted in patients worldwide between 1988 and 2000, corresponding to less than 10% of total hip replacements during the same time period (3). Therefore, the overwhelming majority (over 90%) of total hip arthroplasties currently in service throughout the world include an UHMWPE or a modified UHMWPE component and are based upon Charnley's original concept of hard-on-soft bearing.

Despite the recognized success and worldwide acceptance of total hip arthroplasty, wear of the UHMWPE component is a major obstacle limiting the longevity of these reconstructions. In this type of a total hip replacement, which historically wears at an average rate of approximately 0.1 mm per year, it would take a century to erode through a 10-mm-thick UHMWPE component. However, at this wear rate, 100 million UHMWPE particles (assumed diameter of 1 μm) are liberated into the joint space on a daily basis. It is now well established that particulate debris generated from the articulating surfaces initiates a cascade of adverse tissue response leading to osteolysis and in certain cases loosening of the components (4–8). Extending the longevity of total joint replacements using alternative bearing technologies with improved wear behavior has been the subject of ongoing research in the orthopaedic community.

Since the 1970s, researchers have attempted to improve the tribological characteristics of UHMWPE by modifying the polymer's structure, with the ultimate goal of improving the clinical performance of hip bearings. In the 1970s, carbon fiber–reinforced UHMWPE (Poly-II™) was clinically introduced for its potentially improved wear resistance (9), and a high-pressure recrystallized form of UHMWPE (Hylamer™) was clinically introduced in the 1980s for its improved creep resistance (9). Most recently, in the late 1990s, numerous research centers around the world confirmed that crosslinking of UHMWPE—whether by radiation, peroxide, or silane chemistry— can substantially improve the wear performance of the material in hip joint simulators (10–14). Based on these in vitro analyses, a number of radiation-crosslinked materials have been clinically introduced in the late 1990s.

A. Alternative Bearings for Long-Term Survivorship

Alternative bearings are needed not only to reduce the particulate debris burden and osteolysis but also to improve the survivorship of total joint replacements for younger and more active patients. Charnley originally intended total hip replacement primarily for patients who were disabled by rheumatoid arthritis and severe osteoarthritis (15). The surgery was initially restricted to patients over 65 and middle-aged patients were considered "occasionally" in the case of bilateral arthritis. Despite his restrictions on patient age (and indirectly activity level), Charnley predicted that neither surgeons nor engineers would ever make an artificial hip joint which would last 30 years and at some time in this period enable the patient to engage in athletic activities. However, today total joint arthroplasty is routinely performed on middle-aged patients, and both surgeons and engineers have recognized the need to assess the implications of a wide variety of patient activity levels on the outcome of the total joint arthroplasty. For example, in the UCLA Activity-Level Rating recently proposed by Zahiri and colleagues (16), the maximum score is assigned to patients who "regularly participate in *impact sports*, such as jogging, tennis, skiing, acrobatics, ballet, heavy labor, or backpacking."

In a recent review article describing the multiple factors that can influence wear *in vivo*, Schmalzried et al. (17) noted that "clinical rates of wear have traditionally been expressed with the use of time as the denominator. This has been done for reasons of convenience, not accuracy . . . the wear of a prosthetic hip is a function of use or the number of cycles, it is not simply a function of time." As a result of the difference in activity levels in young and elderly patients, it is not appropriate to compare the wear rates among studies with different patient demographics. Although age, coupled with diagnosis, is a significant predictor of (and surrogate for) activity level, research using pedometers to directly measure the number of steps taken by total hip replacement patients has shown a 40-fold variation in activity level among different patients (17). Therefore, "high demand" patients may be found in both younger and older candidates for total hip replacement.

Even though the demands placed upon total joint replacements by patients have altered considerably since the introduction of the procedure, the aspirations for the longevity of the prosthesis have remained unchanged. Members of the orthopaedic community still strive to create an artificial hip joint that will last 30 years, even for middle-aged patients who want an active lifestyle. However, as recent outcome studies have shown (18,19), the long-term survivorship for total joint replacements decreases after 10 years of implantation. The most broad-based studies of total hip survivorship available in the literature have been conducted using the Swedish Total Hip Replacement Registry. Based on the most recent publication of findings, the register contains the records of 169,419 primary procedures and 13,561 revisions conducted between 1979 and 1998. The registry is used to track the long-term outcome for specific implants, surgeons, surgical centers, and patient groups across Sweden. Researchers have found that "the younger and more active patients are at greater risk [of revision] in all diagnostic groups. This is especially true for patients younger than 55 years of age" (19) (Figure 1).

Therefore, the young, active patient presents a challenge for the conventional CoCr/UHMWPE bearing couple in terms of extending the survivorship into the second decade of service, and most preferably into the third.

B. Overview of Biomaterials and Alternative Bearings

Alternative bearings are intended to significantly reduce or minimize wear at the articulating surface, thereby reducing the risk of debris-mediated bone loss and aseptic loosening. Four classes of bearing materials are discussed throughout this chapter: conventional UHMWPE, UHMWPE with elevated crosslink density (or "highly crosslinked" UHMWPE), CoCr alloys, and ceramics. These four categories of materials are not intended to comprise an exhaustive or all-inclusive list of potentially useful candidates for total hip replacements. A variety of coating and ion implantation technologies are currently under investigation for improved wear resistance in total hip replacements. For a detailed overview of coatings and ion implantation techniques in orthopaedic bearing materials, the reader is referred to a recent comprehensive review (20). However, the majority of these advanced coating materials technologies are still under development. Consequently, we focus our attention in this chapter on the four principal biomaterials used in the articulation of total hip replacements in terms of articulating couples: (a) the conventional articulating couple of CoCr/UHMWPE, (b) UHMWPE with elevated crosslink density articulating with CoCr or ceramic femoral heads, (c) ceramic on conventional UHMWPE and ceramic-on-ceramic articulations, and (d) metal-on-metal articulations. The first material, conventional UHMWPE, will be considered as the reference bearing material with the greatest clinical relevance due to its currently implanted patient base.

II. THE CoCr/UHMWPE ARTICULATION

This section focuses on the development of conventional UHMWPE as the bearing material of choice for total joint replacements.

A. Precursors to the CoCr/UHMWPE Articulation (Pre-1958)

The history of alternative bearings cannot be fully extricated from discussions of biological fixation and the problem of loosening at the bone/implant interface (Table 1). For example, bone-implant fixation was deliberately

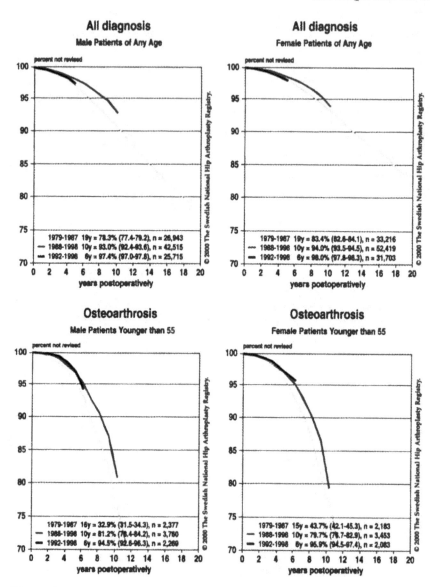

Figure 1 Survivorship of total hip arthroplasty as a function of age, based on the most recent report from the Swedish National Hip Registry. (From Ref. 19.)

avoided in the Smith-Petersen mold arthroplasty developed during the 1920s, which were intended to facilitate bone-implant articulation at the femoral as well as acetabular sides of the component (21). By the 1950s, however, a different school of thought emerged in which bone-implant fixation was now considered an important surgical priority. In 1950, the Judet brothers introduced a hemiarthroplasty consisting of a polymethylmethacrylate ball fixed at the end of a short stem (22). Although these implants provided short-term pain relief, in Charnley's view they ultimately failed after a few years due to a combination of high frictional torque at the articulating surface coupled with inadequate fixation between the short stem and the bone (15).

B. The PTFE Era of Total Hip Replacement: 1958–1962

Charnley's early experiments on joint function were directed at understanding the friction and lubrication of animal and artificial joints (23). Based primarily on a series of pendulum experiments, Charnley proposed in 1959 that polytetrafluoroethylene (PTFE) seemed "ideally suited" as a bearing material for total joint replacement because of its low coefficient of friction and biocompatibility in solid form (23). The chemical structure of PTFE is similar to that of UHMWPE with the exception that the pendant hydrogen atoms on the carbon backbone of the polymer molecule are replaced by flourine (PTFE belongs to the family of fluoropolymers). As a result, PTFE has a density of 2.2 g/cc, as opposed to 0.94 g/cc for UHMWPE. The fluorine atoms on the backbone of the molecular chain render the polymer highly resistant to chemical and thermal degradation.

The PTFE used by Charnley is often (and incorrectly) referred to in the orthopaedics literature as Teflon®, which is the trade name for a family of PTFE resins produced by DuPont (Wilmington, DE) in the United States. Charnley acetabular components were fabricated from Fluon resin produced by Imperial Chemical Industries (ICI) in Great Britain (24). When encountered in Charnley's works, the terms *Teflon, Fluon,* and *PTFE* should be interpreted as synonymous (25).

Despite its excellent lubricity and satisfactory wear performance in vitro, PTFE exhibited two major disadvantages, which were discovered only after implantation in 300 patients (26). First, the PTFE exhibited elevated wear rates in vivo of up to 0.5 mm per month (27). Second, the PTFE wear debris elicited an "intense foreign-body reaction," as Charnley elucidated by injecting two specimens of "finely divided" PTFE into his own thigh (25). Charnley also attempted to use glass-filled PTFE (under the trade name of Fluorosint) as a bearing material for total hip replacements, but despite promising in vitro test results, the composite also performed poorly in vivo (26).

The femoral head in Charnley's CoCr/PTFE implant ranged between 22.25 and 41.5 mm (27). Based on his analysis of wear of the PTFE components, Charnley made the observation that the volume of wear debris increased with the diameter of the femoral head (27). Charnley reasoned that the biological reaction to the debris was related to the wear volume (as opposed to the wear depth or penetration of the femoral head): "It would then follow that the *smallest volume* of particulate matter would be generated by using the *smallest head* which anatomical and mechanical considerations would permit" (27). Consequently, Charnley adopted a 22-mm head size in his future total hip replacement designs to reduce wear and frictional torque generated at the bone/liner interface.

C.   The UHMWPE Era: 1962–Today

UHMWPE produced by Hoechst (Oberhausen, Germany) was first widely adopted in the textile industry and distributed throughout Europe during the 1950s for use in the impact bearings of mechanical looms. Charnley used RCH 1000 for his original acetabular components starting in 1962. RCH 1000 was Hoechst's early trade name for UHMWPE. RCH designated the resin manufacturing location (RuhrCHemie AG, Oberhausen, Germany) and 1000 indicated that the polymer was UHMWPE.

A recent review summarized the evolution of changes in processing and sterilization of UHMWPE (9). Below, we describe the chemical composition and composite microstructure of UHMWPE. We have also reviewed the current trends in the sterilization, shelf life, and in vivo performance of the conventional CoCr/UHMWPE bearing couples.

1.   Chemical Composition

Notwithstanding continual evolutionary changes in the polymerization process, certain basic attributes of the polymer—namely, its excellent wear resistance, low friction, and high impact strength (relative to other polymers), which contributed to its selection for total joint replacement—have not changed substantially during the last four decades (28). UHMWPE, created by the polymerization of ethylene ($CH_2\!=\!CH_2$), is chemically one of the simplest of polymers. UHMWPE itself has the general chemical formula $(-C_2H_4-)_n$, where n is the degree of polymerization, corresponding to the number of repeating units along the polymer chain. In the case of UHMWPE, which is defined according to ISO 11542 specifications as having an average molecular weight of at least 1 million g/mol, the average degree of polymerization (n) is at least 36,000. Among the specific grades of UHMWPE used in orthopaedic applications, the average molecular weight typically ranges from 2 to 6 million g/mol.

2. Composite Microstructure

Polyethylene is a semicrystalline polymer; as such, its mechanical behavior is strongly related to its molecular weight and crystalline morphology. UHMWPE in the solid state is a two-phase material, consisting of domains of crystalline matter embedded within an amorphous phase. The crystalline phase in UHMWPE consists of rows of carbon molecules packed into lamellae, typically 10–50 nm in thickness and on the order of 10–50 μm in length. The amorphous phase consists of randomly oriented and entangled polymer chains from neighboring molecules. The amorphous phase is also traversed by tie molecules, which interconnect remote crystalline domains and provide additional resistance to mechanical deformation. Thus, at a microstructural level, UHMWPE can be considered to be a complex composite material. The complexities in microstructure of UHMWPE give rise to a range in mechanical behavior depending upon the processing, thermal and radiation exposure, storage, and prior mechanical history of the polymer. Today, over 90% of the UHMWPE used in orthopaedics is produced in the form of a fine white powder, or *resin*, which is then consolidated through ram extrusion, slab molding, or direct compression molding methods. The average properties for GUR 1020 and 1050 grades of UHMWPE, which are currently the most widely used in the orthopaedic industry, are summarized in Table 2 based on data collected by a single converter during 441 individual production lots.

3. Current Sterilization and Shelf-Life Trends

As recently as 1995, UHMWPE components were typically sterilized with a nominal dose of 25 to 40 kGy of gamma radiation in the presence of air (9). As described in detail below (Sec. III.B), gamma sterilization leads to the formation of residual free radicals, which are the precursors of oxidation-induced embrittlement (29).

Starting in the 1970s and 1980s, researchers began to document changes in the physical and chemical properties of UHMWPE components following gamma irradiation in air (30–34). Although changes in properties of UHMWPE were observed in these early studies, it was not possible to correlate the observed changes in physical or chemical properties with actual wear performance of acetabular liners in vivo. The association between physical properties and in vivo wear performance of UHMWPE still remains highly controversial, especially with regard to the clinical performance of hip implants (35).

During the 1990s, researchers were able to correlate changes in physical properties of polyethylene, such as density, with degradation of mechanical behavior during in vitro experiments (36–38). Concurrently, a se-

Table 2 Effect of UHMWPE Resin (GUR 1020 vs. GUR 1050) and Conversion Method (Ram Extrusion and Compression Molding) on physical and mechanical properties as specified by ASTM F648[a]

	GUR 1020 Resin			GUR 1050 Resin		
	ASTM F648 (Type 1)	Ram-Extruded	Compression-Molded	ASTM F648 (Type 2)	Ram-Extruded	Compression-Molded
Number of lots tested (1998–2001)		112	91		195	43
Density (kg/m³)	930–940	935 ± 1	935 ± 1	927–938	931 ± 1	931 ± 1
Yield stress (MPa)	21 (minimum)	22.3 ± 0.5	21.9 ± 0.5	19 (minimum)	21.4 ± 0.4	20.9 ± 0.4
Ultimate tensile stress (MPa)	35 (minimum)	53.8 ± 4.2	57.6 ± 4.9	27 (minimum)	51.2 ± 4.0	55.3 ± 4.5
Elongation to failure (%)	300 (minimum)	452 ± 19	458 ± 19	300 (minimum)	398 ± 19	402 ± 18
Izod impact strength, double-notched (kJ/m²)	140 (minimum)	165 ± 17	164 ± 18	73 (minimum)	117 ± 7	116 ± 10

[a]The data summarized here were compiled from a single converter based on the results for 441 individual production lots of UHMWPE produced between 1998 and 2001.

ries of studies were published with the first direct evidence of mechanical degradation in total joint replacement components, especially for knee implants (29,39,40). In light of these studies, by 1998, all of the major orthopaedic manufacturers in the United States were either sterilizing polyethylene using gamma radiation in a reduced oxygen environment (e.g., nitrogen) or sterilizing without ionizing radiation using ethylene oxide or gas plasma (9).

Today, in Europe, a consensus practice of 5-year shelf life has been adopted for medical implants so that sterility can be assured (not for concerns related to oxidation of UHMWPE). Because implants are distributed multinationally, it may be that current packaging for components sold in the United States also stipulates a 5-year shelf life. However, it should be noted that, even today, there is no U.S. standard for shelf life of UHMWPE components after sterilization in air or any other environment.

4. In Vivo Wear Performance of CoCr/UHMWPE

In a clinical setting, UHMWPE wear is typically assessed radiographically, and progresses at an average rate of 0.1 mm/year. However, there is considerable variability in clinical wear rates due to a combination of surgical, patient, and implant-related factors (41). Even when surgical and implant factors are properly controlled in a single-institution study, differences between patients give rise to a wide range in apparent wear behavior. For example, Griffith et al. (42) studied radiographic wear in 491 Charnley prostheses, all with CoCr/UHMWPE articulation and 22-mm head size. After 8.3 years of implantation, the linear wear rate was found to range from 0 mm/year (in 110 patients) to 0.18–0.34 mm/year (in 20 patients), with a mean rate of 0.07 mm/year (42). In a review of 15 clinical studies published between 1975 and 1997 (41), the average in vivo volumetric wear rate for CoCr/UHMWPE was found to be 69 ± 33 mm³/year with a 22-mm femoral head; 85 ± 33 mm³/year with a 28-mm femoral head; and 90 ± 44 mm³/year with a 32-mm femoral head.

The wide variation in clinical wear rates reported historically for CoCr/UHMWPE have led to the recent development of improved methods of radiographic wear assessment. Manual radiographic wear estimation methods were developed by Charnley (43) and Livermore (44). But more recently, semiautomated (computer-assisted) techniques have become widely available to members of the orthopaedic community (45,46). Efforts are currently under way at the American Society for Testing and Materials to standardize computerized radiographic wear measurement techniques and thereby permit improved interinstitutional comparisons of clinical wear.

III. POLYETHYLENES WITH ELEVATED CROSSLINK DENSITY

A. Background

Radiation crosslinking combined with thermal treatment has recently emerged as a technology to improve the wear and oxidation resistance of UHMWPE acetabular components (12–14). The development of this technology during the 1990s led to a series of new alternate polyethylene bearing materials with varying crosslink densities. Crosslinking is certainly not a new technology, as the majority of the conventional UHMWPE bearing surfaces have always been sterilized with gamma irradiation. The typical radiation dose range for gamma sterilization is 25–40 kGy, leading to both product sterility and some crosslinking. Therefore, the majority of UHMWPE acetabular liners used in the past four decades have always been crosslinked to some degree. However, the level of crosslinking achieved through gamma sterilization alone is much lower than what is being realized with the more contemporary methods of radiation crosslinking followed by a thermal treatment step.

B. Radiation Chemistry of Polyethylene

For various industrial or medical applications, peroxide or silane chemistries or ionizing radiation are used to crosslink polyethylene. With all three methods, the recombination reactions of free radicals lead to the formation of crosslinks. Today, for the specific applications in orthopaedics, the manufacturers exclusively use radiation chemistry to crosslink UHMWPE, with either gamma- or electron-beam (e-beam) radiation sources.

When UHMWPE is exposed to gamma or e-beam radiation, carbon-hydrogen and carbon-carbon bonds undergo cleavage leading to the generation of unpaired electrons, so-called free radicals, as shown in Figure 2. The process of carbon-carbon bond cleavage, also referred to as chain scission, leads to a reduction in the molecular weight, hence degradation of the polymer. The primary reaction competing with chain scission is crosslinking, during which two free radicals will react with each other to form an inter-chain covalent bond. The crosslinks are referred to as H-type when the recombination is between two free radicals formed through carbon-hydrogen bond cleavage. When one of the free radicals is originated through chain scission, the crosslinks formed are of Y type, leading to the formation of long-chain branches. Figure 3 shows schematics of H- and Y-type crosslinks. The net effect of ionizing radiation on UHMWPE is crosslinking, as the yield of the crosslinking reactions is about three times larger than that of chain scission (47,48).

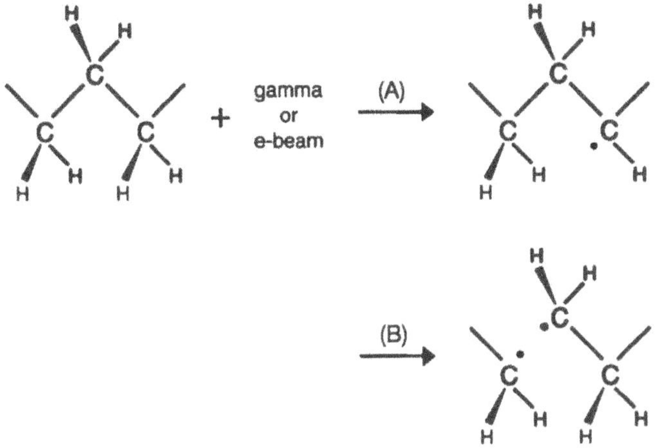

Figure 2 Schematic of the two primary radiolytic reactions leading to the formation of (A) primary free radicals and (B) chain scission. The primary free radicals are formed by the cleavage of a C-H bond, which also liberates a hydrogen free radical. The hydrogen free radicals readily recombine with each other, form hydrogen gas and diffuse out of the polymer. The chain scission is the consequence of the cleavage of the C-C bond along the backbone of the molecular chain resulting in the formation of two terminal free radicals. These free radicals may react with each other to reverse the chain scission, abstract a hydrogen atom from a nearby chain, react with a primary free radical residing on the same chain to form a terminal vinyl, or react with a primary free radical on another chain to form a Y-type long-chain branch crosslink as shown in Figure 3.

Free radical recombination takes place primarily in the amorphous phase of the polymer, where the molecules are in close enough proximity to allow the formation of the interchain carbon-carbon bond that constitutes the crosslink (49,50). In the crystalline phase, because of the increased distance between the molecules, crosslinking is not favored. As a result, the free radicals generated in the crystalline regions are postulated not to take part in the crosslinking reactions and become trapped, mainly in the crystalline/amorphous interfaces (51–53). These *residual* free radicals are the known precursors of oxidation-induced embrittlement secondary to gamma sterilization.

The cascade of events that lead to the oxidation and eventual embrittlement of polyethylene are as follows: (a) Residual free radicals generated by the ionizing radiation react with oxygen to form peroxy free radicals (oxygen-centered radicals), which readily form hydroperoxides by abstracting a hydrogen atom from nearby chains. (b) The abstraction of hydrogen

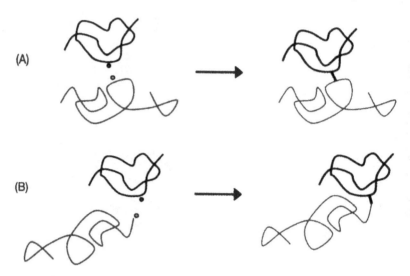

Figure 3 Schematic of the (A) H- and (B) Y-type crosslinks. The H-type crosslinking occurs when two primary free radicals recombine with each other. The Y-type crosslinking occurs when a primary free radical and a chain end free radical react with each other, forming a long-chain branch.

produces a new free radical, which, in turn, takes part in the oxidation cascade. (c) The hydroperoxides are not stable in the long term and/or under high temperatures. This instability results in the decay of the hydroperoxides into carbonyl species, mainly ketones and acids. (d) The formation of acids reduces the molecular weight of the polymer leading to recrystallization, increase in stiffness, and embrittlement of the component.

Considering the significant adverse effects of the residual free radicals to the properties as well as device performance in the long term, there is now a substantial movement towards treating the UHMWPE thermally, following irradiation, to decrease the concentration of the residual free radicals after irradiation (12–14,54). The most effective method of reducing free radicals is to raise the temperature of polyethylene above its peak melting transition (about 137°C) to eliminate the crystalline domains and liberate the trapped, residual free radicals. This allows the rapid removal of the residual free radicals through recombination reactions. Upon cooling down, polyethylene crystallizes, reforming most of the crystalline domains, now in the presence of crosslinks. This slows down the kinetics of crystallization and results in a slight reduction in the crystallinity of polyethylene (55).

Another method for reducing the residual free radical concentration of irradiated UHMWPE is to anneal below its peak melting transition. Because the UHMWPE will be partially molten at the annealing temperature, this method leads to only a partial reduction of the residual free radicals through a series of recombination reactions. The annealing of irradiated UHMWPE is expected to increase the crystallinity, as the thermally activated polymer chains would lead to thickening of the crystalline lamellae.

While the cascade of events that leads to the formation of crosslinks and residual free radicals is identical for both gamma irradiation and e-beam irradiation, there are still important differences between the two irradiation methods, specifically in terms of penetration of the effects of radiation and radiation dose rate achieved. Gamma irradiation sources are commonly based on the artificial isotope of cobalt (^{60}Co) that generates gamma photons. While the penetration of a gamma source into polyethylene has no practical limitations, the activity level of the gamma source limits the radiation dose rate. With an e-beam irradiator, the radiation is in the form of accelerated, charged particles. The penetration of the effects of e-beam radiation is limited by the kinetic energy of the electron beam, measured in millions of electron volts (MeV). With a 10 MeV e-beam incident on a polyethylene surface radiation penetrates about 4–4.5 cm. The radiation dose rate that a commercial e-beam accelerator provides is about two orders of magnitude larger than that from a commercial gamma source.

C. The Effect of Crosslinking on Mechanical Properties of Polyethylene

The changes in the mechanical properties of the radiation- and heat-treated polyethylene are primarily dominated by changes in the crosslink density and crystallinity. The mechanical behavior of UHMWPE in uniaxial tension can be analyzed in two categories. These are the changes in the small- and large-strain mechanical properties, which are mainly governed by the crystallinity and crosslink density of the polymer, respectively. The former group encompasses the elastic behavior and yielding, such as the modulus of elasticity and yield strength of the polymer. The latter includes the ductility, work to failure, and ultimate strength of the polymer. Under multiaxial loading conditions, it is more difficult to separate effects of crystallinity and crosslinking, since both appear to influence the large-strain mechanical behavior in a more complex, synergistic manner (56).

The crystallinity of polyethylene is a function of the radiation dose level and thermal treatment history. Irradiation generates smaller chains with increased mobility, leading to recrystallization and a slight increase in the crystallinity of the polymer. The changes in the crystallinity during the post-irradiation thermal treatment depend on temperature. If the thermal treatment is carried out below the melting transition (<137°C), the chain mobility increases, which, in turn, increases the crystallinity of the polymer. When the thermal treatment is performed at temperatures above the melting transition (>137°C), during cool-down to room temperature, the crystallization of the polymer takes place in the presence of the crosslinks. This leads to a decrease in the crystallinity of the polymer.

The radiation dose level used in the irradiation step determines the crosslink density and thus the large-strain uniaxial mechanical properties of the polyethylene. The crosslink density of the polyethylene limits the ultimate elongation that can be achieved during plastic deformation prior to failure. Therefore, at higher radiation dose levels, the crosslinked polymer exhibits reduced ultimate tensile strength and elongation at break under uniaxial tension. As a result, the work to failure also decreases. As the crosslinking reduces the chain mobility, it also inhibits the active energy-absorbing mechanisms. Therefore, at high uniaxial deformation rates, such as impact loading, the energy absorption before failure decreases, leading to a decrease in the toughness.

Another important variable that affects the mechanical properties of the radiation- and heat-treated polyethylene is the irradiation temperature. When the polymer is irradiated at an elevated temperature (90°C < T < 137°C) the effect of the crosslink density on the large strain mechanical properties decreases significantly (14,57). This may be explained by a non-statistical distribution of the crosslinks resulting at increased irradiation temperatures (14). As a result, the low crosslink-density matrix controls the large-strain mechanical properties. The polyethylenes irradiated at increased temperatures have been reported to exhibit better large-strain mechanical properties than those irradiated at room temperature with identical radiation dose levels (57).

D. Wear Behavior and Mechanisms

The primary mechanism of polyethylene wear in total hip arthroplasty that leads to the generation of sub-micron-size debris is adhesive/abrasive in nature. Elongated fibrils on the articulating surfaces of surgically retrieved acetabular components have been proposed as the precursors for this wear mechanism (58) (Figure 4). The fibrils are postulated (58) to form through large-strain plastic deformation of the articulating surface during in vivo use and are highly oriented in the longitudinal direction of the principal arc of motion of the hip, namely the flexion-extension direction. This orientation leads to strain-hardening of the material in the sliding direction and weakening of the material in the transverse direction. The oriented surface layer is then hypothesized to break up during motions that are at an angle to the principal directions of flexion/extension motion, liberating micron and sub-

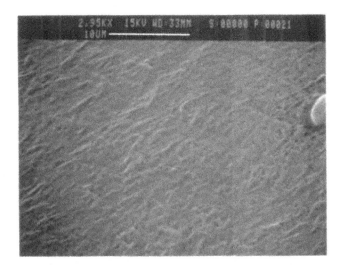

Figure 4 Typical appearance of the articulating surface of a surgically retrieved conventional UHMWPE acetabular liner showing the elongated fibrils. The explant shown was retrieved after 124 months.

micron wear particles (59,60). These crossing motions are induced by the abduction/adduction and internal/external rotation of the hip (61,62). Recent investigations into the effect of crossing motions on adhesive wear of polyethylene (63) and the evolution of polyethylene microstructure near the articulation (64) now provides further evidence for the dominating role of this wear mechanism in the total hip.

The above mechanism of adhesive/abrasive wear is likely to be responsible for the improvement of the wear resistance of polyethylene through crosslinking. In general, the effects of crosslinking and thermal treatment on the mechanical properties of polyethylene might be construed as an indication for increase in wear, presenting a paradox in that wear decreases with crosslinking (13,65). In effect, crosslinking reduces the drawability (ductility) of the polymer chains. Consequently, the large-strain plastic deformation induced by an articulating counterface would also decrease, inhibiting the formation of the elongated fibrils. At high crosslink densities, this effect is more prominent and the wear resistance of the polymer is significantly improved (13,66).

There are numerous investigations on the effects of crosslinking on the wear resistance of polyethylene (12–14). Figure 5A shows the main outcome of a typical investigation (13): the wear rate of polyethylene decreases as a function of increasing radiation dose level, or increasing cross-

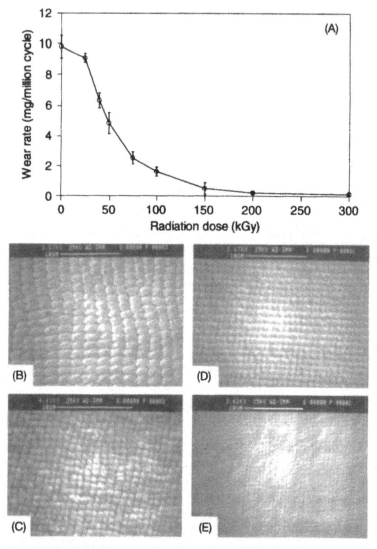

Figure 5 The wear rate, measured gravimetrically, of UHMWPE as a function of radiation dose level is shown in (A). The wear testing was carried out on biaxial pin-on-disk machine with UHMWPE pins. The pins were machined from UHMWPE stock that had been subjected to radiation and melting. (From Ref. 13.) The photomicrographs in (B), (C), (D), and (E) show typical surface morphologies formed at dose levels of 25, 50, 100, and 200 kGy, respectively, following 2 million cycles of bidirectional rubbing action against an implant-finish CoCr disk. Note that the increase in the radiation dose result in an increase in the crosslink density, which leads to a decrease in the amount of surface orientation accumulated during the wear test.

link density. In that study, a bidirectional pin-on-disc machine provided the means for the wear testing of polyethylene pins articulating against CoCr discs with an implant surface finish. The electron microscopy analysis of the articulating surfaces of the pins following 2 million cycles of bidirectional rubbing action presented strong evidence of significant reduction in surface deformation with increasing crosslink density (Figure 5B–E).

Extensive data are also available from hip simulator studies showing the improvement in the wear resistance of polyethylene with crosslinking (12,14,67–69), as shown in Figure 6. In this series, the persistence of the machining marks on the articulating surfaces of the highly crosslinked polyethylene acetabular components after several million cycles of simulated gait offers further evidence of the marked reduction in wear with crosslinking (Figure 7). In contrast, the conventional liners (gamma-sterilized in low oxygen), when subjected to simulated gait cycles, always displayed a highly

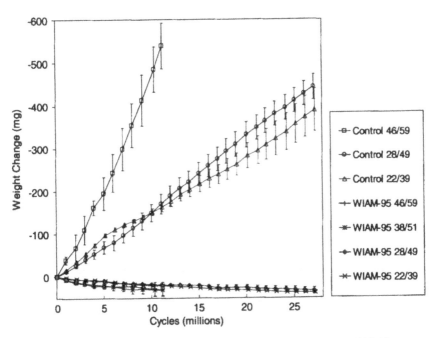

Figure 6 The average weight change of conventional (control) and highly crosslinked (WIAM-95) acetabular liners as tested on a Boston Hip Simulator. The WIAM-95 liners were e-beam irradiated at 125°C with a total dose of 95 kGy and subsequently melted. The inner and outer diameters are specified (From Ref. 172). See Figure 7 for the appearance of the wear surfaces of select test specimens following 7 and 11 million cycles of simulated gait.

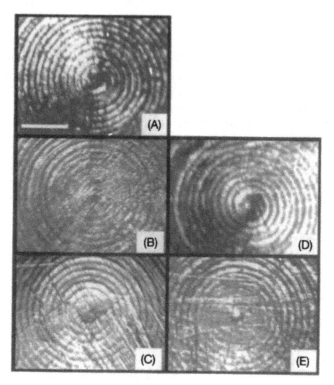

Figure 7 The articulating surface of the highly crosslinked acetabular liners tested in the study shown in Figure 6: The dome of articulation before any testing (A) shows the presence of the machining marks. Following 5 (B and D) and 7 (C and E) million cycles of simulated gait with a femoral head size of 28 mm (B and C) and 38 mm (D and E), the machining marks (average height of 10–30Å) are still present, indicating that the adhesive/abrasive wear is significantly reduced in the highly crosslinked UHMWPE. All photographs follow the 1-mm scale of (A). (From Ref. 172.)

polished appearance, indicating the presence of wear. Furthermore, there is no reported evidence of pitting, cracking, delamination, loss of contour, or fatigue failure during hip simulator testing of either conventional or highly crosslinked polyethylene components.

Another form of wear mechanism in vivo involves the presence of third-body particles, such as bone cement particles, that could increase the roughness of the counterface and accelerate the wear of the polyethylene acetabular liner. Several examples of in vitro hip simulator studies lubricated with bovine serum and added third-body particles (e.g., barium sulfate–

containing bone cement particles) have recently been reported (11,70). These studies provide convincing evidence that the wear rate of the articulating couple of crosslinked polyethylene and CoCr is notably lower than that of conventional articulations (CoCr/UHMWPE).

E. Clinical History

There are a number of historical instances where various investigators have considered the effect of increased crosslink density on the in vitro and in vivo performance of polyethylene acetabular components. The methods included crosslinking polyethylene with high-dose (1000 kGy) gamma radiation in air (71–80), gamma radiation (100 kGy) in the presence of acetylene (81–83), and silane chemistry (84,85). These highly crosslinked polyethylenes were experimental and were not commercially available. Their evaluations were carried out in retrospective clinical studies with limited number of patients. Unfortunately, the studies did not include matched control groups and in some studies a substantial number of the patients were lost to follow-up.

The first study in this historical series was that of Oonishi and co-workers in the early 1970s (80). They implanted UHMWPE acetabular cups that were crosslinked at room temperature using 1000 kGy of gamma radiation. The irradiation was carried in air with no subsequent annealing or melting to reduce the concentration of the residual free radicals. The radiographic wear measurements showed a decreased average rate of femoral head penetration (0.072–0.076 mm/year) for the 1000 kGy–irradiated UHMWPE in comparison with the control UHMWPE (0.098 to 0.25 mm/year), which had been gamma-sterilized in air (78).

The second historical instance of the use of highly crosslinked polyethylenes originated from the efforts of Grobbelaar and DuPlessis in the 1970s (81,82). Grobbelaar implanted polyethylene acetabular liners that were packaged in acetylene gas and gamma-irradiated to a dose level of 100 kGy. The use of acetylene is known to increase the efficiency of crosslinking (86) and reduce the concentration of the residual free radicals. Two different clinical follow-up series have been reported (83). The first is a 14- to 22-year follow-up (average 15.5 years) of 62 patients showing no measurable wear in 56 cases and a total of 1.0–4.0 mm linear penetration in 8 cases. The average wear rate of this series was about 0.011 mm/year. The second series was a 13- to 22-year follow-up (average 15.5 years) of 39 patients with no measurable wear in 30 cases and a total of 0.7–1.5 mm linear penetration in 9 cases. Figures 8A and B show the x-rays of one of the patients from the first series at 6 months and 19 years postoperatively with no signs of wear or interface changes.

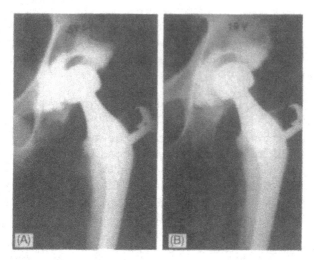

Figure 8 A typical example of the x-ray appearance at 6 months (A) and 19 years (B) postoperative follow-up of one of the patients of Grobbelaar et al., where the acetabular liner was gamma irradiated in the presence of acetylene gas. The images show no detectable wear and no lytic changes at interfaces (From Ref. 83.)

The third example comes from Wroblewski and coworkers (84,85), who reported on the wear behavior of 22-mm diameter, silane-crosslinked polyethylene acetabular components. The clinical and joint simulator studies of Wroblewski showed remarkable agreement in the wear rates of the crosslinked polymer. After an initial "bedding-in" penetration of 0.2–0.4 mm with an average penetration rate of 0.29 mm/year, presumably representing creep, the subsequent average penetration rate (or wear rate) decreased by an order of magnitude to 0.02 mm/year, presumably representing wear. Mean clinical follow-up was 10 years and 6 months, with a total of 14 patients.

The contemporary approaches to crosslinking differ from these historical examples. Today radiation chemistry is the preferred method of crosslinking, and silane chemistry is not used. In addition, postirradiation thermal treatment steps are used in an effort to reduce the residual free radicals and improve the long-term oxidative stability.

F. Current Trends

Table 2 lists the contemporary approaches to improving the wear and oxidation resistance of polyethylene through radiation chemistry for applications in total hip arthroplasty. As shown in Table 3, contemporary modifications to UHMWPE include variations in the radiation source, radiation

Table 3 Current Trends in UHMWPE with Elevated Crosslink Density

	Manufacturer	Radiation Temperature	Radiation Dose (kGy)	Radiation Type	Postirradiation Thermal Treatment	Sterilization Method	Total Radiation Dose Level (kGy)
Longevity™	Zimmer	~40°C	100	E-beam	Melted at 150°C for 6 hr	Gas plasma	100
Durasul™	Sulzer	~125°C	95	E-beam	Melted at 150°C for 2 hr	EtO	95
Marathon™	Depuy/JJ	RT	50	Gamma	Melted at 155°C for 24 hr	Gas plasma	50
XLPE™	Smith & Nephew	RT	100	Gamma	Melted at 150°C (duration unknown)	EtO	100
Crossfire™	Stryker/Osteonics/ Howmedica	RT	75	Gamma	Anneal at 120°C for a proprietary duration	Gamma (30 kGy) in nitrogen	105
Aeonian™	Kyocera	RT	35	Gamma	Annealed at 110°C for 10 hr	Gamma (25–40 kGy) in nitrogen	60–75

dose, radiation temperature, postirradiation thermal treatment, and sterilization methods.

In terms of the radiation dose level used, there are two main approaches. One viewpoint is founded on the argument that a 50-kGy radiation dose level generates sufficient crosslinking to reduce the in vivo production of UHMWPE wear debris below the level of lysis threshold (12). The other viewpoints differ from this approach and advocate the use of higher radiation dose levels, around 100 kGy, to achieve the maximum reduction in the production of polyethylene wear debris (9,14).

In terms of the concentration of residual free radicals, there are also two distinct approaches. One approach aims to prevent oxidation for the lifetime of the implant both on the shelf and in vivo. This is achieved by the postirradiation melting of the polymer in conjunction with a gas sterilization method, which leads to undetectable levels of residual free radicals.

The other approach focuses on preventing the oxidation during the shelf storage of the implants. This is achieved by postirradiation annealing below the melting transition temperature in combination with gamma sterilization and storage in an inert environment, leaving behind residual free radicals. However, there is continued debate on the effects and significance of these residual free radicals after implantation (87).

As the crosslink density and the residual free radical content of the commercially available polyethylenes differ to a certain extent due to the viewpoints described above, differences in their wear and oxidation resistance are expected. With higher crosslink density and a lower concentration of residual free radicals one would expect to achieve an increase in the wear and oxidation resistances, respectively.

With the extensive in vitro demonstration of improved wear achieved with radiation and heat-treated polyethylenes, there is now an opportunity to increase the diameter of the femoral head used in the total hip. Until recent years, 32 mm was the most widely used femoral head diameter in North America. With growing evidence of increased volumetric wear (44) and increased risk for osteolysis (88) in conventional CoCr/UHMWPE articulations with 32-mm femoral heads, there has been a significant shift toward the use of a smaller-diameter femoral head, namely 28, 26, and 22 mm. The highly crosslinked polyethylenes may now reverse this trend and raise the potential for widespread use of larger heads in total hip replacement surgery.

The advantages of using femoral heads of larger diameter in total hip replacement surgery include a greater range of motion, enhanced activities of daily living, a greater intrinsic stability of the implant, a reduced incidence of subluxation, a reduced incidence of dislocation, and less frequent impingement of the femoral neck on the polyethylene. In addition, the greater range of motion available is more forgiving of the inherent errors in acetabular placement, thus providing an increased margin of safety if an error is made in shell placement (89–91).

IV. ARTICULATIONS WITH CERAMICS

A. History

The use of ceramic materials in the total hip was initiated in the 1970s (92). Boutin (92) advanced the approach of ceramic-on-ceramic articulations, while Shikata et al. (80) proposed the use of a ceramic femoral head articulating against an UHMWPE socket. The determinants for these approaches were the high corrosion resistance and biocompatibility of ceramics, along with their superior scratch resistance as compared with metallic alloys. Ceramic-on-ceramic couples were also expected to have better wear resistance compared with the conventional articulation of CoCr/UHMWPE. The initial applications of ceramics in the total hip exclusively used alumina (Al_2O_3). In late 1980s, zirconia (ZrO_2) was introduced for use as a femoral component in ceramic-on-UHMWPE articulations due to its higher strength and toughness as compared with alumina (93).

B. Alumina and Zirconia

Medical-grade alumina is consolidated from a high-purity (>99%) alumina powder through a hot isostatic pressing step (93,94). Modifications to the sintering process over the past three decades have resulted in increased density, hardness, and strength of medical-grade alumina (Table 4). Modifications to the sintering also led to a decrease in the average grain size from 4.5 μm to about 1.8 μm, with a narrower grain size distribution (95). The

Table 4 Various Properties of Alumina and Zirconia Ceramics Used in the Total Hip Reconstruction

Property	Alumina in 1970s	Alumina in 1980s	Alumina in 1990s	Zirconia
Bending strength (MPa)	>450	>500	>550	>900
Fracture toughness (MPa·m$^{1/2}$)	4	4	4	8
Vickers hardness (0.1)	1800	1900	2000	1250
Grain size (micron)	4.5	3.2	1.8	<0.5
Young's modulus (GPa)	380	380	380	210

SOURCES: Refs. 93 and 95.

improved regulation of the grain size did not lead to any noticeable changes in the fracture toughness of alumina (95).

While alumina remains the most widely used ceramic in the total hip, zirconia is also utilized as a replacement for alumina femoral heads, but only for applications where the counterface is UHMWPE. Zirconia is stronger than alumina (Table 4); therefore it can withstand higher stresses, which may be induced when smaller and thinner implants are used.

During deformation, pure zirconia undergoes a crystalline-phase transformation from monoclinic to tetragonal, with the former occupying more space. This transformation adversely affects the mechanical properties of pure zirconia, leading to internal stresses within the deformation zone ahead of propagating cracks. Zirconia can be stabilized with the addition of either magnesium oxide (MgO) or yttrium oxide (Y_2O_3) to avoid the detrimental effects of deformation-induced phase transformation. The medical-grade zirconia is stabilized with the addition of yttrium oxide to maintain a metastable tetragonal crystalline structure that transforms into monoclinic during crack propagation, thereby improving its toughness and resistance to fatigue crack propagation (96).

One significant drawback of ceramic materials is their inherently lower strength and toughness under tension and bending, which are the loading modes that favor the initiation and propagation of cracks. One such adverse loading arises from the mismatch at the taper junction between the metal stem and ceramic head. To prevent this from leading to early fracture, the tolerances at the taper are matched and may be manufacturer-specific. The surgical placement of the components may also predispose the ceramic components to high stresses and initiate fracture. For instance, a third body (bone cement or bone fragment) left in the taper interface (97) or impingement of the femoral component on the rim of the ceramic acetabular liner secondary to malpositioning of the components could also initiate ceramic fracture (98).

Fracture of the ceramic femoral heads when they are articulating against polyethylene or against a ceramic liner is a clinically relevant mode of failure and can occur even with the stronger zirconia ceramic heads (97–104). The revision surgery subsequent to the fracture of a ceramic component may be complicated. It is recommended to revise the polyethylene acetabular liner as well, since the fragments of the fractured ceramic femoral head may have become embedded in the articulating surface and thus could act as third-body particles in the revised articulation (105,106). In addition, the fracture of the ceramic head could damage the Morse taper, which could lead to an adverse loading condition if the femoral head were also revised with a ceramic component. It is now recommended to revise the femoral head with a metallic alloy, such as CoCr, to avoid further catastrophic failure

(101). Another option on the femoral side is to revise the femoral stem and use a ceramic femoral head (101).

C. Ceramic on Polyethylene

While the metallic bearing surfaces can scratch in the presence of a third body and increase the wear of the polyethylene counterface, the hard ceramic bearing surfaces could theoretically remain scratch-free for longer durations in vivo (107–109). There is controversy regarding the benefit of ceramic femoral head components in improving the in vivo wear behavior of polyethylene (106). The in vitro hip simulator studies suggest either a minor (110,111) or no detectable (112) improvement in the wear resistance of polyethylene counterface when a ceramic femoral head is utilized instead of a metallic one. Retrospective in vivo clinical follow-up investigations also show no detectable improvement (113–115). Prospective clinical investigations will be needed to better quantify the effect of the use of ceramic femoral components articulating with polyethylene.

D. Ceramic on Ceramic

In vivo ceramic-on-ceramic articulations use exclusively alumina/alumina, as zirconia has showed extremely high wear rates in laboratory experiments when articulating against itself (116) or against alumina (117). The in vitro laboratory assessment of the alumina-on-alumina couples using hip simulators demonstrated significantly reduced wear rates (two orders of magnitude) when compared with conventional CoCr/polyethylene articulations (118,119). Since the penetration of the femoral head is difficult to measure using radiographic methods, assessment of in vivo wear of the alumina/alumina articulations is limited mainly to the analysis of surgically retrieved components. Such studies have demonstrated in vivo volumetric wear ranging from 3–9 μm/year (120,121) to 1–5 mm^3/year (122). The reported wear rates correspond to a decrease of about one to two orders of magnitude for the in vivo wear rate of alumina/alumina articulations as compared with the conventional CoCr/UHMWPE articulations.

A recently advanced mechanism for the wear of alumina/alumina articulations is postulated to be a consequence of the micro-separation of the head/liner interface during gait (123,124). The femoral head separates from the liner during the swing phase, followed by a rim contact at heel strike and the relocation of the head in the liner during the stance phase. This wear mechanism may provide an explanation for the stripe-like wear marks observed on the articulating surfaces of retrieved alumina femoral heads (124,125).

The significantly low wear rate of alumina-on-alumina bearing surfaces is postulated to be a consequence of elastohydrodynamic lubrication achieved during articulation (126). For this lubrication mode to be operative, the clearance between the acetabular liner and femoral head must be maintained within the theoretical value of $7-10$ μm; therefore precision machining is essential and components from different manufacturers cannot be interchanged (94).

V.   METAL-ON-METAL ARTICULATIONS

A.   History

Prior to 1953, the earliest prototypes of metal-on-metal bearings for total hip replacement were initially fabricated from stainless steel (Table 4) (1,2). Due to in vivo fracture of the prostheses, McKee and Watson-Farrar developed the CoCr/CoCr articulation. A series of 40 implants were implanted between 1956 and 1960 using a screw-type design for acetabular fixation (2). The McKee-Farrar prosthesis evolved to its final design between 1960 and 1965 to accommodate cemented fixation (2). CoCr/CoCr implants of differing designs were also developed by Wilson and Scales (127), Ring (128), Müller (129), and Sivash (130) in the 1960s and 1970s.

Of these designs, only the McKee-Farrar prostheses gained widespread use in the United States (131) until their eventual abandonment in the 1970s in favor of the Charnley design, with its CoCr/UHMWPE articulation (129). Two principal factors have frequently been cited as contributing to the shift from the metal-on-metal to the metal-on-UHMWPE designs: bearing seizure due to comtemporary manufacturing processes and long-term concerns about the health risks associated with metal toxicity and carcinogenicity of the metal debris. More recently, however, Zahiri and colleagues (131) have argued that the femoral stem design, biomechanical factors associated with the joint center, and medialization of the reconstruction as well as surgical implantation technique also contributed to early aseptic loosening of the McKee-Farrar prostheses.

In the 1980s and 1990s, research was published suggesting that the clinical performance of the McKee-Farrar was comparable to that of the Charnley design (132–135). In 1986, August et al. reported on the survivorship of 657 McKee-Farrar prostheses implanted at Norwich, England, corresponding to 81% of the total 808 procedures performed at that institution between 1965 and 1973 (132). At Norwich, the survivorship of the McKee-Farrar decreased by about 1% per year to 84.3% after 14 years; it decreased further to 27.5% after 20 years of implantation. August's radiographic review of 230 unrevised long-term patients (average 14.3 years, range 10–22 years) implanted with the McKee-Farrar in Norwich revealed evidence of acetabular loosening in 51.1% of the cases (132). More recently, in a Scandinavian study of 107 consecutive McKee-Farrar and 70 Charnley total hip arthroplasties, researchers reported no significant difference in 20-year survivorship for aseptic loosening when comparing the metal-metal and CoCr/UHMWPE designs (134).

Consequently, a second generation of metal-on-metal implants was developed starting in the 1980s to address the manufacturing problems that contributed to the early failures of the McKee-Farrar. In 1988, Weber introduced contemporary metal-on-metal bearings into clinical practice in St. Gallen (136), and between 1988 and 2000, around 125,000 of these second-generation metal-on-metal bearings are estimated to have been implanted worldwide (C. Riecker, personal communication, 2001). Intermediate-term clinical reports of these second-generation metal-on-metal implants (up to 7 years in vivo) from the United States and Europe have shown no evidence of osteolysis or radiographic wear (137,138), consistent with the expectation of reduced wear observed with these bearings from recent hip simulator studies (118,139–141).

B.   Composition and Microstructure of CoCr Alloys

Alloys of cobalt, 28% chromium, and 6% molybdenum (Co-28Cr-6Mo, hereafter CoCr) have been used in orthopaedic bearing surfaces since the 1930s, when they were used to fabricate components for the Smith-Petersen mold arthroplasty. CoCr alloys consist of a primary cobalt alloy matrix phase and a secondary metal carbide phase. In the cobalt-based matrix, chromium enhances the mechanical properties of the alloy and promotes the formation of a passive oxide layer, whereas molybdenum is included in the alloy for corrosion resistance (142). The size and distribution of the carbide phase contributes to the hardness and mechanical behavior of the alloy.

The properties of CoCr alloys depend upon their processing history—whether fabricated by investment casting or by a thermomechanical forming process (143). During an investment casting process, a wax replica of the prosthesis is first fabricated and coated with a silicate slurry (144). The replica and slurry are raised above the melting point of the wax (100–150°C) and burned away in a furnace, leaving only the slurry mold with an interior cavity having the dimensions of the replica. The cavity is then filled with molten alloy and, after cooling, the mold is broken to remove the cast implant. Mechanical forming, on the other hand, can be accomplished by a wide range of thermomechanical manufacturing methods, including rolling, forging, swaging, and drawing (142), all of which lead to a *wrought* CoCr alloy. Both cast and wrought CoCr alloys are subjected to annealing heat

treatments for optimization of microstructure and mechanical properties
(142). Historically, the first-generation metal-on-metal components were fabricated by casting, whereas contemporary second-generation metal-on-metal
implants are manufactured from wrought CoCr alloys.

The minimum mechanical properties for cast and wrought CoCr alloys
used in orthopaedic applications are summarized in Table 5, as specified by
current ASTM standards. Wrought CoCr alloys have significantly enhanced
hardness, yield strength, and ultimate properties as compared with cast alloys
(Table 4), resulting from their more uniform carbide microstructure (143).

According to ASTM F75, F799, and F1527, all CoCr alloys used in
orthopaedics contain trace constituents of carbon (0.35%), nitrogen (max
0.25%), nickel (max 1%), iron (max 0.75%), silicon (max 1.0%), and manganese (max 1.0%). Cast CoCr alloys (ASTM F75) may also contain tungsten (max 0.20%), phosphorus (max 0.020%), sulfur (max 0.010%), aluminum (max 0.30%), and boron (max 0.01%). Of these secondary constituents,
the effect of carbon content on CoCr alloys has been examined most closely
by researchers in the orthopaedic community because of the link between
carbon content, carbide formation, and properties of the bearing surface
(139,145–147).

CoCr alloys may be further classified as either low-carbon (<0.05%)
or high-carbon (>0.20%) (145,146). With the exception of certain metal-on-
metal implants produced in Austria, the majority of contemporary metal-on-
metal bearings are fabricated from a high-carbon CoCr alloy (145). Although
the carbon content within this range does not have a substantial effect on
the bulk mechanical properties of wrought CoCr alloy, Varano et al. have
documented significantly greater coefficient of friction for high-carbon alloys
(146). However, in contemporary hip simulator studies, high- and low-car-

Table 5 Minimum Mechanical Properties for Cast, Forged, and Wrought CoCr Alloys,
as Specified by ASTM Standards

Condition	ASTM Standard	Yield Strength (MPa)	Ultimate Tensile Strength (MPa)	Ultimate Elongation (%)	Hardness, HRC, Typical
Casting	F75	450	655	8	NA
Forged	F799	827	1172	12	35
Wrought and annealed	F1537	517	897	20	25
Wrought and hot-worked	F1537	700	1000	12	28
Wrought and warm-worked	F1537	827	1172	12	35

bon CoCr alloys have exhibited comparable wear mechanisms and wear rates (139,148).

C. Design, Lubrication, and Wear of Metal-on-Metal Bearings

Metal-on-metal hip implants have historically been fabricated with very close tolerances between the femoral head and the acetabular socket (2). Minimization of radial clearance at the articulating surface is desirable from the perspective of enhancing lubrication during gait. The thickness of the lubricating fluid film in a metal-on-metal bearing is predicted to increase as the clearance between the head and the socket decreases (126,149,150). Theoretically, no wear can occur when the hard bearing surfaces are continuously separated by a lubricating film of sufficient thickness. Based on elastohydrodynamic lubrication calculations (employing the finite element method), Kothari and colleagues have estimated that the metal surfaces for the McKee-Farrar design could be separated by fluid-film lubrication during the stance phase of gait if the radial clearance were less than 40 μm (150).

In practice, the fluid-film thickness in metal-on-metal joints depends on many other variables, including the elastic properties of the contacting materials, sliding velocity, and viscosity of the lubricant as well as the curvature and roughness of the articulating surfaces (126,149,150). On the other hand, if the radial clearance is too small, it could also prevent the removal of third-body wear debris from the contact area, leading to catastrophic seizure of the bearing, as has been implicated in some of the short-term failures of the McKee-Farrar. As discussed by Chan et al. (139), "the optimal clearance must be a balance between maximizing contact area (smaller clearance) and maximizing the ability for fluid ingress and wear particle egress (larger clearance). Thus, from an engineering standpoint, it may be necessary to accept slightly larger clearances (and slightly more wear) to increase the margin of design safety." Although researchers generally agree that fluid-film lubrication is theoretically possible in metal-on-metal implants, the extent to which it plays a role in the overall wear mechanisms for this class of hard-on-hard bearing surfaces remains the subject of ongoing research (126,149,150).

The presence of detectable wear in retrieved metal-on-metal components attests to the fact that, at some point during the patient's daily duty cycle the articulating surfaces are in intimate contact. In a consensus workshop convened in 1996, orthopaedic researchers generally agreed that the typical long-term in vivo wear rate for first generation metal-on-metal components ranges between 1 and 5 mm^3/year (151). Specific analyses of retrieved first-generation metal-on-metal bearings have reported in vivo volumetric wear rates in the range of 1–23 mm³/year of wear, as compared with 69–90 mm³/year observed with CoCr/UHMWPE bearings (41, 150,152–155).

Design and manufacturing defects, such as a large head-socket clearance, have been hypothesized to contribute to the elevated long-term wear rates observed in certain first-generation metal-on-metal hip implants (151). Clearance has been shown to be related to wear in recent hip simulator testing of second-generation metal-on-metal components (139). However, relationships between head-socket clearance and wear have been difficult to establish from examination of first-generation retrieved components (150,152). For example, in a series of 28 McKee-Farrar components retrieved after 6 to 23 years of implantation, in which the radial clearance was determined to range from 3–112 μm, Kothari and colleagues found no significant relationship between the radial clearance and the total magnitude of volumetric wear in the range of 1–9 mm³/year (150). Scott and Lemons (152) examined 14 retrieved Sivash prostheses implanted for 2 to 22 years with head-socket clearances ranging from 56–115 μm and also observed no correlation between clearance and in vivo wear rate (range: 0.3–27.3 mm³/year). Due to the large number of factors potentially contributing to clinical performance, it remains a challenging task to isolate the effect of specific design and material variables based on the small number of retrieved first generation metal-on-metal components.

The in vivo wear performance of second-generation metal-on-metal bearings has been studied extensively by researchers from Sulzer Orthopedics in Switzerland (156–158). In their most recent report of 111 individual components implanted in 71 patients, Rieker et al. (158) observed a "moderate" initial run-in phase of 25 μm during the first year of implantation, followed by a steady-state wear rate of 5 μm/year (mean follow-up: 23 months; range: 2 to 100 months). These findings have compared favorably with those from the first-generation Muller bearings within a comparable implantation time. The researchers calculated a volumetric wear rate of 0.3 mm³/year during the steady-state phase for the second-generation implants.

D. Short- and Intermediate-Term Failure Mechanisms In Vivo

As discussed by Weber (136), surgeon- and implant-related factors might contribute to short- and intermediate-term failure of second-generation metal-on-metal bearings. For example, in a series of 85 cemented titanium alloy stems implanted between 1988 and 1992 with second-generation metal-on-metal bearings, Weber reported early loosening of 11 titanium stems and 3 metallic cups having a steel mesh outer surface (16% failure rate) after 9 years of follow-up (136). Furthermore, as clinical experience with the McKee-Farrar has shown, use of a metal-on-metal bearing in conjunction with cemented fixation can still lead to long-term osteolysis (159), most likely precipitated by cement debris liberated at the implant-cement interface. Femoral neck impingement with the metal socket, leading to metallosis, is another short-term failure mode that has been documented in a case by Dorr (160) and in another case report by Iida et al. (161) for second-generation metal-on-metal bearings.

E. Biological Implications of Metallic Wear Debris

By virtue of their low wear rates in vivo, second-generation metal-on-metal articulations offer the potential for reducing the incidence of debris-induced osteolysis and long-term aseptic loosening (136–138, 156–158). Although the wear rates in metal-on-metal joints are one to two orders of magnitude less than those of conventional CoCr/UHMWPE bearings, the size of metallic debris ranges between 6 nm and 5 μm, with the majority less than 90 nm (141,162–164). Because of the difference in particle size, metal-on-metal joints have been estimated to liberate about 100 times more wear debris particles than CoCr/UHMWPE bearings (141,163).

The biological implications of long-term exposure to nanometer-sized metallic wear debris is still not fully understood today, but histomorphometric analyses coupled with transmission electron microscopy have shed light on the mechanisms of metallic debris storage. Like UHMWPE debris, metallic debris is transported to the periprosthetic tissues, and because of its small size is readily phagocytosed by histiocytes (163). Transmission electron micrographs by Doorn et al. have shown evidence that the nanometer-sized metallic debris particles can agglomerate intracellularly, which may play a role in decreasing their apparent surface area to the surrounding cytoplasm. From histomorphometric analysis, Doorn et al. have observed that metallic debris elicits less of a histological response than UHMWPE debris, based on counting the number of histiocytes in the periprosthetic tissues (163).

Because of its nanometer size, metallic debris and its degradation products can be bound into proteins and thereby dissolved in body fluids and transported throughout the lymphatic and cardiovascular systems (164–168). Research by Jacobs et al. has documented elevated chromium and cobalt concentrations in the serum and urine of patients implanted long-term with McKee-Farrar prostheses relative to controls who were given CoCr/UHMWPE implants (165,167). In a prospective, randomized, short-term study of patients implanted with second-generation metal-on-metal, ceramic-on-ceramic, and metal-on-polyethylene components, Brodner et al. (168)

detected a median serum cobalt concentration of 1.1 μm/L in patients implanted with metal-on-metal implants 1 year after surgery, whereas the concentrations for the other bearing couples were below the detection limit. Although researchers have elucidated a mechanism whereby the body is capable of eliminating cobalt and chrome via urine, the effects and significance of long-term systemic exposure to heavy metals remains an ongoing clinical concern, particularly with regard to carcinogenesis.

Epidemiological studies have not demonstrated a significantly increased risk for cancer after first generation metal-on-metal total joint replacements (159,169), but the uncertainty (confidence intervals) associated with these risk assessments is considerable. For example, in a recent meta-analysis of eight previous epidemiological studies, Tharani and colleagues found that the risk factor for cancer after metal-on-metal total hip replacement was 0.95, with a 95% confidence interval of 0.79–1.13; the risk factor for hematopoeitic cancers was 1.59, with a 95% confidence interval of 0.82–2.77 (169). Due to the small cohort of 579 Finnish patients previously analyzed with McKee-Farrar components (159), the cancer risk assessments conducted to date have not conclusively addressed all of the long-term biological issues related to the products of metal-on-metal articulation in the much larger population of patients worldwide with second-generation implants.

VI. SUMMARY

Orthopaedic surgeons are now presented with a wide range of choices when selecting an implant configuration for a particular patient. In the United States, contemporary ceramic-on-ceramic implants are approved only for investigational clinical trials, so the selection of alternative bearings is restricted to metal-on–crosslinked UHMWPE and metal-on-metal solutions, whereas surgeons in Europe, Asia, and Japan have ready access to current ceramic-on-ceramic designs.

As we have discussed throughout this chapter, all three families of alternative bearings—that is, metal on metal, ceramic and ceramic, and metal on crosslinked UHMWPE—represent a second generation of technology that incorporates successful elements from previous designs to provide significantly lower wear than their historical predecessors, as was shown through in vitro simulator investigations and in vivo clinical studies. All three of these orthopaedic bearing solutions are anticipated to lead to a lower incidence of osteolysis and ultimately fewer revisions during the second and third decades of service.

The alternative bearing solutions are not without their risks or uncertainties. For bearing couples containing a ceramic component, one risk is that of implant fracture. In metal-on-metal bearings, the risk pertains to the effects of long-term systemic exposure to metal wear debris. With the cross-linked UHMWPE-on-metal bearings, extensive in vitro analyses have been performed by several centers; and researchers have not been able to identify their relative risks with respect to those of conventional UHMWPE-on-metal bearings. Consequently, the clinical and research communities continue to track the in vivo performance of these alternative bearings with vigilance and anticipation.

REFERENCES

1. Wiles P. The surgery of the osteo-arthritic hip. Br J Surg 1957; 45:488–497.
2. McKee GK and Watson-Farrar J. Replacement of arthritic hips by the McKee-Farrar prosthesis. J Bone Joint Surg [Br] 1966; 48(2):245–259.
3. Smith RC, Geier MA, Reno J, and Sarasohn-Kahn J, eds. Orthopaedic products. In: 1999–2000 Medical & Healthcare Marketplace Guide, New York: IDD Enterprises 1998:265–272.
4. Willert HG, Bertram H, and Buchhorn GH. Osteolysis in alloarthroplasty of the hip. The role of ultra-high molecular weight polyethylene wear particles. Clin Orthop 1990; 258(258):95–107.
5. Willert H. Reactions of the articular capsule to wear products of artificial joint prostheses. J Biomed Mater Res 1977; 11:157–164.
6. Willert H. Tissue reactions to plastic and metallic wear products of joint endoprostheses. Gschwend N and Debrunner H, eds. In: Total Hip Prosthesis. Huber: Bern: Huber, 1976.
7. Goldring SR, Jasty M, Roueke CM, Bringhurst FR, and Harris WH. Formation of a synovial-like membrane at the bone-cement interface. Its role in bone resorption and implant loosening after total hip replacement. Arthritis Rheum 1986; 29(7):836–842.
8. Jasty M, Floyd WEI, Schiller AL, Goldring SR, and Harris WH. Localized osteolysis in stable, non-septic total hip replacement. J Bone Joint Surg 1986; 68A:912–919.
9. Kurtz SM, Muratoglu OK, Evans M, and Edidin AA. Advances in the processing, sterilization, and crosslinking of ultra-high molecular weight polyethylene for total joint arthroplasty. Biomaterials 1999; 20(18):1659–1688.
10. Shen F, McKellop H, and Salovey IR. Morphology of chemically crosslinked ultrahigh molecular weight polyethylene. J Biomed Mater Res 1998; 40:71–78.
11. McKellop H, Shen F-W, DiMaio W, and Lancaster JG. Wear of gamma-crosslinked polyethylene acetabular cups against roughened femoral balls. Clin Orthop Rel Res 1999; 369:73–82.

12. McKellop H, Shen F-W, Lu B, Campbell P, and Salovey R. Development of an extremely wear resistant ultra-high molecular weight polyethylene for total hip replacements. J. Orthop Res 1999; 17(2):157–167.

13. Muratoglu OK, Bragdon CR, O'Connor DO, Jasty M, Harris WH, Gul R, and McGarry F. Unified wear model for highly crosslinked ultra-high molecular weight polyethylenes (UHMWPE). Biomaterials, 1999; 20(16):1463–1470.

14. Muratoglu OK, Bragdon CR, O'Connor DO, Jasty M, and Harris WH. A novel method of crosslinking UHMWPE to improve wear, reduce oxidation and retain mechanical properties. J Arthrop 2001; 16(2):149–160.

15. Charnley J. Arthroplasty of the hip: A new operation. Lancet 1961; 1:1129–1132.

16. Zahiri CA, Schmalzried TP, Szuszczewicz ES, and Amstutz HC. Assessing activity in joint replacement patients. J Arthrop 1998; 13(8):890–895.

17. Schmalzried TP, Shepherd EF, Dorey FJ, Jackson WO, dela Rosa M, Fávae F, McKellop HA, McClung CD, Martell J, Moreland JR, and Amstutz HC. The John Charnley Award. Wear is a function of use, not time. Clin Orthop 2000; 381:36–46.

18. Malchau H, Herberts P, and Ahnfelt L. Prognosis of total hip replacement in Sweden. Follow-up of 92,675 operations performed 1978–1990. Acta Orthop Scand 1993; 64:497–506.

19. Malchau H, Herberts P, Söderman P, and Odén A. Prognosis of total hip replacement: Update and validation of results from the Swedish National Hip Arthroplasty Registry, 1979–1998. 67th Annual Meeting of the American Academy of Orthopaedic Surgeons, Scientific Exhibition, 2000.

20. Dearnaley G. Diamond-like carbon: A potential means of reducing wear in total joint replacements. Clin Mater 1993; 12(4):237–244.

21. Smith-Petersen MN. Evolution of mould arthroplasty of the hip joint. J Bone Joint Br 1948; 30-B(1):59–75.

22. Judet J and Judet R. The use of an artificial femoral head for arthroplasty of the hip joint. J Bone Joint Br 1950; 32-B(2):166–173.

23. Charnley J. The lubrication of animal joints. Institution of Mechanical Engineers: Symposium on Biomechanics, 1959; 17:12–22.

24. Li S and Burstein AH. Ultra-high molecular weight polyethylene. The material and its use in total joint implants. J Bone Joint Surg Am 1994; 76(7):1080–1090.

25. Charnley J. Tissue reaction to the polytetrafluoroethylene. Lancet 1963; 2:1379.

26. Charnley J. Low friction principle. In: Low Friction Arthroplasty of the Hip: Theory and Practice. Berlin: Springer-Verlag. 1979:3–16.

27. Charnley J, Kamangar A, and Longfield MD. The optimum size of prosthetic heads in relation to the wear of plastic sockets in total replacement of the hip. Med Biol Eng 1969; 7(1):31–39.

28. Polyethylene resins. In: Modern Plastics Encyclopaedia for 1962. New York: McGraw-Hill, 1961:251–268.

29. Sutula LC, Collier JP, Saum KA, Currier BH, Currier JH, Sanford WM, Mayor MB, Wooding RE, Sperling DK, Williams IR, et al. Impact of gamma

sterilization on clinical performance of polyethylene in the hip. Clin Orthop 1995; 319:28–40.

30. Rose RM, Goldfarb EV, Ellis E, and Crugnola AN. Radiation sterilization and the wear rate of polyethylene. J Orthop Res 1984; 2(4):393–400.

31. Eyerer P and Ke YC. Property changes of UHMW polyethylene hip cup endoprostheses during implantation. J Biomed Mater Res 1984; 18(9):1137–1151.

32. Eyerer P, Kurth M, McKellop HA, and Mittlmeier T. Characterization of UHMWPE hip cups run on joint simulators. J Biomed Mater Res 1987; 21(3): 275–291.

33. Grood ES, Shastri R, and Hopson CN. Analysis of retrieved implants: Crystallinity changes in ultrahigh molecular weight polyethylene. J Biomed Mater Res 1982; 16(4):399–405.

34. Roe RJ, Grood ES, Shastri R, Gosselin CA, and Noyes FR. Effect of radiation sterilization and aging on ultrahigh molecular weight polyethylene. J Biomed Mater Res 1981; 15(2):209–230.

35. Gomez-Barrena E, Li S, Furman BS, Masri BA, Wright TM, and Salvati EA. Role of polyethylene oxidation and consolidation defects in cup performance. Clin Orthop 1998; 352:105–117.

36. Kurtz SM, Rimnac CM, Li S, and Bartel DL. A bilinear material model for ultra-high molecular weight polyethylene total joint replacements. In: Transactions of the 40th Orthopedic Research Society. 1994. New Orleans, LA.

37. Kurtz SM, Rimnac CM, Santner TJ, and Bartel DL. Exponential model for the tensile true stress-strain behavior of as-irradiated and oxidatively degraded ultra high molecular weight polyethylene. J Orthop Res 1996; 14(5):755–761.

38. Kurtz SM, Rimnac CM, and Bartel DL. Predictive model for tensile true stress-strain behavior of chemically and mechanically degraded ultrahigh molecular weight polyethylene. J Biomed Mater Res 1998; 43(3):241–248.

39. Collier JP, Sperling DK, Currier JH, Sutula LC, Saum KA, and Mayor MB. Impact of gamma sterilization on clinical performance of polyethylene in the knee. J Arthrop 1996; 11(4):377–389.

40. White SE, Paxson RD, Tanner MG, and Whiteside LA. Effects of sterilization on wear in total knee arthroplasty. Clin Orthop 1996; 331:164–171.

41. Sauer WL and Anthony ME. Predicting the clinical wear performance of orthopaedic bearing surfaces. In: Jacobs JJ and Craig TL, eds. Alternative Bearing Surfaces in Total Joint Replacement. West Conshohocken, PA: American Society for Testing and Materials, 1998:1–29.

42. Griffith MJ, Seidenstein MK, Williams D, and Charnley J. Socket wear in Charnley low friction arthroplasty of the hip. Clin Orthop 1978; 137:37–47.

43. Charnley J and Halley DK, Rate of wear in total hip replacement. Clin Orthop 1975; 112:170–179.

44. Livermore J, Ilstrup D, and Morrey B. Effect of femoral head size on wear of the polyethylene acetabular component. J Bone Joint Surg [Am] 1990; 72(4):518–528.

45. Devane PA, Bourne RB, Rorabeck CH, Hardie RM, and Horne JG. Measurement of polyethylene wear in metal-backed acetabular cups. I. Three-dimensional technique. Clin Orthop 1995; 319:303–316.

46. Martell JM and Berdia S. Determination of polyethylene wear in total hip replacements with use of digital radiographs. J Bone Joint Surg Am 1997; 79(11):1635–1641.

47. Guven OE. Crosslinking and scission in polymers. In: Guven O, ed. NATO ASI Series, Mathematical and Physical Sciences vol 292. Boston: Kluwer, 1988.

48. Brandrup J and Immergut EH. Polymer Handbook, 3rd ed. New York: Wiley, 1989.

49. Dole M. Crosslinking and crystallinity in irradiated polyethylene. Polym Plast Technol Eng 1979; 13(1):41–64.

50. McGinniss V. Crosslinking with radiation. In: Brandrup J and Immergut EH, eds. Polymer Handbook. New York: Wiley, 1989:418–449.

51. Jahan MS and Wang C. Combined chemical and mechanical effects on free radicals in UHMWPE joints during implantation. J Biomed Mater Res 1991; 25:1005–1017.

52. Kashiwabara H, Shimada S, and Hori Y. Free radicals and crosslinking in irradiated polyethylene. Radiat Phys Chem 1991; 37(1):43–46.

53. Randall JC, Zoepfl FJ, and Silverman J. A 13C NMR study of radiation-induced long-chain branching in polyethylene. Makromol Chem Rapid Commun 1983; 4:149–157.

54. Muratoglu O, Bragdon CR, O'Connor D, Skehan H, Delaney J, Jasty M, and Harris W. Effect of temperature on radiation crosslinking of UHMWPE for use in total hip arthroplasty. 46th Annual Meeting. Orlando, FL: ORS, 2000.

55. Dijkstra DJ, Hoogsteen W, and Pennings AJ. Cross-linking of ultra-high molecular weight in the melt by means of electron beam irradiation. Polymer 1989; 30:866–873.

56. Edidin AA and Kurtz SM. Development and validation of the small punch test for UHMWPE used in total joint replacements. In: Soboyejo W, ed. Functional Biomaterials. Winterthur, Switzerland: Trans Tech Publications, 2000.

57. Muratoglu O, Bragdon C, O'Connor D, Jasty M, and Harris W. The effect of irradiation temperature on the crosslinking of UHMWPE. In: 1999 Society for Biomaterials 25th Annual Meeting Transactions. Providence, RI: 1999.

58. Jasty MJ, Goetz DD, Lee KR, Hanson AE, Elder JR, and Harris WH. Wear of polyethylene acetabular components in total hip arthroplasty. An analysis of 128 components retrieved at autopsy or revision operation. J Bone Joint Surg 1997; 79(A):349–358.

59. Pooley CM and Tabor D. Friction and molecular structure: The behavior of some thermoplastics. Proc R Soc Lond 1972: 329:251–274.

60. Bragdon C, O'Connor D, Lowenstein J, Jasty M, and Syniuta W. The importance of multidirectional motion on the wear of polyethylene. Proc Inst Mech Eng [H] 1996; 210:157–165.

61. Ramamurti BS, Bragdon CR, O'Connor DO, Lowenstein JD, Jasty M, Estok DM, and Harris WH. Loci of movement of selected points on the femoral

head during normal gait. Three-dimensional computer simulation. J Arthrop 1996; 11(7):845–852.

62. Ramamurti BS, Estok DM, Jasty M, and Harris WH. Analysis of the kinematics of different hip simulators used to study wear of candidate materials for the articulation of total hip arthroplasties. J Orthop Res 1998; 16:365–369.

63. Wang A, Sun DC, Stark C, and Dumbleton JH. Wear mechanisms of UHMWPE in total joint replacements. Wear 1995; 181–183:241–249.

64. Edidin AA, Pruitt L, Jewett CW, Crane DJ, Roberts D, and Kurtz SM. Plasticity-induced damage layer is a precursor to wear in radiation-cross-linked UHMWPE acetabular components for total hip replacement. Ultra-high-molecular-weight polyethylene. J Arthrop 1999; 14(5):616–627.

65. Muratoglu OK, Bragdon CR, O'Connor DO, Merrill EW, Jasty EM, and Harris WH. Electron beam crosslinking of UHMWPE at room temperature, a candidate bearing material for total joint arthroplasty. 23rd Annual Meeting of the Society for Biomaterials. 1997. New Orleans.

66. Kurtz SM, Pruitt LA, Jewett CW, Foulds JR, and Edidin AA. Radiation and chemical crosslinking promote strain hardening behavior and molecular alignment in ultra high molecular weight polyethylene during multi-axial loading conditions. Biomaterials 1999; 20(16):1449–1462.

67. Bragdon C, O'Connor D, Weinberg E, Skehan H, Muratoglu O, Lowenstein J, and Harris W. The role of head size on creep and wear of conventional vs. highly cross-linked polyethylene acetabular components. Society for Biomaterials 25th Annual Meeting Transactions. Providence, RI: 1999.

68. McKellop H and Shen F. Wear of surface gradient crosslinked UHMWPE cups against damaged femoral balls. 46th Annual Meeting, ORS (Session 5, Implant Wear I). 2000. Orlando, Florida.

69. McKellop H, Shen F-W, Lu B, Campbell P, and Salovey R. Effect of sterilization method and other modifications on the wear resistance or acetabular cups made of ultra-high molecular weight polyethylene. J Bone Joint Surg 2000; 82-A(12):1708–1725.

70. Bragdon CR, Muratoglu OK, O'Connor DO, Lowenstein JD, Skehan H, Lozynski A, Jasty M, and Harris WH. Resistance of a highly crosslinked polyethylene to third body wear. In: Annual Meeting of Orthopaedic Research Society, Orlando, FL: 2000.

71. Oonishi H, Igaki H, and Takayama Y. Long-Term Clinical Wear Rates for Irradiation Sterilized UHMWPE THR Cups and Laboratory Correlation. in 35th Annual Meeting, Orthopaedic Research Society. Las Vegas, NV: 1989.

72. Oonishi E and Stuji E. SEM Observation on the clinically used gamma-irradiated reinforced HDP socket in total hip replacement. Adv Biomater 1990; 9:379–385.

73. Oonishi H and Takayama Y. The effects of gamma-irradiation on wear resistance of polyethylene socket in total hip prostheses—Wear test and clinical results. In: The 17th Annual Meeting of the Society for Biomaterials. Scottsdale, AZ: 1991.

74. Oonishi H, Takayama Y, and Tsuji E. Improvement of polyethylene by irradiation in artificial joints. Radiat Phys and Chem 1992; 39(6):495–504.

75. Oonishi H. Long term clinical results of THR. Clinical results of THR of an alumina head with a cross-linked UHMWPE cup. Orthop Surg Traumatol 1995; 38(11):1255–1264.

76. Oonishi H, Takayama Y, and Tsuji E. The low wear of cross-linked polyethylene socket in total hip prostheses. In: Wise DL, Trantolo DJ, Altobelli DE, Yaszemski MJ, Gresser JD, and Schwartz ER, eds. Encyclopedic Handbook of Biomaterials and Bioengineering. Part A: Materials. New York: Marcel Dekker, 1995:1853–1868.

77. Oonishi H, Saito M, and Y K. Wear of high-dose gamma irradiated polyethylene in total joint replacement—Long term radiological evaluation. 44th Annual Meeting, Orthopaedic Research Society March 16–19 New Orleans, LA: 1998.

78. Oonishi H, Igaki H, and Takayama Y. Wear resistance of gamma-ray irradiated UHMW polyethylene socket in total hip prostheses—Wear test and long term clinical results. The Third World Biomaterials Congress, 1998:588.

79. Oonishi H, Kadoya Y, and SM. Gamma-irradiated cross-linked polyethylene in total hip replacements—Analysis of retrieved sockets after long-term implantation. J Biomed Mater Res 2001; 58(2):167–171.

80. Shikata T, Oonishi H, Hashimato Y, and al e. Wear resistance of irradiated UHMW polyethylenes to Al2O3 ceramics in total hip prostheses. Transactions of the 3rd Annual Meeting of the Society for Biomaterials, 1977:118.

81. DuPlessis TA, Grobbelaar CJ, and Marais F. The improvement of polyethylene prostheses through radiation crosslinking. Radiat Phys Chem 1977; 9: 647–652.

82. Grobbelaar CJ, Du Plessis TA, and Marais F. The radiation improvment of polyethylene prostheses: A preliminary study. J Bone Joint Surg 1978; 60-B(3):370–374.

83. Grobbelaar CJ, Weber FA, Spirakis A, DuPlessis TA, Cappaert G, and Cakic JN. Clinical experience with gamma irradiation-crosslinked polyethylene-A 14 to 20 year follow-up report. S Afr Bone Joint Surgery 1999; XI(3):140–147.

84. Wroblewski B, Siney P, and Fleming P. Low-friction arthroplasty of the hip using alumina ceramic and cross-linked polyethylene. A ten-year follow-up report. J Bone Joint Surg 1999; 81-B(1):54–55.

85. Wroblewski BM, Siney PD, Dowson D, and Collins SN. Prospective clinical and joint simulator studies of a new total hip arthroplasty using alumina ceramic heads and cross-linked polyethylene cups. J Bone Joint Surg 1996; 78B:280–285.

86. Klein PG, Gonzalez-Orozco JA, and Ward IM. Structure and morphology of highly oriented radiation crosslinked polyethylene fibres. Polymer 1991; 32(10):1732–1736.

87. Muratoglu O, Bragdon CR, O'Connor D, Skehan H, Delaney J, Jasty M, and Harris WH. Comparison of wear behavior of four different types of crosslinked acetabular components. 46th Annual Meeting, ORS. Orlando, FL: 2000.

88. Frankel A, Balderston R, Booth R, and Rothman R. Radiographic demarcation of the acetabular bone-cement interface. The effect of femoral head size. J Arthrop 1990; 5(suppl):1–3.

89. Jaramaz B, Nikou C, and DiGioia AM. Effect of cup orientation and neck length in range of motion simulation. Transactions of 43rd Annual Meeting of ORS. 1997:286.

90. Jaramaz B, Nikou C, and DiGioia AM. Sensitivity of impingement limits to error in cup placement. Transactions of 44th Annual Meeting of ORS. 1998: 402.

91. Jaramaz B, Nikou C, and DiGioia AM. Effect of combined acetabular/femoral implant version on hip range of motion. Transactions of 45th Annual Meeting of ORS. 1999:926.

92. Boutin P. [Alumina and its use in surgery of the hip. (Experimental study)]. Presse Med 1971; 79(14):639–640.

93. Willmann G, Ceramics for total hip replacement—What a surgeon should know. Orthopedics 1998; 21(2):173–177.

94. Boutin P, Christel P, Dorlot JM, Meunier A, de Roquancourt A, Blanquaert D, Herman S, Sedel L, and Witvoet J. The use of dense alumina-alumina ceramic combination in total hip replacement. J Biomed Mater Res 1988; 22(12):1203–1232.

95. Willmann G. Ceramic femoral head retrieval data. Clin Orthop 2000; 379: 22–28.

96. Christel P, Meunier A, Heller M, Torre JP, and Peille CN. Mechanical properties and short-term in-vivo evaluation of yttrium- oxide-partially-stabilized zirconia. J Biomed Mater Res 1989; 23(1):45–61.

97. Hummer CD, 3rd, Rothman RH, and Hozack WJ. Catastrophic failure of modular zirconia-ceramic femoral head components after total hip arthroplasty. J Arthrop 1995; 10(6):848–850.

98. Heck DA, Partridge CM, Reuben JD, Lanzer WL, Lewis CG, and Keating EM. Prosthetic component failures in hip arthroplasty surgery. J Arthrop 1995; 10(5):575–580.

99. Peiro A, Pardo J, Navarrete R, Rodriguez-Alonso L, and Martos F. Fracture of the ceramic head in total hip arthroplasty. Report of two cases. J Arthrop 1991; 6(4):371–374.

100. Michaud RJ and Rashad SY. Spontaneous fracture of the ceramic ball in a ceramic-polyethylene total hip arthroplasty. J Arthrop 1995; 10(6):863–867.

101. Krikler S and Schatzker J. Ceramic head failure. J Arthrop 1995; 10(6):860–862.

102. Holmer P and Nielsen PT. Fracture of ceramic femoral heads in total hip arthroplasty. J Arthrop 1993; 8(6):567–571.

103. Higuchi F, Shiba N, Inoue A, and Wakebe I. Fracture of an alumina ceramic head in total hip arthroplasty. J Arthrop 1995; 10(6):851–854.

104. Callaway GH, Flynn W, Ranawat CS, and Sculco TP. Fracture of the femoral head after ceramic-on-polyethylene total hip arthroplasty. J Arthrop 1995; 10(6):855–859.

105. Kempf I and Semlitsch M. Massive wear of a steel ball head by ceramic fragments in the polyethylene acetabular cup after revision of a total hip prosthesis with fractured ceramic ball. Arch Orthop Trauma Surg 1990; 109(5):284–287.

106. Fritsch EW and Gleitz M. Ceramic femoral head fractures in total hip arthroplasty. Clin Orthop Rel Res 1996; 328:129–136.

107. Lancaster JG, Dowson D, Isaac GH, and Fisher J. The wear of ultra-high molecular weight polyethylene sliding on metallic and ceramic counterfaces representative of current femoral surfaces in joint replacement. Proc Inst Mech Eng [H] 1997; 211(1):17–24.

108. Cuckler JM, Bearcroft J, and Asgian CM. Femoral head technologies to reduce polyethylene wear in total hip arthroplasty. Clin Orthop 1995; 317(317): 57–63.

109. Barbour PSM, Stone MH, and Fisher J. A hip joint simulator study using new and physiologically scratched femoral heads with ultra-high molecular weight polyethylene acetabular cups. Proceedings of the Institution of Mechanical Engineers, 2000, Part H. J Eng Med 2000; 214(H6):569–576.

110. Wang A, Essner A, Polineni VK, Stark C, and Dumbleton JH. Lubrication and wear of ultra-high molecular weight polyethylene in total joint replacements. Tribol Int 1998; 31(1–3):17–33.

111. Wright K and Scales J. The use of hip joint simulators for the evaluation of wear of total hip prostheses. In: Writer G, Lerey J, and DeGrosst K, eds. Evaluation of Biomaterials. New York: Wiley, 1980:135.

112. McKellop H, Lu B, and Benya P. Friction, lubrication, and wear of cobalt-chromium, alumina, and zirconia hip prostheses compared on a joint simulator. In: Trans 38th ORS. Washington DC: 1992.

113. Sugano N, Nishii T, Nakata K, Masuhara K, and Takaoka K. Polyethylene sockets and alumina ceramic heads in cemented total hip arthroplasty. A ten-year study. J Bone Joint Surg Br 1995; 77(4):548–556.

114. Cales B. Zirconia as a sliding material: Histologic, laboratory, and clinical data. Clin Orthop 2000; 379:94–112.

115. Sychterz CJ, Engh CA Jr, Young AM, Hopper RH Jr, and Engh CA. Comparison of in vivo wear between polyethylene liners articulating with ceramic and cobalt-chrome femoral heads. J Bone Joint Surg Br 2000; 82(7):948–951.

116. Willmann G, Fruh HJ, and Pfaff HG. Wear characteristics of sliding pairs of zirconia (Y-TZP) for hip endoprostheses. Biomaterials 1996; 17(22):2157–2162.

117. Fruh HJ, Willmann G, and Pfaff HG. Wear characteristics of ceramic-on-ceramic for hip endoprostheses. Biomaterials 1997; 18(12):873–876.

118. Clarke IC, Good V, Williams P, Schroeder D, Anissian L, Stark A, Oonishi H, Schuldies J, and Gustafson G. Ultra-low wear rates for rigid-on-rigid bearings in total hip replacements. Proc Inst Mech Eng [H] 2000; 214(4):331–347.

119. Nevelos JE, Ingham E, Doyle C, Nevelos AB, and Fisher J. The influence of acetabular cup angle on the wear of "BIOLOX Forte" alumina ceramic bear-

ing couples in a hip joint simulator. J Mater Sci Mater Med 2001; 12(2):141–144.

120. Dorlot JM, Christel P, and Meunier A. Wear analysis of retrieved alumina heads and sockets of hip prostheses. J Biomed Mater Res 1989; 23(A3 suppl): 299–310.

121. Bizot P, Nizard R, Lerouge S, Prudhommeaux F, and Sedel L. Ceramic/ceramic total hip arthroplasty. J Orthop Sci 2000; 5(6):622–627.

122. Nevelos JE, Ingham E, Doyle C, Fisher J, and Nevelos AB. Analysis of retrieved alumina ceramic components from Mittelmeier total hip prostheses. Biomaterials 1999; 20(19):1833–1840.

123. Lombardi AV, Mallory TH, Dennis DA, Komistek RD, Fada RA, and Northcut EJ. An in vivo determination of total hip arthroplasty pistoning during activity. J Arthrop 2000; 15(6):702–709.

124. Nevelos J, Ingham E, Doyle C, Streicher R, Nevelos A, Walter W, and Fisher J. Microseparation of the centers of alumina-alumina artificial hip joints during simulator testing produces clinically relevant wear rates and patterns. J Arthrop 2000; 15(6):793–795.

125. Dorlot J. Long-term effects of alumina components in total hip prostheses. Clin Orthop 1992; (282):47–52.

126. Jin ZM, Dowson D, and Fisher J. Analysis of fluid film lubrication in artificial hip joint replacements with surfaces of high elastic modulus. Proc Inst Mech Eng [H] 1997; 211(3):247–256.

127. Wilson JN and Scales JT. The Stanmore metal on metal total hip prosthesis using a three pin type cup. A follow-up of 100 arthroplasties over nine years. Clin Orthop 1973; 95(95):239–249.

128. Ring PA. Complete replacement arthroplasty of the hip by the ring prosthesis. J Bone Joint Surg Br 1968; 50(4):720–731.

129. Muller ME. The benefits of metal-on-metal total hip replacements. Clin Orthop 1995; 311(311):54–59.

130. Sivash KM. The development of a total metal prosthesis for the hip joint from a partial joint replacement. Reconstr Surg Traumatol 1969; 11:53–62.

131. Zahiri CA, Schmalzried TP, Ebramzadeh E, Szuszczewicz ES, Salib D, Kim C, and Amstutz HC. Lessons learned from loosening of the McKee-Farrar metal-on-metal total hip replacement. J Arthrop 1999; 14(3):326–332.

132. August AC, Aldam CH, and Pynsent PB. The McKee-Farrar hip arthroplasty. A long-term study. J Bone Joint Surg Br 1986; 68(4):520–527.

133. Djerf K and Wahlstrom O. Total hip replacement comparison between the McKee-Farrar and Charnley prostheses in a 5-year follow-up study. Arch Orthop Trauma Surg 1986; 105(3):158–162.

134. Jacobsson SA, Djerf K, and Wahlstrom O. Twenty-year results of McKee-Farrar versus Charnley prosthesis. Clin Orthop 1996; 329(suppl):S60–S68.

135. Jacobsson SA, Djerf K, and Wahlstrom O. A comparative study between McKee-Farrar and Charnley arthroplasty with long-term follow-up periods. J Arthrop 1990; 5(1):9–14.

136. Weber BG. METASUL from 1988 to today. In: Rieker CB, Windler M, and Wyss U, eds. Metasul: A Metal-on-Metal Bearing. Bern: Huber, 1999:23–28.

137. Wagner M and Wagner H. Medium-term results of a modern metal-on-metal system in total hip replacement. Clin Orthop 2000; 379:123–133.

138. Dorr LD, Wan Z, Longjohn DB, Dubois B, and Murken R. Total hip arthroplasty with use of the Metasul metal-on-metal articulation. Four to seven-year results. J Bone Joint Surg Am 2000; 82(6):789–798.

139. Chan FW, Bobyn JD, Medley JB, Krygier JJ, and Tanzer M. The Otto Aufranc Award. Wear and lubrication of metal-on-metal hip implants. Clin Orthop 1999; 369:10–24.

140. Firkins PJ, Tipper JL, Ingham E, Stone MH, Farrar R, and Fisher J. Influence of simulator kinematics on the wear of metal-on-metal hip prostheses. Proc Inst Mech Eng [H] 2001; 215(1):119–121.

141. Firkins PJ, Tipper JL, Saadatzadeh MR, Ingham E, Stone MH, Farrar R, and Fisher J. Quantitative analysis of wear and wear debris from metal-on-metal hip prostheses tested in a physiological hip joint simulator. Biomed Mater Eng 2001; 11(2):143–157.

142. Lemons JE. Metals and alloys. In: Petty W, ed. Total Joint Replacement. Philaldelphia: Saunders, 1991:21–27.

143. Dearnley PA. A review of metallic, ceramic and surface-treated metals used for bearing surfaces in human joint replacements. Proc Inst Mech Eng [H] 1999; 213(2):107–135.

144. Park JB. Metallic biomaterials. In: Bronzino JD, ed. The Biomedical Engineering Handbook. Boca Raton, FL: CRC Press, 1995:537–551.

145. Poggie RA. A review of the effects of design, contact stress, and materials on the wear or metal-on-metal hip prostheses. In: Jacobs JJ and Craig TL, eds. Alternative Bearing Surfaces in Total Joint Replacement. West Conshohocken, PA: American Society for Testing and Materials, 1998:47–54.

146. Varano R, Yue S, Bobyn JD, and Medley J. Co-Cr-Mo alloys used in metal-metal bearing surfaces. In: Jacobs JJ and Craig TL, eds. Alternative Bearing Surfaces in Total Joint Replacement. West Conshohocken, PA: American Society for Testing and Materials, 1998:55–68.

147. Chan FW, Bobyn JD, Medley JB, Krygier JJ, Yue S, and Tanzer M. Engineering issues and wear performance of metal on metal hip implants. Clin Orthop 1996; 333:96–107.

148. Park SH, McKellop H, Lu B, Chan FW, and Chiesa R. Wear morphology of metal-metal implants: Hip simulator tests compared with clinical retrievals. In: Rieker CB, Windler M, and Wyss U, eds. Metasul: A Metal-on-Metal Bearing. Bern: Huber, 1999:73–81.

149. Chan FW, Medley JB, Bobyn JD, and Krygier JJ. Numerical analysis of time-varying fluid film thickness in metal-metal hip implants in simulator tests. In: Jacobs JJ and Craig TL, eds. Alternative Bearing Surfaces in Total Joint Replacement. West Conshohocken, PA: American Society for Testing and Materials, 1998:111–128.

150. Kothari M, Bartel DL, and Booker JF. Surface geometry of retrieved McKee-Farrar total hip replacements. Clin Orthop 1996; 329(suppl):S141–S147.

151. Amstutz HC, Campbell P, McKellop H, Schmalzreid TP, Gillespie WJ, Howie D, Jacobs J, Medley J, and Merritt K. Metal on metal total hip re-

placement workshop consensus document. Clin Orthop 1996; 329(suppl): S297–S303.

152. Scott ML and Lemons JE. The wear characteristics of Sivash/SRN Co-Cr-Mo THA articulating surfaces. In: Jacobs JJ and Craig TL, eds Alternative Bearing Surfaces in Total Joint Replacement. West Conshohocken: American Society for Testing and Materials, 1998:159–172.

153. Willert HG, Buchhorn GH, Gobel D, Koster G, Schaffner S, Schenk R, and Semlitsch M. Wear behavior and histopathology of classic cemented metal on metal hip endoprostheses. Clin Orthop 1996; 329(suppl):S160–S186.

154. McKellop H, Park SH, Chiesa R, Doorn P, Lu B, Normand P, Grigoris P, and Amstutz H. In vivo wear of three types of metal on metal hip prostheses during two decades of use. Clin Orthop 1996; 329(suppl):S128–S140.

155. Willert HG and Buchhorn GH. Retrieval studies on classic cemented metal-on-metal hip endoprostheses. In: Rieker CB, Windler M, and Wyss U, eds. Metasul: A Metal-on-Metal Bearing. Bern: Huber, 1999:39–60.

156. Schmidt M, Weber H, and Schon R. Cobalt chromium molybdenum metal combination for modular hip prostheses. Clin Orthop 1996; 329(suppl):S35–S47.

157. Sieber HP, Rieker CB, and Kottig P. Analysis of 118 second-generation metal-on-metal retrieved hip implants. J Bone Joint Surg Br 1999; 81(1):46–50.

158. Riecker CB, Köttig P, Schön R, Windler M, and Wyss U. Clinical tribological performance of 144 metal-on-metal hip articulations. In: Rieker CB, Windler M, and Wyss U, eds. Metasul: A Metal-on-Metal Bearing. Bern: Huber, 1999: 83–92.

159. Visuri T, Pukkala E, Paavolainen P, Pulkkinen P, and Riska EB. Cancer risk after metal on metal and polyethylene on metal total hip arthroplasty. Clin Orthop 1996; 329(suppl):S280–S289.

160. Dorr LD, Hilton KR, Wan Z, Markovich GD, and Bloebaum R. Modern metal on metal articulation for total hip replacements. Clin Orthop 1996; 333:108–117.

161. Iida H, Kaneda E, Takada H, Uchida K, Kawanabe K, and Nakamura T. Metallosis due to impingement between the socket and the femoral neck in a metal-on-metal bearing total hip prosthesis. A case report. J Bone Joint Surg Am 1999; 81(3):400–403.

162. Doorn PF, Campbell PA, Worrall J, Benya PD, McKellop HA, and Amstutz HC. Metal wear particle characterization from metal on metal total hip replacements: Transmission electron microscopy study of periprosthetic tissues and isolated particles. J Biomed Mater Res 1998; 42(1):103–111.

163. Doorn PF, Campbell P, and Amstutz H. Particle disease in metal-on-metal total hip replacements. In: Rieker CB, Windler M, and Wyss U, eds. Metasul: A Metal-on-Metal Bearing. Bern: Huber, 1999:113–119.

164. Fisher J, Ingham E, Stone M, Wroblewski BM, Besong AA, Tipper JL, Firkins PJ, Minakawa H, Matthews JB, and Green T. Wear particle morphologies in artificial hip joints: Particle size is critical to the response of macrophages.

In: Rieker CB, Windler M, and Wyss U, eds. Metasul: A Metal-on-Metal Bearing. Bern: Huber, 1999:121–124.

165. Jacobs JJ, Skipor AK, Doorn PF, Campbell P, Schmalzried TP, Black J, and Amstutz HC. Cobalt and chromium concentrations in patients with metal on metal total hip replacements. Clin Orthop 1996; 329(suppl):S256–S263.

166. Jacobs JJ, Skipor AK, Patterson LM, Hallab NJ, Paprosky WG, Black J, and Galante JO. Metal release in patients who have had a primary total hip arthroplasty. A prospective, controlled, longitudinal study. J Bone Joint Surg Am 1998; 80(10):1447–1458.

167. Jacobs JJ, Hallab NJ, Skipor AK, Urban RM, Mikecz K, and Glant TT. Metallic wear and corrosion products: biological implications. In: Rieker CB, Windler M, and Wyss U, eds. Metasul: A Metal-on-Metal Bearing. Bern: Huber, 1999:125–132.

168. Brodner W, Bitzan P, Meisinger V, Kaider A, Gottsauner-Wolf F, and Kotz R. Elevated serum cobalt with metal-on-metal articulating surfaces. J Bone Joint Surg Br 1997; 79(2):316–321.

169. Tharani R, Dorey FJ, and Schmalzried TP. The risk of cancer following total hip or knee arthroplasty. J Bone Joint Surg Am 2001; 83-A(5):774–780.

170. Charnley J. Total hip replacement by low-friction arthroplasty. Clin Orthop 1970; 72:7–21.

171. Ring PA. Five to fourteen year interim results of uncemented total hip arthroplasty. Clin Orthop 1978; 137:87–95.

172. Muratoglu O, Bragdon C, O'Connor D, Perinchief R, Estok D, Jasty M, and Harris W. A New Concept: Larger Diameter Femoral Heads Used in Conjunction with a Highly Crosslinked UHMWPE. ms-submitted to JOA (2001).

2
Cementless Femoral Stem Design

Robert B. Bourne
University of Western Ontario, London, Ontario, Canada

End-stage arthritic conditions of the hip rob patients of their quality of life. Total hip arthroplasty has been a salvation to these patients, relieving pain and restoring function. Total hip arthroplasty has been demonstrated to be one of the most cost-effective and cost-saving medical interventions known (Figure 1) (1,2). Indeed, total hip arthroplasty has been one of the truly remarkable medical advances of the past 40 years. Limitations of early designs prompted surgeons to offer total hip arthroplasty to elderly patients over the age of 70 for whom a resection arthroplasty would be a viable option (3–10). The success of total hip arthroplasty in these individuals has led to a continual expansion of these indications. Most patients offered total hip arthroplasty are over 60 years of age; but in institutions such as ours, 20% of total hip arthroplasties are now performed in patients less than 55 years of age. Continuous improvements in total hip replacement design, metallurgy, fixation, and bearing surfaces has allowed this expansion of indications for total hip arthroplasty.

The fixation of total hip arthroplasties has followed two distinct paths —namely, cemented or cementless fixation (Figure 2A and B). Most forms of fixation have undergone continuous improvement. The Swedish Hip Arthroplasty Register has clearly demonstrated the benefits of this stepwise improvement in cemented hip arthroplasties. Since 1979, there has been a stepwise reduction in cumulative revision rates (5). Indeed, for cemented total hip replacements, the majority of orthopaedic surgeons would now utilize lavage of the bony surfaces, a cement restrictor, a cement gun, a proximal pressurizer, and a femoral stem with a rounded-rectangular cross section that allows at least 2 mm of cement mantle. Our results using this technique have been stellar, with 97% success at 10 to 15 years (11).

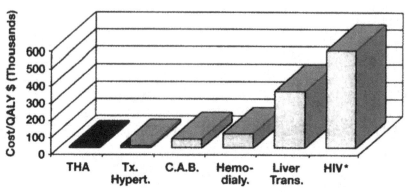

* Cost/Additonal Life Saved

Figure 1 Cost per quality adjusted life year (QALY) of total hip replacement compared with the medical treatment of moderate hypertension—coronary artery bypass, hemodialysis, liver transplantation, and universal precautions for human immunovirus (HIV). Treatments under $20,000 are the most cost effective (type A interventions). Total hip replacement falls within type A interventions at $7000/ QALY.

The evolution of cementless femoral stems has been similar. Many of the deficiencies of earlier cementless stems have been overcome, and durable fixation with 97–100% survivorship has been demonstrated (12–23). Our own clinical studies have demonstrated 95% survival of cementless anatomic stems and 99.5% survival of cementless tapered stems at more than 10 years follow-up (24). Three main types of cementless stems have evolved: tapered, anatomic, and cylindrical distal fixation types. In the past, the younger, more active patient with a funnel-shaped femur and a diagnosis of osteoarthritis has been considered the ideal candidate for this type of fixation. In the Swedish Hip Arthroplasty Registry, cementless femoral stem fixation has proven superior to cemented fixation in patients less than 60 years of age (17). With the success of cementless femoral stems, there has been a gradual upward creep in terms of the age of patients offered this type of fixation. For many surgeons, the shape of the proximal femoral medullary canal has been important. Some 85% of patients have so-called Dorr A or B femoral morphology, in which there is a funnel-shape (24). These patients seem ideal for cementless fixation. Some surgeons offer cementless femoral stems to all patients, even if they have cylindrical Dorr type C femoral morphology (Figure 3). The results in this group seem very durable as well, but with the price of proximal femoral stress shielding. Many surgeons also offer ce- mentless femoral stems to patients with inflammatory arthritic conditions

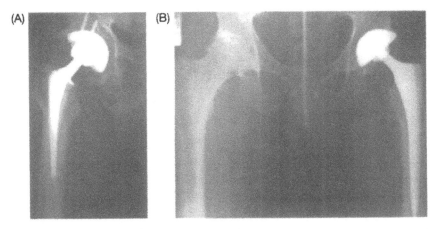

Figure 2 Contemporary hybrid (cementless socket, cemented stem) (A) and cementless (B) total hip replacements. (From Synergy, Smith & Nephew, Memphis, TN.)

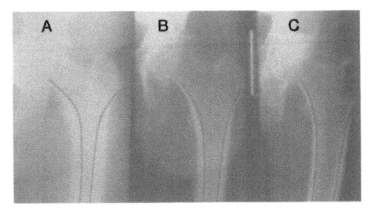

Figure 3 Radiographic examples of Dorr type A, B, and C proximal femoral morphologies. Some 85% of patients have type A or B femurs—morphologies ideal for cementless fixation.

such as rheumatoid arthritis. Once again, excellent results have been reported (13,14,16).

Several controversies still exist with regard to cementless femoral stems. Good results have been reported with the use of ongrowth grit-blasted surfaces, hydroxyapatite surfaces and various porous ingrowth surfaces (i.e. sintered beads, sintered wire mesh and plasma spray) (12,14,16–18,21–

23,25–28). Differentiating features have included the prevalence of thigh pain and stress shielding. Various stems also have substantial differences in terms of head and neck design that affect range of motion without impingement and the ability of various stems to reproduce femoral head offset.

I. HISTORIC OVERVIEW

A. First-Generation Cementless Stems

Cementless femoral stems became possible when strong, biologically inert metal alloys were discovered. The Austin-Moore implant represents a prototype in this class of implants (Figure 4). These implants lacked any ingrowth surface to enhance implant fixation. Rather, they depended upon a wedge fit principal for fixation. Often a bone plug was placed within a hole that passed from front to back in the proximal aspect of the Austin-Moore prosthesis in the hope that this bone plug would heal anteriorly and posteriorly to the femoral canal and enhance fixation. The surgeon had a limited size selection to choose from, and—not surprisingly—pain in the thigh and loss of fixation were not uncommon problems. More recently, this type of cementless femoral stem was used quite successfully with more size options in endoprostheses such as the Bateman bipolar implant.

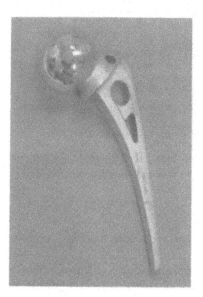

Figure 4   An example of a retrieved Austin Moore prefitted femoral stem (Howmedica, East Rutherford, NJ).

In the early 1970s, several investigators attempted to enhance femoral component fixation by exploring the use of various porous ingrowth surfaces. Cameron, Pilliar, and Macnab utilized a single-size implant in the same shape as the Austin-Moore device, but this time coated with a sintered bead porous ingrowth surface. Lunceford and Engh improved upon this implant, increasing the number of sizes available to enhance diaphyseal fixation (Figure 5A). A similar approach was utilized by Lord, but in this instance a cast madreporic ingrowth/ongrowth surface was developed (Figure 5B). These implants provided excellent femoral fixation but also introduced the new clinical problems of thigh pain and stress shielding. In addition, these implants proved difficult to extract in cases of deep sepsis or femoral stem fracture.

In the early 1980s, anatomic cementless femoral stems emerged. Porous Coated Anatomic (PCA) total hip replacement would represent the prototype in this regard (Howmedica, East Rutherford, NJ). The PCA THR was fabricated from cobalt chromium alloy and featured a proximal sintered bead porous ingrowth surface and an anteriorly curved femoral stem (Figure 6). Excellent biological fixation was achieved with this implant, and indeed, in our hands, a 95% stem survivorship at 10 or more years follow-up was achieved. Pain in the thigh was found in more than 22% of our PCA total hip replacement patients in studies published at 2, 5, and 10 years follow-up (16).

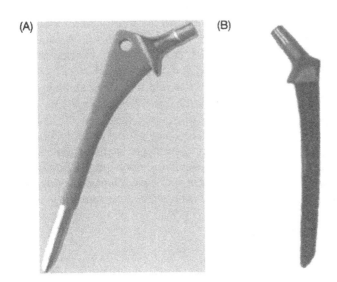

(A)   (B)

Figure 5   Examples of early-distal-fixation "biologic ingrowth" femoral stems, the Anatomic Medullary Locking (AML; DePuy, Warsaw, IN) (A), and Lord (Howmedica, East Rutherford, NJ) femoral stems (B).

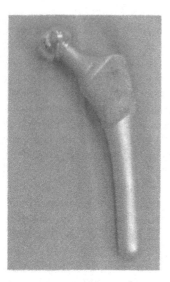

Figure 6 The Porous Coated Anatomic (PCA; Howmedica, East Rutherford, NJ), anatomic femoral stem.

The other approach to cementless femoral stem fixation was the emergence of taper design implants (Figure 7A, B, and C) (1,2,7,12,13,21,25–27,29,30). Most of these taper devices featured a three degree medial to lateral and often anterior to posterior taper of the femoral stem. A common feature of these devices was a three-point fixation visible on true lateral radiographs (Figure 8A and B). The femoral component touched the cortical bone proximally and posteriorly, anteriorly at the metaphyseal-diaphyseal junction, and posteriorly at its distal tip. Some cementless taper design femoral stems depended upon a grip-blasted plus some supplemental fixation (i.e., squared corners or proximal ridges). The Zweymueller and Canal Locking System (CLS) total hip replacements are prototypes in this regard. Other cementless taper designs featured a proximal ingrowth/ongrowth surface made up either of sintered beads or a plasma spray. Excellent clinical results for 10 or more years have been achieved with cementless tapered femoral components.

II. DIFFERENTIATING FEATURES

A. Thigh Pain

Pain in the thigh following cemented total hip replacements is infrequent. Our studies have demonstrated that only 3% of cemented femoral stems are

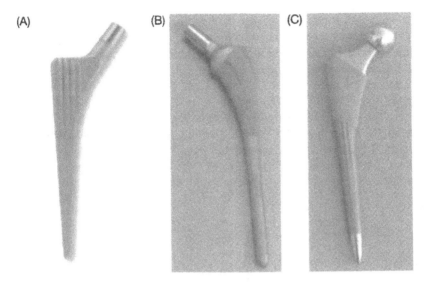

Figure 7 Examples of cementless tapered femoral components, the Canal Locking System (CLS; Sulzer, Winterhur, Switzerland) (A), the Mallory Head (Biomet, Warsaw, IN) (B), and the Synergy (Smith & Nephew, Memphis, TN) (C).

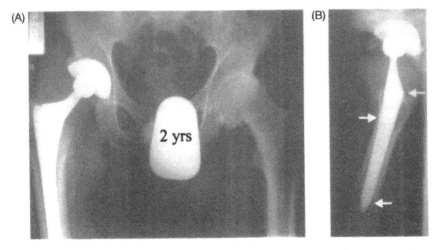

Figure 8 Anteroposterior and lateral radiographs of a cementless Synergy total hip replacement (Smith & Nephew, Memphis, TN). Note the "three-point fixation" on the lateral radiograph.

associated with thigh pain (Figure 9). Unfortunately, some cementless femoral stem designs are associated with greater prevalence of pain in the thigh following total hip replacement surgery (Table 1). Our studies of the PCA total hip replacement have demonstrated a 22% prevalence at 2 years, a 26% prevalence at 5 years, and a 23% prevalence at 10 years of follow-up (16). Typically, this thigh pain was activity-related and mild to moderate in intensity. The thigh pain was rarely severe enough to warrant revision surgery. Pain in the thigh has also been a problem for cementless distal-fixation cylindrical-type stems. Various authors have reported a prevalence of significant thigh pain ranging from 8–15% when such devices are used (14). In contrast, we conducted a randomized clinical trial comparing cemented

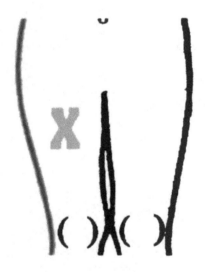

Figure 9 Pain drawing used to collect data on pain in the thigh plate after total hip replacement.

Table 1 Prevalence of Pain in the Thigh with Various Total Hip Replacement Stems

Cemented	3%
Cementless tapered	3%
Cementless anatomic	22%
Cementless distal fixation	10%

total hip replacements to cementless tapered total hip replacements. The prevalence of pain in the thigh was only 3% for the cementless tapered and cemented femoral components (1,2). This thigh pain was always mild (i.e., 1–3 on a 10-point visual analogue scale). Cementless tapered femoral components appear to have some advantages in terms of minimizing pain in the thigh following total hip arthroplasty.

B. Stress Shielding

Some element of stress shielding always accompanies total hip replacements in which the femoral neck is osteotomized and the femur loaded through the endosteal canal. Patient and implant factors have been found to be important in the development of stress shielding. Patients with severe osteoporosis have been shown to be more vulnerable in terms of developing stress shielding. In addition, implant stiffness has proven to be important. Bobyn et al. demonstrated that stress shielding was more frequent with an extensively coated cobalt chromium femoral component larger than 13.5 mm in

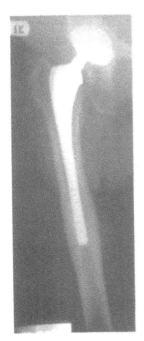

Figure 10 An example of new periosteal bone formation in Gruen zones 3 and 5 ten years after insertion of a Mallory Head cementless tapered total hip replacement (Biomet, Warsaw, IN).

(A)

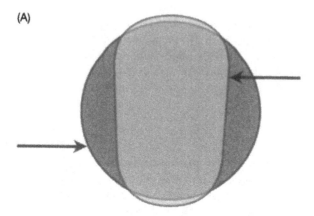

(B)

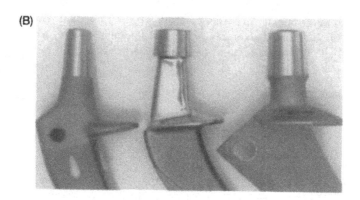

(C)

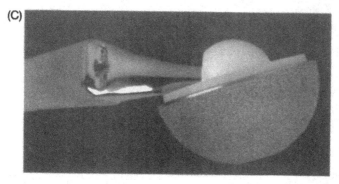

Figure 11 Contemporary developments in THR femoral neck design to enhance range of motion. These include a rounded trapezoid neck (A), a shortened Morse taper (B) and improved acetabular chamfer design (C).

diameter. Tapered cementless total hip replacements have an advantage in this regard. First, the tapered shape presents a less stiff femoral component to the bone due to the smaller stem cross section. Second, most cementless tapered femoral components are manufactured from titanium alloy, which is one-half the stiffness of cobalt chrome alloys. Third, most cementless tapered femoral components rely on proximal fixation and therefore load the proximal femur more proximally than distal fixation devices. Fourth, long-term follow-ups of several cementless tapered femoral components have revealed actual bone buildup and cortical hypertrophy in Gruen zones 4 and 5 in up to 50% of patients (Figure 10).

C. Range of Motion

As cementless femoral components have evolved, more importance has been directed toward better Morse taper and femoral neck design to minimize impingement of the femoral neck on the acetabular components and to reduce impingement related wear. There has been a move away from rounded femoral neck designs in favor of rounded trapezoidal designs that increase range of motion before impingement occurs. This also helps the surgeon adopt a head-to-neck ratio of two or more, a factor that has been shown to be important in minimizing dislocation. In keeping with this concept, the

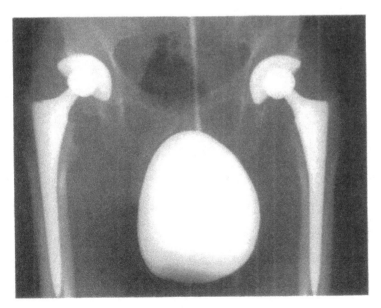

Figure 12 A total hip replacement with good restoration of femoral neck offset.

length of the Morse tapers have been shortened and the use of skirted femoral heads discouraged so as to reduce impingement and enhance range of
motion (Figure 11A, B, and C).

D. Soft Tissue Balancing of the Hip

Most contemporary cemented and cementless total hip replacements have
directed more attention to the concept of soft tissue balancing of the hip
(31,32). Proper positioning of the center of rotation of the femoral head and
restoration of femoral head offset have proved important in restoring abductor strength, thereby reducing the prevalence of limp and the need for
walking aids (Figure 12). This soft tissue balancing has also been demonstrated to have an important effect in reducing the resultant forces across
the hip and thereby minimizing polyethylene wear. Finally, proper soft tissue
balancing of the hip has been shown to be important in enhancing hip stability and minimizing the potential for dislocation.

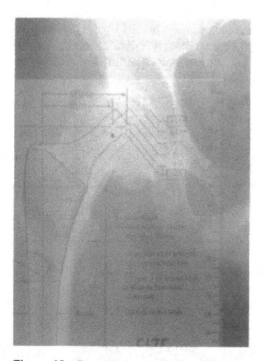

Figure 13 Preoperative templating of an arthritic hip to determine whether a standard or high-offset femoral component should be used as well as what size of component should be selected and the level at which the femoral neck should be cut.

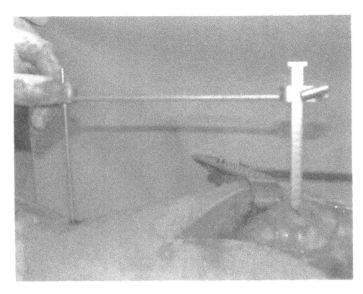

Figure 14   A useful device to assess leg length and offset restoration intraoperatively (Smith & Nephew, Memphis, TN).

Proper soft tissue balancing of the hip begins with preoperative templating, not only to determine femoral stem size but also to guide acetabular component positioning and to predict the potential need for a high offset femoral stem (Figure 13). The use of intraoperative leg length/offset measuring guides before dislocation of the hip and after insertion of the trial or definitive implants is of great benefit in restoring proper hip biomechanics (Figure 14). Finally, the surgeon needs some intraoperative flexibility to restore proper soft tissue balancing. This would include the use of standard or high-offset femoral stems combined with the use of standard or lateralized acetabular polyethylene liners (Figure 15A and B). Our studies have demonstrated that, using these techniques, offset restoration can be obtained in more than 90% of patients. This is a definitive improvement over historical design, where offset was restored in only about 40% of patients.

III.   AUTHOR'S PREFERRED TECHNIQUE

Based on the preceding data, the author has preferred to use cementless tapered total hip replacements since 1987. We have recently reported on the performance of 307 consecutive cementless tapered total hip replacements with 10–13 years follow-up (11). Only two femoral stems were revised, one for sepsis and one for a periprosthetic fracture. Encouraged by these clinical

(A)

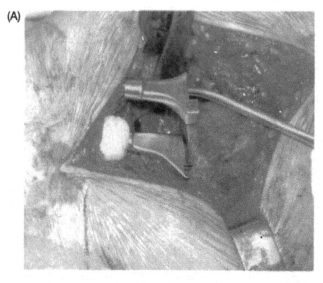

(B)

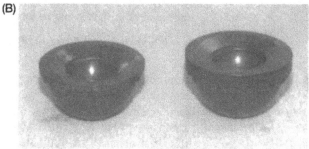

Figure 15 The use of dual-offset femoral stems (A) and lateralized acetabular liners (B), give the surgeon flexibility to "soft tissue balance the hip" intra-operatively.

results, we continue to advocate the use of cementless tapered total hip replacements in 85% of patients. The shape of the proximal femoral med-ullary canal is the most important selection criterion. Cementless tapered femoral components are ideally suited to so-called Dorr type A and B funnel-shaped proximal femoral morphologies (23). This femoral shape is present in 85% of patients. Cementless femoral components can be used in Dorr type C cylindrical femurs, but the implants needed are large and stiff, often resulting in significant stress shielding. In the past, cemented femoral com-ponent fixation was advocated in elderly patients, such that they could be fully weight-bearing immediately. Contemporary cementless tapered total hip replacements allow such immediate weight bearing, so this impediment, too, no longer exists.

REFERENCES

1. Bourne RB, Rorabeck CH, Laupacis A, Tugwell P, Wong C, Bullas R. Total hip replacement. The case for non-cemented femoral fixation because of age. Can J Surg 38:1:567, 1995.
2. Rorabeck CH, Bourne RB, Laupacis A, et al. A double blind study of 250 cases comparing cemented to cementless total hip arthroplasty. Cost effectiveness and its impact on health related quality of life. Clin Orthop 298:156–164, 1994.
3. Clarke IC, Gruen T, Matos M, Amstutz HC. Improved methods for the quantitative radiographic evaluation with particular reference to total hip arthroplasty. Clin Orthop 121:83–91, 1976.
4. Gruen JA, McNeice GM, Amstutz HC. Modes of failure of cemented stem-type femoral components. A radiographic analysis of loosening. Clin Orthop 141:17–27, 1979.
5. Malchau H, Herberts, P, Ahnfelt L. Prognosis of total hip replacement in Sweden. Follow-up of 92,675 operations performed 1978–1990. Acta Orthop Scand 64(5):497–506, 1993.
6. Older J. Low friction arthroplasty of the hip. Clin Orthop 211:36–42, 1986.
7. Schmalzried TP, Jasty M, Harris WH. Periprosthetic bone loss in total hip arthroplasty. Polyethylene wear debris and the concept of the effective joint space. J Bone Joint Surg 74A:849–863, 1992.
8. Stauffer RN. Ten year follow-up study of total hip replacement. J Bone Joint Surg 64A:983–990, 1982.
9. Sutherland CJ, Wilde AH, Borden LS, Marks KE. A ten year follow-up of 100 consecutive Muller curved stem total hip replacement arthroplasties. J Bone Joint Surg 64A:970–982, 1982.
10. Willert HG, Bertram H, Buchhorn GH. Osteolysis in alloarthroplasty of the hip. The role of ultra-high molecular weight polyethylene wear particles. Clin Orthop 258:95–107, 1990.
12. Bourne RB, Rorabeck CH, Patterson J, Guerin J. Tapered Titanium Cementless Total Hip Replacements: a 10–13 year follow-up study. Proceedings of the Hip Society, CORR, December 2001.
13. Delauncy C, Kapandji AI. Ten year survival of Zweymuller total prostheses in primary uncemented arthroplasty of the hip. Rev Clin Orthop Repar Appar Mot 84:759–761, 1998.
14. Engh CA Jr, Culpepper WJ II, Engh CA. Long term results of use of the anatomic medullary locking prosthesis in total hip arthroplasty. J Bone Joint Surg 79A:177–184, 1997.
15. Hellman EJ, Capello NN, Feinberg JR. Omnifit cementless total hip arthroplasty. A 10-year average follow-up. Clin Orthop 364:164–174, 1999.

16. Kawamura H, Dunbar M, Murray P, Bourne R, Rorabeck C. The porous coated anatomic total hip replacement: A ten to fourteen year follow-up of a cementless total hip arthroplasty. J Bone Joint Surg, September 2001. In press.

17. Malchau H, Herberts P, Soderman P. Prognosis of total hip replacement in Sweden. Presented at Canadian Orthopaedic Association Meeting, June 2, 2001.

18. McLaughlin JR, Lee KR. Total hip arthroplasty with an uncemented femoral component. Excellent results at ten-year follow-up. J Bone Joint Surg 79B: 900–907, 1997.

19. McLaughlin JR, Lee KR. Total hip arthroplasty in young patients. 8 to 13 year results using an uncemented stem. Clin Orthop 373:153–163, 2000.

20. Puolakka TJ, Pajamaki KJ, Pulkkinen PO, Nevalainen JK. Poor survival of cementless Biomet total hip: A report on 1,047 hips from the Finnish Arthroplasty Register. Acta Orthop Scand 70:425–429, 1999.

21. Sakalkale DP, Engh K, Hozack WJ, Rothman RH. Minimum 10 year results of a tapered cementless hip replacement. Clin Orthop 362:138–144, 1999.

22. Schram M, Keck F, Hohmann D, Pitto RP. Total hip arthroplasty using a cemented femoral component with taper design. Outcome at 10-year follow-up. Arch Orthop Trauma Surg 120:7–8, 2000.

23. Xenos JS, Callaghan JJ, Heeken RD, et al. The porous coated anatomic total hip prothesis, inserted without cement. A prospective study with a minimum of ten year of follow-up. J Bone Joint Surg 81A:74–82, 1999.

24. Dorr L, Faugere M, Mackel A. Structural and cellular assessment of bone quality. Bone 14:231–242, 1993.

25. Bourne RB, Rorabeck CH. A critical look at cementless stems. Taper designs and when to use alternatives. Clin Orthop 355:212–223, 1998.

26. Mulliken BD, Bourne RB, Rorabeck CH, Nayak, NN. A tapered titanium femoral stem inserted without cement in a total hip arthroplasty. Radiographic evaluation and stability. J Bone Joint Surg 78A:1214–1225, 1996.

27. Mulliken, BD, Bourne RB, Rorabeck CH, Nayak NN. Results of the cementless Mallory Head primary total hip arthroplasty: A 5 to 7 year review. Iowa Orthop J 16:20–34, 1996.

28. Wykman A, Lundberg, A. Subsidence of porous coated noncemented femoral components in total hip arthroplasty. A roentgen stereophotogrammetric analysis. J Arthrop 7:197–200, 1992.

29. Emerson RH Jr, Sanders SB, Head WC, Higgins L. Effect of circumferential plasma-spray porous coating on the rate of femoral osteolysis after total hip arthroplasty. J Bone Joint Surg 81A:1291–1298, 1999.

30. Lombardi AV Jr, Mallory TH, Vaughn BJ, Drouilliard P. Aseptic loosening in total hip arthroplasty secondary to osteolysis induced by wear debris from titanium-alloy modular femoral heads. J Bone Joint Surg 71A:1337–1342, 1989.

31. Davey JR, O'Connor DO, Burke DW, Harris HW. Femoral component offset. Its effect on strain in bone cement. J Arthrop 8:23–26, 1993.

32. McGrory BJ, Morrey BF, Cahalan TD, An KN, Cabanela ME. Effect of femoral offset on range of motion and abductor muscle strength after total hip arthroplasty. J Bone Joint Surg 77B:865–869, 1995.

3
Cemented Stems

Steven M. Dellose, Andrew H. Kim, and Raj K. Sinha
University of Pittsburgh Medical Center, Pittsburgh, Pennsylvania

I. INTRODUCTION

The aging population is growing rapidly, and persons 60 years or older are the fastest growing group of patients (1). Today, the choice between cemented and noncemented fixation of femoral stems remains controversial.

In the 1960s, Sir John Charnley introduced low-friction cemented total hip arthroplasty (THA). Cement fixation had been the mainstay of femoral fixation throughout that era. Some studies showed survival rates at 20 years of close to 90%. Despite this fact, there is a continued push to improve techniques and materials in the hope of increasing the longevity of THA.

In light of the confusing results in the literature, it has become more difficult to draw informed conclusions concerning hip implants. Variations in patient selection, femoral component materials, cement composition, implantation technique, and design have made it almost impossible to decide the ultimate performance of cemented femoral components (1). Careful scrutiny of individual studies and the literature as a whole is necessary to draw accurate conclusions concerning cemented stems and noncemented stems (Figure 1).

II. HISTORICAL EVOLUTION OF CEMENTED STEMS

Hip arthroplasty surgery was first attempted almost five decades ago. Early attempts were fraught with failure and frustration.

In the 1950s, Austin Moore popularized the long-stem prosthesis. It was an uncemented design that was inserted loosely in the bone. The stem

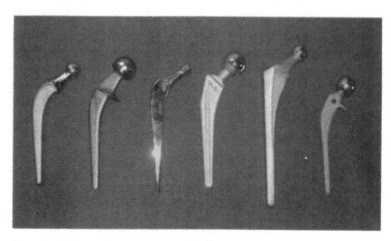

Figure 1 Examples of cemented stems. From left to right: Charnley, titanium monoblock, Exeter, Sulzer CLS cemented, Osteonics Omnifit, Zimmer Precoat.

was fenestrated and would self-lock within the bone. Ingrowth or ongrowth of the bone to the stem was possible and subsequently led to advances in noncemented stem design.

Sir John Charnley, in the 1960s, experimented with many variations of prosthetic design. Initially, he used cemented femoral stems with a low friction polytetrafluoroethylene (PTFE, or Teflon) articulation. Although PTFE did well in experimental studies, PTFE showed very poor wear characteristics within the body and had to be abandoned in 1961. After catastrophic failures, the articulating segment was changed to a high-molecular-weight polyethylene (HMWP). The wear characteristics of HMWP were 500–1000 times better than those of PFTE (2). The low-friction arthroplasty that was used by Dr Charnley is still being produced and implanted today.

Charnley borrowed from the dental community a form of acrylic cement suitable for orthopaedic surgery—namely, polymethylmethacrylate. This substance was not actually used to bond the prosthesis to the bone but primarily as a grout to occupy the space between the bone and the implant.

Dr Charnley's results are the standard for comparison for almost all implant designs. European and American results often differ with identical implants and techniques. For instance, Wroblewski et al. reported excellent survivorship of Charnley stems in 1998 (3). Using revision as an endpoint, stem survival was 94% at 17 years in 63 hips. Garrellick et al. also produced an excellent survivorship of 93.2% using the Charnley cemented prosthesis at a minimum 10-year follow-up (4). In a report by Fender in 1999, results of the Charnley prosthesis used across a single health region in England were less favorable, with a revision rate of almost 10% at 5 years (5). Charnley reported only a 0.21% revision rate in 1978 from a series of 10,913 low-friction arthroplasties (LFA) performed between 1966 and 1976 (23 revisions), with a 2–12 year follow-up (2).

Initially, failure was identified inaccurately as cement debonding or cement failure and was thought to be primarily a problem with the cement. This phenomenon was most commonly seen in younger, more active patients. *Cement disease* was the term coined for this loosening of the femoral stem and was often associated with marked bony destruction (1). Today, the term *cement disease* is not used, as we now know that the most common form of failure is from aseptic loosening (1) (Figure 2).

In analyzing reports, it is important to keep in mind how failure is defined. The definition of failure differs among surgeons. Pain, osteolysis, need for a revision surgery, and radiographic loosening have all been used to define failure and may contribute to the varied results among authors.

Design changes and stem characteristics continued to evolve over time in an effort to improve the longevity of the joint replacement. As the initial results appeared favorable, the indications for surgery were expanded. Unfortunately, as the limits of material characteristics were challenged, failures followed and consequently contributed to even more design changes. Some features proved beneficial while others led to catastrophic failures.

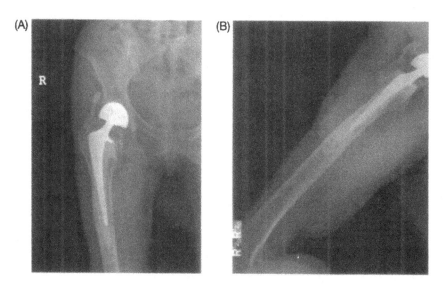

Figure 2   Loose cemented bipolar stem. Note radiolucencies at cement-bone interface, subsidence of stem and cement, and cortical remodeling.

The National Institutes of Health recently released its recommendations on total hip arthroplasty, citing that cemented femoral fixation provides excellent, reliable long-term results (6). A hybrid design was considered the standard. Using a well-designed prosthesis and proper cementing techniques, there does not seem to be a significant difference between cementless and cemented femoral fixation in the young and the very old (6).

III. STEM FIXATION

A. Prosthesis–Cement Interface

The main purpose of the cement mantle is to provide stability to the implant while dispersing the forces equally from the hip to the endosteal bone. The joint reactive force of the hip is transmitted down the metal prosthesis through the cement to the bone. The ideal prosthesis should be sized to fit with enough room for an adequate cement mantle. The finish of the prosthesis can be variable and different designs perform differently within the cement. The amount of surface roughness of the prosthesis determines the initial interdigitation at the implant–cement interface. With increased roughness, there is more initial bonding strength. The polymethylmethacrylate acts primarily as a grout to stabilize the implant and occupies the area between the peaks and valleys of a rough implant and the bone, with no distinctive adhering properties.

B. Cancellous Bone Interdigitation

It is necessary to prepare the canal properly. A stable level of cancellous bone is needed for proper interdigitation of the cement during pressurization. The cement flows into the cancellous portion of the bone initially via pressure from the insertion of the cement. Pressurization can be performed with finger packing or other commercially available methods, such as a pressurizing gun. With the cement inserted into the canal, the prosthesis is introduced and additional pressurization of the cement into the cancellous bone helps provide the additional trabecular interdigitation needed for a strong cement–bone interface.

C. Cement Drying

During cementation, a thin layer of cement is dragged from the entrance point of the prosthesis to the distal tip. This thin layer surrounds the entire prosthesis and centralizer (7). Voids in the cement can occur during this stage and care must be taken to introduce the stem properly into the cement (Figure 3).

Optimal alignment of the stem is imperative for proper mechanics of the hip. Alignment also is important to ensure proper cement mantle thickness in all areas around the prosthesis. Proper mantle thickness in all areas should be a minimum of 2 mm (8).

A matching precementing trial is also a necessity. A system that has an adequate variation of sizes allows the use of a biomechanically stronger implant with adequate cement thickness in all areas. Using a stem that is too large will decrease the available area for the cement mantle. Weakening of the cement mantle in those specific areas causes fatigue and failure where the cement is thin. The implant should be a minimum of 2 mm smaller circumferentially than the trial.

Care also must be taken not to disturb the prosthesis while the cement is hardening, which would create a gap between the cement and the prosthesis. This will cause instability and allow direct access of particles to all areas of the stem–cement interface.

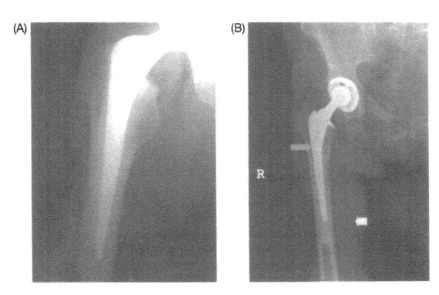

Figure 3   (A) A grade cement mantle. There are no voids or radiolucencies, and the stem is well-centered. (B) C2 grade cement mantle. The green arrow indicates a region devoid of cement, and the white arrow indicates a region where the mantle is extremely thin and the prosthesis is touching cortical bone.

IV. BIOMECHANICS

Polymethylmethacrylate (PMMA) is a type of acrylic cement. The reaction
of the PMMA is produced by the addition of a liquid to a solid. The solid
is a granular form of the polymer of methylmethacrylate along with an
activator. The liquid contains the initiator and the monomer form of the
methylmethacrylate. There is a spontaneous exothermic reaction upon the
mixture of these compounds in which heat is dissipated through the prosthesis and the wet bone (9). There is some expansion in the volume, with
subsequent shrinkage of the cement during cooling. The final volume change
is roughly a 3–5% increase in size from the initial induction of the liquid
phase (9).

The properties of the cement are dictated by varying the molecular
weight and distribution of monomer and polymer. Mechanical properties
such as elongation have large ranges (0.8–2.5%) and the typical modulus
ranges between 1.1 and 4.1 GPa. In general, PMMA is more ductile than
brittle and displays some viscoelastic properties and creep. PMMA is strongest in compression and weakest in shear and tensile strain. Antibiotics may
also alter the biomechanical properties of bone cement (10).

The biomechanics of the fixation are dependent on the cement–prosthesis interface and the cement–bone interface. In smooth, collarless stems,
subsidence is appreciated. This may be due to "creep" of the cement and
the viscoelastic properties it possesses; it may actually support the longevity
of a stable cemented implant.

There is no question that using a matted stem achieves greater initial
pullout strength compared to a smooth stem, but longevity is a question that
is not answered clearly (11). It is not known which method of fixation is
more desirable. There are studies suggesting that each method can achieve
good, long-lasting results.

A. Modes of Cement Failure

Many different factors contribute to a long-lasting implant. Early loosening
of a cemented stem is a multifactorial process (1). Debonding of the cement–prosthesis interface has been implicated as the initial step in femoral
loosening (12). The inciting event seems to be related to mechanical stress
and can be increased by a multitude of different factors (Table 1).

There is an interplay of events starting with mechanical stress of the
cement mantle. Proximal bone resorption can increase the mechanical stress
felt by the proximal cement mantle. Proximal loosening and increased micromotion can cause the cement mantle to fail. This produces a pathway for
wear debris to gain access to the effective joint space. Some authors have

Table 1 Factors Contributing to Loosening

Larger stem	Increased offset	Younger active patients
Stiffer stem	Varus positioning	Heavy patients
Thin cement	Poor bone quality	

described an increased fluid pressure driving the particles between the interfaces of the prosthesis, bone, and cement. Wear debris promotes tissue response and further third-body wear (13). The wear debris then incites the histological response leading to osteolysis and further bone loss.

Failure of the prosthesis–cement interface is dependent on characteristics of the stem and possibly surgical technique. Different stem finishes and designs behave differently in the cement and thus may fail in different circumstances (14). Migration at the cement–prosthesis interface may be advantageous in some stem designs. Subsidence of the stem may reinforce the bone–cement interface by expanding the cement mantle (15). The use of power reaming has been implicated in failures of the cement–bone interface (1). Stone et al. reported a 12% failure rate at 5.5 years in cases where power reaming was used (16). This was shown to dramatically decrease the shear strength of the cement–bone interface.

Shepard looked at precoated stems with early failures (12). Since there was increased cement–precoat bonding in cement times below 6 min, they concluded that increased stresses were being seen at the cement–bone interface. However, failure of the precoat stems occurred at the precoat–prosthesis interface (12). Ong et al. reported failure at the implant–cement interface in precoat stems (1,17). Dowd et al. reported the failure occurring at the bone–cement interface (1,18). Middleton reported that most of the revisions in his small series (66%) had loosening at both interfaces (13).

Elasticity of the stem can contribute to loosening. Increased elasticity of titanium causes increased peak stresses in the cement mantle, increased micromotion of the stem, and increased loosening. Micromotion and corrosion were postulated culprits of the osteolysis (19). Micromotion also increases with thinner cement mantles (1,19). Stiffer stem designs made of chromium cobalt may not allow transfer of stress to be seen at the calcar and can lead to bone resorption and loosening (20,21).

Subsidence of the stem is a sensitive indicator of early failure, especially in shape-closed designs (1). Results published by Howie et al. support the fact that subsidence can occur in certain designs without loosening, specifically force-closed designs (14). These, as opposed to shape-closed designs, rely on some subsidence to ensure a secure fit. Others debate this opinion, concluding that any subsidence greater than 1.2 mm within the first 2 years of follow-up has been associated with a higher rate of revision surgery (15).

Radiographic failure and evaluation of stability have been described by Gruen et al. (22). A system was devised that separates the areas of the femur into seven zones on radiographs. Radiolucent lines within certain zones can be quantified. However, agreement on which zones and lines depict loose implants is still under discussion. Subsidence, pedestal formation, and cement fracture are also suspicious signs of loosening (15,19,23).

Harris defined three scenarios depending on the extent of radiolucency at the cement prosthesis interface. Subsidence, cement fracture, and pedestal formation with a radiolucency surrounding 100% of the prosthesis constituted the "definitely loose" fraction of patients. Patients with radiolucencies between 50 and 99% were described as the "probably loose" group, and patients with less than 50% radiolucency were described as the "possibly loose" group (22) (Figure 4).

B. Cement Technique

Aseptic loosening appears to be dependent on cement technique (24). Three generations of cementing technique have been described (Table 2).

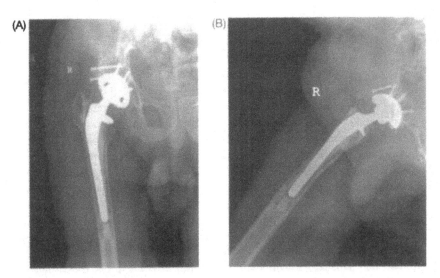

Figure 4   Example of a loose precoated stem with subsidence and endosteal osteo-lysis.

Table 2 Generations of Cement Technique

First (Before 1975)	Second (Begins 1975)	Third (Begins 1982)
Cement finger packing	Cement gun (1971)	Porosity reduction
No formal canal preparation	Pulsatile lavage	Pressurization
Sharp edges	Canal brush	Centralizer
Cast stem	Round medial border	Stem precoat or rough surface
No pressurization	Cement restrictor	
No cement restrictor		

Barrack (1) as well as Suominen (24) published evidence of improved results using advanced cementing techniques. Suominen reported a 300% increased failure rate without the use of a cement restrictor (24). Of 113 cases of cemented total hip replacement, 25 cases without a cement plug were diagnosed as radiographically loose, as compared with only 6 cases in which a cement plug was used. Careful cementing technique has lead to more successful and predictable results (24). With second- and third-generation cemented stems, fixation has been more reliable; failures via stem loosening less than 10 years after implantation are rare (1). No significant difference between second- and third-generation techniques has been well established (6). Many different aspects may affect the eventual longevity of the implant. Different aspects of bone and cement preparation are discussed below.

C. Cement Preparation

Some of the advances in cement technique are related to the preparation of the cement. There are a variety of methods of mixing the polymer. Some methods include hand mixing, closed-system mixers, vacuum reduction, and centrifugation. Early in the history of THA, first-generation cement handling techniques were used. These cements were mixed by hand in an open environment that allowed the incorporation of air into the cement and an increased porosity.

Mixing of cement using contemporary methods with vacuumed porosity reduction has not necessarily led to stronger cement. Reported increases of 44% ultimate tensile strength have been reported over hand-mixing methods (25). However, vacuum mixing may actually be a relative risk factor for stem failure. Dowd et al. showed better results in a series implanted in nonvacuumed cement as compared with centrifugation (18). There is no convincing evidence to say that differences between second- and third-generation techniques have made a substantial difference (1). Other advances in cement preparation, such as pressurization and adequate cement mantle thickness, have led to increases in survival rates (7).

D. Timing of Cementation

The actual timing of the cementation may also be important. Using wetter cement may allow for more interdigitation. Shepard et al. showed increased interdigitation with rough stems with wet cement versus dryer, doughy cement. The authors in this study recommended altering the time of cementation depending on the specific roughness of the prosthesis being used: that is, to cement rough stems earlier than smoother stems (12). The cement–prosthesis interface does not seem to be influenced by cement timing when using smooth stems (1). It is easier to maintain the alignment and orientation of the stem using a doughy form of cement, and this is therefore recommended with smooth stems (12).

E. Cement Restriction

Second-generation techniques include the use of cement restrictors to conceptually convert an open system to a closed space. This allowed for retrograde filling of the canal (8). The concept of a distal cement plug to allow adequate pressurization of the cement is now well accepted. The pressurization allows trabecularization of the cement into the bone, providing a stronger cement–bone interface (7). Retrograde filling and pressurization was possibly the biggest advance in second-generation cementing techniques (Figure 5).

Intramedullary pressures during pressurization using a cement restrictor and retrograde filling approach 35–75 lb/in^2. Noble et al. tested cement restrictors and documented the percentage of failure for each of five different plugs at 50 lb/in^2. There is tremendous variability between the commercially available plugs (7) (Table 3).

Finger packing of cement reaches values of only 10 lb/in^2 or less. Manual packing can also add blood and foreign particles to the cement, thereby potentially weakening the polymer (7). In the Swedish National Hip Arthroplasty Register, over 134,000 hip arthroplasties were studied. Finger packing was associated with double the rate of aseptic loosening compared to delivery with a syringe (7).

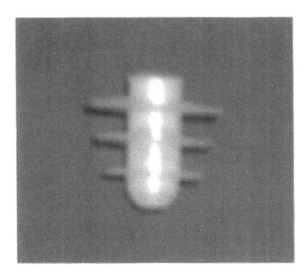

Figure 5 Example of a commercially available cement restrictor.

F. Cement Mantle

Achieving a proper cement mantle is of paramount importance. The rate of loosening is lower with a circumferential cement mantle between 2.5 and 5 mm and a distal cement mantle of 2 mm or more. Proximal medial cement mantles should be a minimum of 3 mm, and distally the stems should occupy less than 80% of the width of the canal (8). Noble showed that the ideal mantle is not uniform but ranges from 3–7 mm and is greater than 2 mm in every area (7). Cement is significantly weaker with a mantle of less than 2 mm (7). Peak stresses at the cement–prosthesis interface are dramatically increased with mantles less than 1 mm and can lead to cement mantle fail-

Table 3 Comparison of Current Cement Restrictors

Type of Plug	% of Plugs Resisting 50 lb/in^2
Sidel	24
Dow	37
Buck	62
Umbrella	84
ADG	94

ures (26). There is also an association with increased motion in the areas of less than 1 mm, in contrast to areas that are 3–4 mm (1,26). Typically, thin cement mantles occur at the level of the medial femoral neck or distally at the tip (7). Absence of proximal medial cement has been linked to some stem failures (1) (Table 4).

G. Canal Preparation

Proper interdigitation into stable cancellous bone must occur. The use of power reaming and conical reamers may destroy the stable layer of cancellous bone between the stiff component and the stiff cortical bone (16). Without this cancellous bone, the strength of the cement–bone interface may be jeopardized (1).

Clearing the particles of bone, debris, and blood prior to cementation has been an advancement in cement technique. Many different methods have been used to approach the drying of the canal, including epinephrine, thrombin, or hydrogen peroxide–soaked sponges.

Wroblewski et al. described clearing of the femoral calcar cancellous bone to allow proper cement mantle thickness (27). A review of 330 patients without calcar femorale debridement had a failure rate of 4.8% while 111 patients with calcar bone removal had a failure of 0.9%. These authors recommend clearing of the calcar bone routinely.

H. Centralization

Proper alignment of the stem in the canal helps to ensure a proper cement mantle (28). In an attempt to control the alignment, proximal and distal centralizers have been developed. Goldberg et al., using proximal and distal centralizers on the prosthesis, were able to achieve 91% satisfactory alignment with optimal cement mantles (8). Centralizer fracture at the time of implantation occurred in a small percentage of cases (6 out of 7 of the misaligned stems) but had no effect on the 4- to 8-year survival (8). Noble compared the use of proximal and distal centralization to a single centralizer

Table 4   Evaluation of Cement Mantle

A	Complete whiteout
B	Slight radiolucency
C1	Radiolucency of 50–99% of the cement-bone interface
C2	Mantle defect
D	Grossly poor cement mantle

distally and to no centralizers (7). He found that with the use of both a proximal and distal centralizer, he could align all his prostheses without any malalignment. With use of a single distal centralizer, he reported a 3% distal malalignment and a 19% proximal malalignment. Without any centralizer, his results deteriorated: 49% distal and 35% proximal malalignment (7).

There have been some reported concerns with the use of distal centralizers. Voids can occur around the distal end of the centralizer (8). Cement voids can occur up to 42% of the time (7). Centralizer fracture occurred in a small percentage of patients but had no long-term effect on the 4- to 8-year survival (8) (Figure 6).

I. Precoated Femoral Stems

Precoating the proximal portion of the stem with an extruded layer of prefabricated cement is a way to proximally centralize the prosthesis as well as increase the mechanical pullout strength. The precoat may be at least the minimum desired thickness of cement mantle (7). Shepard et al. reinforced the thought that precoating has a substantial effect on increasing the tensile

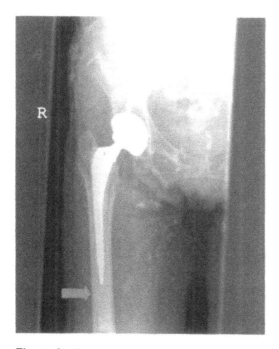

Figure 6 Cemented stem with air bubble in the distal portion of the mantle.

and shear stress of the initial bonding of the cement (12). The precoat cement undergoes repolymerization if mixed with a wetter form of cement (less than 6 min). The prosthesis precoat bond fails prior to the cement–precoat bond in pullout trials (1). Dowd et al. examined 154 rough precoat stems and reported that the failure occurred at the cement bone interface (1,18). Early failure with osteolysis was reported in 15% of the stems (1). Precoating of stems is also thought to decrease the amount of subsidence (Figure 7).

J. Different Cements

There are basically two different forms of cement available: low-viscosity injectable cement and high-viscosity cement (10). Many different commercial cements are available, each displaying a different biomechanical portfolio. For instance, the toughness of Palacos cement can be almost double that of Simplex or Zimmer Regular (10).

Experimentation with new cements should be performed with caution. Catastrophic failures have occurred with new cements. For example, a cement called BONELOC (Polymers Reconstructive Ace-S, Ferum, Denmark) was pulled from the market after its introduction led to failures (1).

K. Alignment

The association of varus stem alignment with suboptimal results of cemented femoral stems is well known (8). Goldberg et al. demonstrated good results in stems that were found to have less than 2 degrees of malalignment and a cement mantle of 3 mm. Second- and third-generation techniques cannot overcome the problems associated with malalignment of the stem. Increased stresses are seen with the thin cement mantle resulting from malalignment. In addition, increased joint-reactive forces from varus malposition can increase stresses on the cement (Figure 8).

V. STEM DESIGN

Many early stem designs functioned well. More recently, stem design changes have been associated with early failure. Subtle changes in stem design have led to a wide variety of results and difficulty interpreting the literature. Geometry, collar additions, and finish have a significant effect on rates of failure.

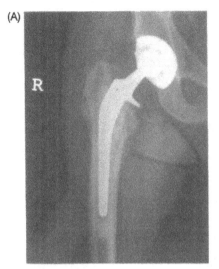

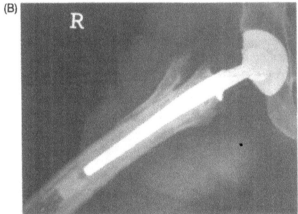

Figure 7 Appearance of a precoated stem with probable loosening. (A) On the AP view, there is an area of focal osteolysis in Guren Zone 7 and of linear osteolysis in Zone 3. Also, there is debonding of the lateral shoulder of the prosthesis from the cement. (B) On the lateral view, there is a radiolucency in Zone 11, anterior and distal to the stem tip.

A. Geometry

The geometry of the stem has been implicated in some THA failures (1). Different shaped stems exhibit different stress and strain patterns. Chang et al. determined that use of a rectangular stem reduced stresses on the cement

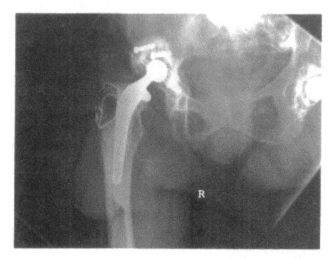

Figure 8 A well-functioning stem placed in a varus position.

mantle (1,29). However, circular stems had less torsional resistance. Wan et al. discovered that debonding occurred more often in triangular stems (21). Rectangular stems with smooth edges fared best. The distal taper does not seem to be as important as the proximal fit or fill of the prosthesis for a particular canal size (21).

B. Fixation Site

The site of fixation also determines the stress strain patterns of stems. Woolson et al. described the fractures of 10 chromium cobalt stems (1,30). Early proximal loosening and a cantilever fatigue-type failure of the implants were demonstrated in these stems. The site at which the stems fractured was convincing evidence that increased strains were generated on the anterior surface of the stem. Anterior stem pressures seem to be higher than posterior surface pressures.

C. Force-Closed Fixation Versus Shape-Closed Fixation

Force-closed fixation relies upon subsidence of the stem over time to achieve permanent stability. Force-closed systems should have a polished or smooth stem to allow for adequate subsidence and stabilization. They rely on cement creep (13). Conversely, shape-closed implants depend upon initial stability by virtue of the stem design, in particular shape and presence of a collar (1).

It may be beneficial to have enhanced interdigitation by increasing stem roughness. This increases the initial stabilization and is found in shape-closed designs (11). With cemented matted stems, the amount of particulate debris generated once the stem became loose was higher. The rough surface was thought to account for this process (13) (Figure 9).

D. Stem Length and Size

Most modern systems have increased the number of sizes available. Smaller sizes should be used only when warranted by the patient's size. Santore demonstrated a high failure rate with stems less than 100–110 mm in size (1). The ideal stem size has not yet been determined. Graduation of stem length varies with stem size (1). Picking a proper stem size allows for a proper cement mantle. Stuffing the canal with an oversized component from underbroaching leads to an inadequate cement mantle. Preoperatively, offset

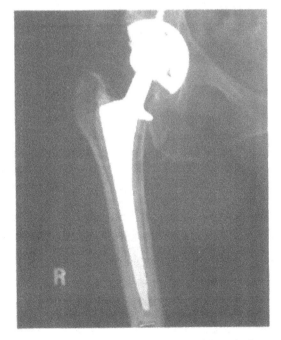

Figure 9 A rough textured stem with early loosening as demonstrated by radiolucency along most of the cement–bone interface.

should be determined. Increasing the offset can increase the transfer stress across the cement mantle. It is important to template preoperatively to determine the correct stem size, alignment, and offset in order to restore proper hip mechanics.

E. Stem Surface

Charnley states in his book, written in 1972, that there is "no need to roughen the surface of the stem in hope of enhancing the mechanical bond between the metal and the cement..." (2). Stem surface has been shown to have an important effect on stem survival (1). For example, Middleton showed that stem surface and finish had a profound effect on loosening rates (13). Using the same Exeter stem with different finishes, they were able to demonstrate a markedly higher rate of loosening in the matt-finished stem compared to the polished stem. Modularity did not play a role in loosening rates.

There is no clear agreement as to which mode of fixation is preferred. Rough stems initially form a stronger bond. With any early loosening, an increased amount of debris generation occurs as compared with smooth stems. It is thought that the motion of the rough surface can accelerate osteolysis (1). The present literature is inconclusive concerning the long-term results of surface finish (12).

F. Patient Selection

As there are many controversies surrounding cemented femoral stems, patient selection may be the most important factor. Increased cycles and fatigue stresses can be seen in younger patients. Initially, Charnley's patient selection was very strict. Older, more sedentary, less obese patients underwent low-friction arthroplasty. Over the years, indications were stretched to include younger, heavier, and more active patients. For instance, Hozack et al. reported that heavy men are at greatest risk for failure (1,31). Harrington et al. determined that body weight had four times the effect of offset in increasing cement strains (1,32).

It is generally accepted that younger patients with good bone quality are better candidates for noncemented prostheses. A consensus on the use of cement fixation for younger patients may never be apparent (1). One conclusion can be made: with increased variability in patient selection, it will inevitably become more difficult to compare results among different researchers.

G. Biomechanics of the Stem and Bone Resorption

Kim et al. concluded that close proximal fit of a stem reproduces normal magnitudes of strain, in contrast to a distal fit that decreases proximal loading (33). Disuse atrophy causing bone resorption follows the principle of Wolfe's law. Thus, reproducing anatomical strain patterns in the femoral neck should reduce the amount of bone resorption. Multiple variations in stem design and materials have been developed.

First, the stiffness of the stem has been changed. Different metal alloys have been used with varying degrees of elasticity. Titanium stems with higher elasticity can transfer more energy between the stem and the cement mantle. This may reduce the amount of stress shielding for bone, but cement mantle stress is increased and can lead to mantle failure (19).

Also, crevice corrosion in the titanium alloy was correlated with a radiographic osteolysis pattern. Histological sections confirmed the foreign-body reaction. This was thought to contribute to the early loosening (19). In a different study, a stiffness of less than 0.33 was consistent with less stress shielding proximally (21). Somewhere in the spectrum between a stiff implant that decreases the transfer of stress to the cement and a more elastic implant that will decrease the proximal bone loss is the ideal implant.

VI. RESULTS OF MODERN CEMENTED FEMORAL STEMS

This chapter has so far discussed the evolution of the cemented femoral stem. The multitude of factors that may contribute to the longevity of cemented total hip replacement has been mentioned. These factors include cementing technique, patient selection, stem design, surface finish, and metallurgy. This section examines the results of total hip replacement with a cemented femoral stem in light of these factors.

Current cementing technique, more so than any other change, has contributed significantly to improving the longevity of cemented femoral stems. As previously mentioned, first-generation cementing technique refers to the finger-packing of doughy cement into the unplugged femoral canal. Second-generation cementing technique included plugging the medullary canal, the canal with pulsatile lavage, and inserting the cement in a retrograde fashion using a cement gun. Third-generation cementing technique includes all second-generation techniques plus porosity reduction, via centrifugation or vacuum mixing, with pressurization of the cement mantle and stem centralization (Table 2).

In order to fully appreciate the success of second-generation cementing technique, results of first-generation cementing technique are discussed first. Long-term results of third-generation cementing technique are still undetermined.

Most long-term results of the first-generation cementing technique are not very good. Sutherland et al. (34) reported on 53 hips followed over 10 years. A 28% incidence of migration of the femoral component was noted. Combining the radiographically loose stems with the clinically loose stems, the overall incidence of aseptic loosening was 40% for the femoral component. Stauffer et al. (35) also reported poor results in their review of the Mayo Clinic experience during the years 1960–1970. A 10-year follow-up of 231 hips revealed a radiographic loosening rate of 29.9% for femoral components and a revision rate of 6.1% because of stem loosening. Wroblewski (3) in 1986 published his 15 to 21-year results in 116 Charnley hips. He reported subsidence of the stem or the stem-cement complex in 29% and fracture of the femoral cement in 14.7%.

Several studies exhibit good results of first-generation cementing technique. For example, Schulte et al. (36) reported good results in their 20-year follow-up of 322 Charnley hips. These authors reported a 2% (8 of 322) revision rate because of aseptic loosening of the femoral component and 3% revision rate in the 98 hips of living patients. When the rates of radiographic loosening and aseptic loosening confirmed at revision were combined, 6% of all 322 femoral components and 7% of the 98 femoral components in living patients had loosened.

Superior results of second-generation cementing technique have been demonstrated clearly in the literature. Such improvement has led some surgeons to promote cemented femoral fixation in all primary total hip replacements (22,37). Barrack et al. (38) reported excellent results in their 12-year follow-up of 50 cemented hips using a collared and rectangular cross-sectioned stem with round corners made of cobalt chrome. No femoral stems were revised and only one stem was loose radiographically at a 12-year follow-up. These results occurred despite the fact that the average patient age was less than 50 at the time of total hip replacement. The authors attributed this success to better stem design and especially to improvement in cementing technique. Mulroy et al. (39) also reported good results. In their 15-year-average follow-up study of 162 hips, only 4 femoral components (2%) were revised because of aseptic loosening. Of the 90 patients (102 hips) who were alive 14 or more years after total hip replacement, only 2 hips (2%) had revisions because of aseptic loosening, and 7 (7%) exhibited femoral component loosening radiographically. These authors also attributed their excellent results mostly to improvement in cementing technique. Based on their results, Mulroy et al. recommended insertion of a femoral component with second-generation cementing technique for all standard primary total hip replacements. Smith et al. (40) reported a 5% revision rate because of aseptic loosening of the femoral component in 161 hips over an 18-year average follow-up. Of the 84 hips in the 73 patients who had survived 17–20 years after the index operation, the prevalence of revision of the femoral component because of aseptic loosening was 7%. Clearly, there has been a significant improvement in the results of second-generation cement technique over those of first-generation cement technique.

Patient selection is also very important in the longevity of total hip replacement. Presumably, younger patients are more active and put more cyclic loading on the cemented total hips. The patient group of less than 50 years of age is particularly interesting. Both Dorr et al. (41) and Chandler et al. (42) have reported on their poor results with the use of cemented femoral stems. Since then, there have been numerous other studies with good results in patients younger than age 50, using cemented femoral stems. Barrack's (38) excellent results have already been mentioned. Ballard et al. (25) reported on forty-two hips at an average 11-year follow-up. Two femoral components (5%) were revised for aseptic loosening. Additionally, five femoral components (12%) were found to be definitely loose radiographically. These authors concluded that excellent fixation of the femoral component can be accomplished using improved cementing technique. Sullivan et al. (43) reported their 18-year follow-up of 84 cemented Charnley stems. All patients were less than 50 years of age. Two hips (2%) were revised because of aseptic loosening of the femoral component, and 5 stems (6%) were radiographically loose.

Implant designs have also evolved over the years in the hope of improving the cemented femoral stems. When cement fatigue was identified as one of the major factors for early loosening of cemented femoral stems, designs that created high stresses in the cement mantle were discontinued. For example, Mueller stems are no longer popular because of their thin, sharp design, which results in large compressive stress, leading to poor results (34). Crowninshield et al. (44) concluded, in a finite element analysis, that the maximum cement compressive stress is related to the anteroposterior dimension of the medial surface of the stem. Cross sections with a relatively small anteroposterior dimension on the medial surface result in large compressive stresses. The design of the Charnley stem had a round-cornered rectangular cross section with uniform anteroposterior dimension and tapered from medial to lateral. This stem was polished and made of stainless steel. Results with this type of stem are well documented in the literature, and it is considered the benchmark for cemented total hip replacement. Cemented femoral stems that were used in studies by Mulroy et al. (39) and by Barrack et al. (38) had a rectangular cross section with rounded corners and broad medial borders. These stem designs, along with second-generation cementing technique, produced excellent results. There are other cemented femoral stem designs that have also showed good clinical results, such as the Wrightington FC, Spectron, and Lubinus hips.

Sochart et al. (45) reported their comparison of the Wrightington FC hip with the Charnley hip in their 10- to 15-year follow-up. The Wrightington stem is rectangular proximally, becoming circular in cross section as it tapers from top to bottom and has four longitudinal depressions that are described as derotation flutes. Using revision for aseptic loosening as the criterion, the Kaplan-Meier survival of the femoral implant at 5, 10, and 15 years was 100, 99, and 98%, respectively in the Wrightington FC group and 100, 99, and 87% in the Charnley group. This favorable results for the Wrightington FC femoral stem was partly attributed to the stem's maximal proximal fill with its rectangular shape, the stem's ability to resist shear load via longitudinal flutes in the conical stem, and the strong resistance to mediolateral and anteroposterior bending due to the circular cross section. Another example of a cemented femoral stem design with good results is the double-tapered, polished Exeter stem. This design takes advantage of the creeping property of PMMA; therefore, subsidence of an Exeter stem should not be interpreted as loosening. This geometry is designed to transfer load onto the proximal femur. Fowler (23) reported excellent result of only 7 (1.64%) cases of aseptic loosening out of the original 426 Exeter stems in 11–16 year follow-up. Howie et al. (14) supported Fowler et al.'s result that stem-cement subsidence can occur without loosening. Howie et al. reported that there were no revisions secondary to aseptic loosening of Exeter stems in their 9-year follow-up of 20 hips. Other examples of good modern stems are the Lubinus (46) and Spectron (4) hip prostheses.

The use of a collar may be one of the most controversial topics in stem design. Harris (47) and other supporters of collars claim that collars help increase load transfer to the proximal medial bone, which decreases calcar resorption and reduces the strain in the cement in the proximal medial cement. Oh and Harris (48) reported in their in vitro testing that transfer of load directly to the calcar through a larger collar in direct contact with the cortical bone restored 30 to 40% of the normal strain to the femoral calcar. On the other hand, zero or near-zero strain was recorded when the femoral component did not have collar-calcar contact. Lewis et al. (20) more recently reported that a titanium stem with a collar allows creation of calcar stresses of 80% of the anticipated normal levels. A cobalt chrome stem creates calcar stress of 67% of these normal values. Kelley et al. (49) compared 44 collared versus 40 collarless stems in a randomized, prospective study with average follow-up of 4.6 years. Clinically, there was no difference in Harris hip scores and in femoral subsidence. The major radiographic finding was the loss of endosteal height of the femoral neck in the collarless group. Also, there was a decrease in the incidence in the radiolucent lines in the Gruen zones II and VII in the collared group. These authors demonstrated that it is possible to stress the proximal medial femur with collared prostheses. Meding et al. (50) also showed similar results. Their results showed that the collarless group lost significantly more medial femoral neck bone, and had a higher incidence of radiolucent lines in Gruen zone VI. Both groups showed the same aseptic loosening rate.

Studies reporting good clinical results using collarless cemented stems are also numerous. Barrack et al. (38) and Mulroy et al. (39) reported their encouraging results using collared stems, as already mentioned. Opponents of using collared cemented stems question the reproducibility of collar-calcar contact as well as the maintainance of collar-calcar contact over subsequent years. Ling (51) points out several detrimental aspects of the collar. These include debris production secondary to fretting between the undersurface of the collar and either the subjacent cement or the bone. Ling also points out that it is only with collared stems that the calcar pivot phenomenon occurs. The best clinical example of a successful collarless cemented stem is the Exeter hip. Fowler and Ling (23) reported an aseptic loosening rate of only 1.64% of the 426 original Exeter cemented stems in their 11- to 16-year follow-up.

The effects of surface finish in the cemented femoral stem are inconclusive. There are conflicting results in the literature. Smith et al. (40) and Mulroy et al. (39) reported their excellent long-term results using roughened cemented femoral stems with second-generations cementing technique. In contrast, a study by Schulte et al. (36) is an example of a good result using a polished Charnley stem despite using first-generation cementing technique. A study done by Meding et al. (52) also supports the use of polished femoral stems. In their study, these authors used two different stems: a T-28, which was highly polished stainless steel with a trapezoidal shape distally; and a TR-28 was forged cobalt chrome with a roughened surface finish and rectangular distal shape. In their long-term follow-up study of 171 T-28 hips and 158 TR-28 hips, they found no statistical difference when considering revision for aseptic femoral loosening as the endpoint for failure. When considering radiographic criteria for loosening, there was an 11.1% failure in the T-28 group versus a 15.8% failure in the TR-28 group. This was statistically significant. However, this result is difficult to interpret, because two different stem designs and stem materials were used. A smaller but better study by Howie et al. (14) compared the result of matt versus polished cemented femoral stems. Except for the surface finish, the same stem design, surgical technique, and cementing technique were used. Howie et al. reported a 9-year follow-up of 20 Exeter femoral stems with a matt surface finish and 20 polished Exeter femoral stems. They reported that after 9 years, four matt but no polished stems had been revised for aseptic loosening. It was concluded that the matt surface was responsible for increased loosening in the double-tapered stem design.

The metallurgy of cemented femoral stems has also evolved. The original Charnley stems were made of stainless steel. Today, realizing that cement fatigue is one of the major factors in the failure of cemented femoral stems, manufacturers routinely use a stiffer material such as cobalt chrome. Successful results using cemented femoral stems made of either stainless steel (23,36) or cobalt chrome (36,38) have been well documented in the literature. Results of titanium cemented femoral stems have not been so favorable. The rationale for using titanium was based on its good biocompatibility, lower modulus of elasticity to deliver more load to bone, and high corrosion resistance. Although the use of titanium stems was supported by in vitro testing (20), clinical results of cemented titanium femoral stems have been poor. The results of Witt et al. (53) with the McKee Farrar titanium alloy stem was poor. Sixty-six cemented titanium stems were implanted between 1985 and 1987. Thirteen stems were revised secondary to either painful hip or radiographic loosening at average of 2-year follow-up. These authors attributed this failure rate to a change in metallurgy from cobalt-chrome to titanium. Scholl et al. (21) looked at their experience of 132 cemented titanium femoral stems at mean follow-up of 6.6 years. Thirty percent of the stems showed clear signs of radiologic osteolysis in the proximal femur. Six stems (4.5%) had already been revised, and another seven stems (5.3%) were loose clinically and radiographically. The authors attributed these early failures to titanium's high modulus of elasticity, leading to micromotion at the stem–cement interface, and corrosion of titanium alloy initiating an inflammatory foreign-body reaction.

Thus far, results of cemented total hip replacement with regard to modern cementing technique, patient selection, stem design, surface finish, and metallurgy have been examined. Results of some of these factors are clear, while results of others are controversial. In the face of such controversy— along with so many implant choices in the market as well as implant techniques—it becomes very difficult to sort out how to achieve the best results in cemented total hip replacements. Patient selection is important. Good results can be achieved in younger patients; however, there are many more successful clinical results of cemented femoral stems in older patients in the literature. Modern cementing technique is crucial. Achieving an adequate cement mantle with good stem alignment while minimizing cement defects requires practice of modern cementing techniques. Implant choice cannot be overlooked. There are many successful implant designs. Collared versus collarless stems and surface finish are controversial issues. However, successful implants have a few things in common. Most successful implants have polished surfaces to minimize particulate debris production, and round corners with broad medial and lateral borders and a tapered geometry to minimize focal cement stress. The majority of these stems are made of stiffer material, such as cobalt-chrome or stainless steel.

The authors' preferred technique of cemented femoral stem implantation is as follows. Broaching the femoral canal, without reaming, to appropriate size in relation to the actual stem size is essential. This mismatch must be enough to create adequate space for cement mantle. The femoral canal is lavaged, then packed with an epinephrine or a hydrogen peroxide–soaked gauze to minimize further bleeding. Cement is prepared with vacuum mixing for porosity reduction and inserted in a retrograde fashion using a cement gun. For pressurization, a cement restrictor is used distally and digital pressurization is generally practiced proximally. A distal, without proximal, centralizer is used for good alignment of the femoral stem and also to help achieve a cement mantle at least 2 mm thick. Finally, the author's implant of choice is a collarless, tapered, and polished stem, with rounded corners, made of cobalt chrome.

REFERENCES

1. Barrack R. Early failure of modern cemented stems. Arthrop 15(8):2000.
2. Charnley J. Low Friction Arthroplasty of the Hip: Theory and Practice. New York: Springer-Verlag, 1979.
3. Wroblewski BM. Fifteen- to twenty-year results of the Charnley low-friction arthroplasty. CORR 211:30–35, 1986.
4. Garellick G, Malchau H, Regner H, Herberts P. The Charnley versus the Spectron hip prosthesis. J Arthro 14(4):414–425, 1999.
5. Fender D, Harper WM, et al. Outcome of Charnley total hip replacement across a single health region in England. J Bone Joint Surg (Br), 81:577, 1999.
6. Harris W. Options for primary femoral fixation in total hip arthroplasty. Clin Orthop Rel Res 344:118–123, 1997.
7. Noble PC. Pressurization and centralization enhance the quality and reproducibility of cement mantles. Clin Orthop Rel Res 355:77–89, 1998.
8. Goldberg BA. Proximal and distal femoral centralizers in modern cemented hip arthroplasty, Clin Ortho Rel Res 349:163–173, 1998.
9. Charnley J. Acrylic Cement in Orthopedic Surgery. Edinburgh and London: Churchill Livingstone, 1972.
10. Buckwalter JA. Orthopedic Basic Science. 2d ed.: American Association of Orthopaedic Surgery, 2000.
11. Huiskes R. Migration, stem shape, and surface finish in cemented total hip arthroplasty. Clin Orthop Rel Res 355:103–112, 1998.

12. Shepard MF. Influence of cement technique on interface strength of femoral components. Clin Orthop Rel Res 381:26–35, 2000.
13. Middleton RG. Effects of design changes on cemented tapered femoral stem fixation. Clin Orthop Rel Res 355:47–56, 1998.
14. Howie DW, Middleton RG, Costi K. Loosening of matt and polished cemented femoral stems. J Bone Joint Surg 80B:573–576, 1998.
15. Alfaro-Adrian J. Cement migration after THR. J Bone Joint Surgey (Br), 18(1): 1999.
16. Stone KD, Lewallen DG, Ilstrup DM. Femoral loosening following third generation cemented total hip arthroplasty. J Arthrop 11:228, 1996.
17. Ong A, Wong KL, Lai MC, et al. Early failure of precoated femoral components in primary total hip arthroplasty: One surgeon's experience. AAOS, New Orleans, 1998.
18. Dowd JE, Cha CW, Trakru S, et al. Failure of total hip arthroplasty with a precoated femoral prosthesis: 4 to 11 year results. Clin Orthop 355:70, 1998.
19. Scholl E, Eggli S, Ganz R. Osteolysis in cemented titanium alloy hip prosthesis. J Arthrop 15:570–575, 2000.
20. Lewis JL, Askew MJ, Wixon RL, Kramer GM, Tarr RR. The influence of prosthetic stem stiffness and of a calcar collar on stresses in the proximal end of the femur with a cemented femoral component. J Bone Joint Surg 66A; 280–286, 1984.
21. Wan ZN. Effect of stem stiffness and bone stiffness on bone remodeling in cemented total hip replacement. J Arthrop 14(2):1999.
22. Harris W. The case for cementing all femoral components in total hip replacement. CJS 38(suppl 1):1995.
23. Fowler JL, Lee AJC, Ling RSM. Experience with the exeter total hip replacement since 1970. Orthop Clin North Am 19(3):1988.
24. Suominen S. Femoral component fixation with and without intramedullary plug. Arch Trauma Surg 115:276–279, 1996.
25. Ballard WT, Callaghan JJ, Sullivan PM, Johnston RC. The results of improved cementing techniques for total hip arthroplasty in patients less than fifty years old. J Bone Joint Surg 76A:959–964, 1994.
26. Ramaniraka NA, et al. The fixation of the femoral cemented component: Effects of stem stiffness, cement thickness and roughness of the cement-bone surface. J Bone Joint Surg (Br) 82:297, 2000.
27. Wroblewski BM. The Calcar femorale in cemented stem fixation in total hip arthroplasty. J Bone Joint Surg (Br) 28(6):2000.
28. Koster HG. Centralization of the femoral component in cemented hip arthroplasty using guided stem insertion. Orthop Trauma Surg 117:425–429, 1998.
29. Chang PB, Mann KA, Bartel DL. Cemented femoral stem performance: Effects of proximal bonding, geometry and neck length, Clin Orthop 355:90, 1998.
30. Woolson ST, Milbauer JP, et al., Fatigue fracture of a modern forged cobalt chrome alloy femoral component: A report of ten cases. J Bone Joint Surg 79: 1842, 1997.
31. Hozack WJ, Rothman RH, Booth RE Jr, et al. Twenty year survival of 1,157 Charnley cemented total hip arthroplasties. J Arthrop 12:219, 1997.

32. Harrington M, O'Connor DO, Lozynsky AJ, et al. Factors associated with the stability of cemented femoral stems. Harvard Orthop J 1:53, 1999.
33. Kim YH. Strain distribution in the proximal human femur. J Bone Joint Surg (Br) 83B(2), 2001.
34. Sutherland CJ, Wilde AH, Borden LS, Marks KE. A Ten-year follow-up of one hundred consecutive Muller curved stem total hip replacement arthroplasties. J Bone Joint Surg 64A:970–982, 1982.
35. Stauffer RN. Ten-year follow-up study of total hip replacement. J Bone Joint Surg 64A:983–990, 1982.
36. Schulte KR, Callaghan JJ, Kelley SS, Johnston RC. The outcome of Charnley total hip arthroplasty with cement after a minimum twenty-year follow-up. J Bone Joint Surgery 75A:961–975, 1993.
37. D'Lima DD, Oishi CS, Petersilge WJ, Colwell CW, Walker RH. 100 cemented versus 100 noncemented stems with comparison of 25 matched pairs. Clin Orthop Rel Res 348:140–148, 1998.
38. Barrack RL, Mulroy RD, Harris WH. Improved cementing techniques and femoral component loosening in young patients with hip arthroplasty. J Bone Joint Surg 74B:385–389, 1992.
39. Mulroy WF, Estok DM, Harris WH. Total hip arthroplasty with use of so-called second-generation cementing techniques. J Bone Joint Surg 77A:1845–1852, 1995.
40. Smith SW, Estok DM, Harris WH. Total hip arthroplasty with use of second-generation cementing techniques. J Bone Joint Surg 80A:1632–1640, 1998.
41. Dorr LD, Takei GK, Conaty P. Total hip arthroplasties in patients less than forty-five years old. J Bone Joint Surg 65A:474–479, 1983.
42. Chandler HP, Reineck FT, Wixson RL, McCarthy JC. Total hip replacement in patients younger than thirty years old. J Bone Joint Surg 63A:1426–1434, 1981.
43. Sullivan PM, MacKenzie JR, Callaghan JJ, Johnston RC. Total hip arthroplasty with cement in patients who are less than fifty years old. J Bone Joint Surg 76A:863–869, 1994.
44. Crowninshield RD, Brand RA, Johnston RC, Milroy JC. The effect of femoral stem cross-sectional geometry on cement stresses in total hip reconstruction. Clin Orthop Rel Res 146:71–77, 1980.
45. Sochart DH, Hardinge KH. Comparison of the Wrightington FC hip with the Charnley low-friction arthroplasty. J Bone Joint Surg 80B:577–584, 1999.
46. Alho A, Lepisto J, Ylinen P, Paavilainen T. Cemented Lubinus and Furlog total hip endoprostheses: A 12-year follow-up of 175 hips comparing the cementing technique, Arch Orthop Trauma Surg 120:276–280, 2000.
47. Harris WH. Is it advantageous to strengthen the cement-metal interface and use a collar for cemented femoral components of total hip replacement? Clin Orthop Rel Res 285:67–72, 1992.
48. Oh I, Harris WH. Proximal strain distribution in the loaded femur. J Bone Joint Surg 60A:75–85.
49. Kelley SS, Fitzgerald RH, Rand JA, Ilstrup DM. A prospective randomized

study of a collar versus a collarless femoral prosthesis. Clin Orthop Rel Res 294:114–122, 1992.

50. Meding JB, Nassif JM, Ritter MA. Long-term survival of the T-28 versus the TR-28 cemented total hip arthroplasties. J Arthrop 1(5):928–933, 2000.

51. Ling RS. The use of a collar and precoating on cemented femoral stems is unnecessary and detrimental. Clin Orthop Rel Res 285:73–83, 1992.

52. Meding, JB. A comparison of collared and collarless femoral components in primary cemented total hip arthroplasty. J Arthrop 14(2):1999.

53. Witt JD, Swann M. Metal wear and tissue response in failed titanium alloy total hip replacements. J Bone Joint Surgery 73B:559–563, 1991.

4
Acetabular Component Design

Hugh U. Cameron
University of Toronto, Toronto, Ontario, Canada

I. CEMENTED ACETABULAR COMPONENTS

A. Polymethylmethacrylate

Cemented acetabular components are held in place by polymethylmethacrylate (PMMA). Bone cement comprises powder and liquid components. The powder is made up of granules of prepolymerized methacrylate with 2% benzoyl peroxide. The liquid is methylmethacrylate monomer with 1–2% dimethyl paratoluidine and a very small amount of a polymerizing inhibitor, such as hydroxyquinone. On mixing the powder and liquid, a growing chain of methacrylate molecules forms. This material, in various proprietary forms, has in essence remained unchanged for more than 20 years. Various efforts, over the years, to improve bone cement have failed, some dramatically.

B. Implantation of Bone Cement

Fixation of bone cement to bone is by mechanical interlock. There is no adhesion. To achieve interlock, the bone surface must be rough and irregular. This explains the common experience of early clinical failure in attempting to recement implants, as the original periimplant interface left from the previously failed components is quite smooth and therefore does not allow interlock.

To achieve interlock, the bone surfaces should be clean and the trabecular spaces open. The rotating reamers may produce a smooth surface because they press in the bone debris and fat. Blood clots and debris on the surface will leave gaps between cement and bone. In animal experiments, it has been shown that this will reduce the strength of the bone cement interface by 50% (1). Such a surface reduces not only the sheer strength of the interface but also the tensile resistance, potentially leaving gaps between cement and bone as the bone cement undergoes some volumetric shrinkage during polymerization. If the cement is centrifuged to reduce the number of voids and hence increase the fracture toughness, the shrinkage will increase from 3–5%. Vacuum mixing has become popular to reduce voids in the cement and because of concerns about the possible toxic effects of the monomer. A recent study, however (2), has failed to demonstrate any improvement in strength of fixation by so doing.

To clean the bone, a brush was developed by Miller, and Ling and Lee developed a pulsatile saline jet lavage (3). Lee and Ling (4) also developed a device to allow the cement to be pressurized into bone. All three of these devices are now part of standard practice in cementation technique.

C. Acetabular Preparation

The acetabulum is reamed with circular reamers to known outer diameter. The articular cartilage is removed and the acetabulum deepened enough to ensure reasonable cup coverage. Screiber et al. (5) demonstrated in cadaver studies that leaving the subchondral bone plate intact was of value. However, my own studies of a decade ago (6) showed that if the subchondral plate was left intact and only the three classic antirotation holes were drilled in 39 Mueller-type cups, the initial postoperative x-rays showed lucency in one zone in 69% of cases, in two zones in 18%, and in three zones in 21%. In 104 cups with pods to prevent bottoming out, 65% of cases showed lucency in one zone in the initial postoperative x-rays, 25% in two zones, and 28% in three zones. These x-rays were perhaps overread, as no lucency was noted in the cement that had been forced into the antirotation holes. Alarmed by these findings, I changed techniques to drill multiple 4.5 μm holes through the subchondral plate. This dramatically reduced the incidence of lucency in the initial postoperative x-rays. However, this may be an artifact as the cement on entering the holes may simply obscure the lucency which remains.

Should the subchondral plate, therefore, largely be removed to allow access to more of the cancellous space? The answer to this is not yet clear, as cancellous bone is mechanically weak and less able to withstand the stresses transmitted by the cemented component. In animal experiments under ideal conditions, Linders and Ivarson (7) showed that an osseous interface could be produced between cement and cortical bone but not with cancellous bone. Linders (8) points out that a cartilaginous interface is usually seen in the acetabulum, where presumably most of the subchondral plate has been removed. Branemark (9) demonstrated that early loading tends to result in soft tissue formation. It is for this reason that dentists inserting posts into the jaw leave the post unloaded for months. In theory, therefore, patients who have had a hip replacement, whether cemented or uncemented, should be kept non–weight bearing for some time. The problem is, however, that even rolling over in bed can put a load of three times body weight through the hip, so that non–weight bearing reduces the peak loads (one-leg stance loads the hip to five times body weight) but does not eliminate load. Bed rest in traction for a couple of months is therefore theoretically desirable but practically impossible.

Willert (10) has categorized the response of bone to cement into three phases. Phase 1 occurs in the first 2–3 weeks postimplantation. Tissue necrosis is the dominant finding. Phase 2 is a reparative phase, which lasts up to 2 years, and phase 3 is a stable implant bed. The initial bone response is an infarct with marrow necrosis. The dead marrow is then replaced by fibrous tissue. The fractured bone trabeculae heal as normal fracture healing. The necrotic bone trabeculae are removed by osteoclastic resorption and new bone forms within the fibrous tissue. Osteoid and later mineralized bone may fill the irregular surface of the bone cement, but the osteoid may fail to calcify. Willert found that less than 20% of the bone cement in the acetabulum was in contact with bone. In other areas, a connective tissue membrane occurred with foreign-body giant cells. In the stable situation, the number of giant cells diminished.

Fornasier (11), in a postmortem study of well-fixed hips more than 5 years postimplantation, found an active membrane with varying degrees of fibrohistiocytes. This membrane was similar to that found in loose asymptomatic total hip replacements. The density of the histiocytes correlated with the thickness of the membrane, the number of polyethylene particles, and the time after implantation. He therefore proposed an inevitable loosening cascade. The histiocytes have the ability to ingest and participate in bone resorption directly or through osteoclastic activation. Birefringent polymeric wear-debris particles were found in the cytoplasm of the histiocytes, indicating that they were phagocytosed and probably ingested into the phagolysosomes. Phagolysosomes contain proteolytic enzymes for the digestion of foreign materials. If this debris is not capable of being digested, it is ejected from the cells into the intercellular space.

This ejecta can dissolve the tissue cement substance of the intercellular space as well as act as a chemotactic agent, resulting in further histiocytic cellular migration and activation. This material can also activate osteoclasts. The debris is again phagocytosed and the cycle repeated endlessly.

Willert described the semistable state when constant micomotion occurs. This stage is categorized by scar formation within the fibrous tissue with the formation of a synovial-like membrane, which can easily be disturbed and become necrotic. In an unstable state, there is a progressive replacement of bone and bone marrow by granulation tissue, and discrete expansion of the membrane can occur, giving rise to focal osteolysis.

D. Factors Affecting the Interface

1. Heat

Cement liberates heat during curing. The threshold temperature for impaired regeneration was found by Eriksson (12) to be in the range of 44–47°C for 1-min exposure. Tossing-Larsen and Franzen (13) found that the mean maximum cement curing temperature was 43°C. However, in 5 of 28 readings, it was above 44°C. There was no correlation between the size of the cement mass and temperature rise. Precooling of the cement or components was of little value. I found that the use of a cemented ceramic socket, which is a much better "heat sink" than polyethylene, did not influence the development of a radiolucent line (14). Moberg et al. (15) found, using RSA, that the majority of acetabulae that migrate do so in the first 4 months; they postulated that this might be as a result of heat injury or insufficient mechanical support by weak cancellous bone.

2. Creep

Bone cement is a thermoplastic polymer that can undergo "creep." Polymers are affected by a temperature called the glass transition temperature (TG). Below the TG, the polymer is a glass and a brittle elastic solid. Above the TG, it is a viscous liquid. Lee et al. (16) have indicated that the body temperature of 310k is close to the TG of PMMA, which is 373k. The temperature in the loaded joint is 2–3 degrees higher than the normal body temperature of 37°C, which may have some impact in allowing cement to act as a viscoelastic solid. The application of load causes a small elastic deformation followed by continuous deformation (creep). Releasing the load causes slow reverse creep. Different cements creep at different rates due to differing porosities, and water facilitates creep by acting as an internal lubricant.

It is difficult to see separation between an all-polyethylene acetabular component and the cement mantle. However, in examining cemented ceramic components (14), I was able to detect separation between the ceramic prosthesis and the cement mantle in zone 3 in many cases and occasionally in zone 2 without any obvious fracture of the cement bed. This slow deformation obviously changes the loading of the cement/implant interface. In this study, separation or debonding was seen in components in which the cement grooves were shallow and not undercut. This was not seen when threaded components were cemented in place, as presumably the thread depth gave much better resistance to tensile loads in zone 3. This obviously suggests that deep undercut grooves are of value in preventing cement/implant debonding. Unfortunately, the corollary is that this will produce increased tensile loads on the cement/bone interface in zone 3.

On examining this issue, Chiu and I (17) reviewed long-term (i.e. more than 7-year) follow-up on three distinct series: a cemented Mueller-type cup with no cement pods and no undercut grooves; an all-polyethylene Spectron cup with undercut grooves, pods to prevent the cup from bottoming out, and a small lip; and a similar cup that was metal-backed.

There were 130 Mueller-type cups, 174 polyethylene Spectron cups, and 60 metal-backed Spectron cups. Follow-up was 7–18 years. We graded lucency into single-zone, partial, and complete lucency. Linear wear was also examined using a simple Mueller-type protractor. With this technique, wear of less than 1 mm, which was felt acceptable, cannot be measured accurately, as minimal wear is of little significance.

We found that sex was not related to lucency or wear. Metal and ceramic heads did not affect lucency but did affect wear. Of those with ceramic heads, 10.3% showed acetabular wear, compared to 27.7% of those with metal heads. Age did not relate to wear but, surprisingly, it did to lucency. Of those under age 65, 20.9% showed some lucency, as did 28.9% of those between 65 and 75 and 45% of those over age 75. Length of follow-up related to lucency and wear. Of patients with a follow-up of less than 10 years, 38.2% showed some lucency, compared with 50% with over 10 years of follow-up, while 14% of those with less than 7 years of follow-up showed some wear, compared with 20.6% of those with more than 8 years. Original disease did not affect wear but did affect lucency. A total of 21.9% of OA (osteoarthritis) cases showed some lucency, 16.7% of RA (rheumatoid arthritis) cases, 44.4% of CDH (congenital dislocation hip) cases, and 25% of posttraumatic cases. Cup size was not related to wear or lucency and cup type did not affect wear. Surprisingly and counterintuitively—in view of the fact that Ritter (18) has stated that 100% of his acetabular cups that loosened showed early lucency in zone 1—lucency seen in the first postoperative x-ray did not affect final outcome, as 49.5% of those with no initial lucency developed it and 41% of those with some lucency had progression. At the longest data point, 63.9% of Mueller cups showed some lucency and 24.6% complete lucency. Furthermore, 83.3% of polyethylene Spectrons showed some lucency and 41.9% complete lucency, while 77.3% of metal-backed Spectrons showed some lucency and 37.8% complete lucency. The overall number of revisions for acetabular loosening was quite small. At 11–12 years, where the data still contains reasonable numbers, 93.3% of Mueller cups survived, as did 93.7% of polyethylene Spectron cups and 90.12% of metal-backed Spectron cups. Beyond these data points, the numbers become so small that caution must be used in interpreting them (Tables 1 to 3).

3. Wear Debris

Any articulating bearing will produce some wear debris. The body can tolerate a certain amount of wear debris, but when the volume reaches a certain mass or time limit, which may be patient-specific, osteolysis occurs. One theory of osteolysis is that the particles in and of themselves induce a bone-destroying granuloma. Another theory, put forward by Schmalzreid, is that wear debris particles produce a synovitis that results in increased fluid production and also leads to capsular scarring. As the pseudocapsule surrounding the joint becomes more scarred, it becomes thicker and less compliant. This means that the fluid pressure produced by the movement of the joint will go up to as much as 700 mmHg. This produces a hydraulic ram effect. Osteolysis, therefore, occurs as a result of this hydraulic ram acting on any exposed bone, such as the calcar and greater trochanter on the femoral side or the periphery of the acetabulum on the acetabular side. Lucent lines imply that at best a fibrous interface is present, which may be part of the effective joint space, thus explaining the appearance of dome osteolysis in cups with no holes.

Obviously, therefore, reduction of wear debris is desirable. Sir John Charnley postulated that the smaller the femoral head, the less the friction and therefore the less likelihood of loosening. For years, 32-mm heads were used as it was felt that they posed less risk of dislocation, although in reality dislocation has less to do with head size than with the difference between head/neck diameter. Livermore et al. (19) showed that linear wear was greater with small heads and volumetric wear greater with larger ones. He felt that a 28-mm head was a reasonable compromise.

Schuller and Marti (20) found that the use of ceramic heads as compared with metal heads reduced polyethylene wear, but they did not find that it reduced the number of radiographically suspected acetabular loosenings. They did find that the cases with proven loosening had a higher than average wear rate. Chiu and I also examined ceramic versus metal heads. We found that they did not affect lucency rates but did affect wear, with 10.3% of cups with ceramic heads showing obvious wear as well as 27.7% of those with metal heads. No difference, however, was found in less than 7 years of follow-up.

The degree of polishing of metal heads is now much better than it was previously. The bearing properties of metal heads can be improved by ion implantation, but this is only a few angstrom units thick and the effect is therefore transitory. Coatings such as titanium nitrate and black diamond

Table 1 Life-Table Analysis: Mueller

Year since operation (x to x + 1) yr	Number at start	Number removed	Number withdrawn	Number at risk	Probability of removal	Standard error	Probability of survival	Cumulative survival rate	Survival rate after x year
0–1	116	0	2	115	0	0	1	100	100
1–2	114	0	1	113.5	0	0	1	100	100
2–3	113	1	10	108	0.0092	0.0092	0.9908	99.08	100
3–4	102	0	9	97.5	0	0	1	99.08	99.08
4–5	93	0	6	90	0	0	1	99.08	99.08
5–6	87	2	11	81.5	0.0245	0.0171	0.9755	96.65	99.08
6–7	74	0	2	73	0	0	1	96.65	96.65
7–8	72	1	7	68.5	0.0146	0.0145	0.9854	95.24	96.65
8–9	64	0	10	59	0	0	1	95.24	95.24
9–10	54	1	10	49	0.0204	0.0202	0.9796	93.30	95.24
10–11	43	0	7	38	0	0	1	93.30	93.30
11–12	33	0	6	29.5	0	0	1	93.30	93.30
12–13	26	0	7	23	0	0	1	93.30	93.30
13–14	20	0	7	16.5	0	0	1	93.30	93.30
14–15	13	2	4	11	0.1818	0.1163	0.8182	76.34	93.30
15–16	7	0	6	4	0	0	1	76.34	76.34
16–17	1	0	0	1	0	0	1	76.34	76.34
17–18	1	0	1	0.5	0	0	1	76.34	76.34

Plot of Cumulative survival rate % (y-axis, 0–100) versus Year (x to x+1) (x-axis, 0–18).

Table 2 Life-Table Analysis: Poly. Spectron

Year since operation (x to x + 1) yr	Number at start	Number removed	Number withdrawn	Number at risk	Probability of removal	Standard error	Probability of survival	Cumulative survival rate	Survival rate after x year
0–1	177	0	4	175	0	0	1	100	100
1–2	173	0	0	173	0	0	1	100	100
2–3	173	0	20	163	0	0	1	100	100
3–4	153	1	8	149	0.0067	0.0067	0.9933	99.33	100
4–5	144	0	12	138	0	0	1	99.33	99.33
5–6	132	0	9	127.5	0	0	1	99.33	99.33
6–7	123	0	16	115	0	0	1	99.33	99.33
7–8	107	2	12	101	0.0198	0.0139	0.9802	97.36	99.33
8–9	93	1	7	89.5	0.0111	0.0111	0.9889	96.28	97.36
9–10	85	1	4	83	0.0120	0.0120	0.9880	95.12	96.28
10–11	80	1	18	71	0.0141	0.0140	0.9859	93.78	95.12
11–12	61	0	7	57.5	0	0	1	93.78	93.78
12–13	54	1	11	48.5	0.0206	0.0204	0.9794	91.85	93.78
13–14	42	1	7	38.5	0.0260	0.0256	0.9740	89.46	91.85
14–15	34	1	22	23	0.0435	0.0425	0.9565	85.57	89.46
15–16	11	0	8	7	0	0	1	85.57	85.57
16–17	3	0	3	1.5	0	0	—	85.57	85.57

Table 3 Life-Table: Metal

Year since operation (x to x + 1) yr	Number at start	Number removed	Number withdrawn	Number at risk	Probability of removal	Standard error	Probability of survival	Cumulative survival rate	Survival rate after x year
0–1	45	0	0	0	0	0	—	100	100
1–2	45	0	0	0	0	0	—	100	100
2–3	45	0	2	44	0	0	—	100	100
3–4	43	0	3	41.5	0	0	—	100	100
4–5	40	1	5	37.5	0.0267	0.0263	0.9733	97.33	100
5–6	34	0	0	34	0	0	—	97.33	97.33
6–7	34	0	1	33.6	0	0	—	97.33	97.33
7–8	33	0	6	30	0	0	—	97.33	97.33
8–9	27	0	1	26.5	0	0	—	97.33	97.33
9–10	26	0	5	23.5	0	0	—	97.33	97.33
10–11	21	0	6	18	0	0	—	97.33	97.33
11–12	15	1	3	13.5	0.0741	0.0713	0.9249	90.12	97.33
12–13	11	2	6	8	0.2500	0.1531	0.7500	67.59	90.12
13–14	3	0	3	1.5	0	0	—	67.59	67.59

may also help, but they tend to be somewhat scratch-sensitive. It is impossible to completely eliminate three-body wear in an artificial joint, as bone dust, cement particles, and metallic particles all exist and may be drawn into the bearing during separation in swing phase.

Original polyethylene has been improved by better manufacturing practices—i.e., a reduction of fusion defects, removal of calcium stearate, and ensurance of less variability of crosslinking. Gamma radiation of polyethylene in air to sterilize it results in an increase of free radicals, which, in turn, leads to oxidative degradation of the polyethylene. Ethylene oxide sterilization or gamma radiation in the inert gas does not produce this effect. With time, more oxidative degradation occurs if polyethylene is stored in air. The shelf life of polyethylene is therefore finite, and inert gas packaging obviously extends it.

The number of crosslinks in the polyethylene chain can be increased by adding energy, e.g., e-beam or gamma radiation. In joint simulators, the resulting materials show significantly better adhesive and abrasive wear resistance over conventional polyethylene. One major problem in testing materials for bearings, however, are the tests themselves. Conventional pin-and-disc tests are of little value. Simulators are better than they were, but they too lack validation. Many simulators use a single vector, whereas it is well known that there are multiple vectors of load in the hip. Even fewer simulators use stop/start and virtually none simulate impact, which some patients certainly produce when the components separate in the swing phase of gait. The ductility and fracture toughness of this heavily crosslinked polyethylene is reduced. Those who remember the "new" polyethylenes—such as heat-pressed, carbon fiber–reinforced polyethylene and hylamer, which promised so much and delivered so little—must view any change to polyethylene with a certain degree of misgiving and realize that it may take many years to determine whether this advance is really an advance or a sideways step.

4. Alignment

It is generally agreed that the cup should be inserted at 45 degrees to the vertical. If the cup is too vertical, the head articulates with the lateral edge of the cup rather than the dome. This may predispose to a dislocation. It is difficult to demonstrate this conclusively, but it is my impression that cup wear is accelerated with a vertical cup (Figure 1). This tends to be more of a problem with a noncemented cup as surgeons, in an attempt to get full bony coverage, may insert the cup at 55 degrees—the anatomical axis of the true acetabulum minus the limbus. It is then necessary to use a liner with a lip to hold the head in place. Extended lips are meant for added

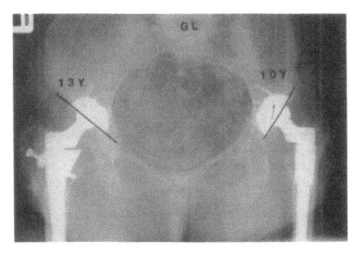

Figure 1 Identical components were used in this CDH case. At 10 years, the cup, that was inserted vertically shows more wear than the cup that was in place for 13 years.

stability and not for load bearing, and they can both wear and break. If a cup is inserted too horizontally, there is no posterior wall support; it may also predispose to dislocation.

Most cups are inserted in some degree of anteversion, as is the femoral component. Many would agree that the combined anteversion of cup and femur should be 30–40 degrees. Care must be taken during trialing that the hip is stable and the neck does not impinge in extension.

A neutral cup with no extended lip can be inserted with any pusher. If an extended lip is present in a monoblock cup, however, it is impossible to determine both vertical angle and version by eye and an inserter that will allow the extended lip to be neutralized by the inserter head is therefore necessary. If an inserter locks tightly to a cup, then any movement of the inserter during curing of the cement will tend to rock the cup. For that reason, once the cup has been inserted at the appropriate angle, the inserter must be removed and a pusher substituted. The ball on the pusher must be smaller than the internal diameter of the acetabulum. This means that the ball rests on the polar position of the cup and rocking of the pusher will not rock the cup.

5. Polyethylene Thickness

It is generally accepted that an all-polyethylene cemented cup should have about 8 mm of polyethylene to prevent deformation and cold flow, which can accelerate wear and lead to abnormal stresses on the cement mantle. This means that for smaller sockets, a 22-mm head is preferable. For example, a 44-mm-diameter cup will have a potential wall thickness of 11 mm. However, cement grooves will reduce this to about 8 mm. It follows, therefore, that cups smaller than 42 mm in outer diameter probably should not be cemented. A 39-mm offset bore cup used to be available and perhaps still is. The wall thickness in zone 3 in this cup is vastly reduced to allow greater superior thickness. Franz Weber (Weber, personal communication) reports good long-term results with this cup; on the one occasion that I used it, it was pretty durable. It is, however, a frightening thing to be able to deform a cup with one's fingers, like a soft Ping-Pong ball, and then contemplate putting this in a young person.

Metal backing was introduced to allow liner exchange. It was felt that it would smooth out the stresses. Reported results with cemented metal-backed cups have not been good (21), but many of these cups had an unstable porous metal layer at the back. Our experience with metal-backed Spectron cups which were not porous has not been bad, but equally it has not been better than that with a similar all polyethylene cup.

If one incorporates all of the laboratory data, therefore, an all-polyethylene cemented cup should be at least 8 mm thick, have a lip to allow cement compression, pods to prevent bottoming out, and undercut grooves. The differences, however, between this "high-tech" and expensive cup and the simple Mueller-type cup with circumferential grooves is marginal at 12 years of follow-up.

Literature reviews of the results of various implants are fraught with difficulties. The main difficulty is the adoption by the orthopaedic world of the so-called survivorship analysis. All this measures is revision. If the patient with a loose joint is not actually revised, then he or she is reported as if the operation had been a success. Once the follow-up is over 10–15 years, the number of patients left is generally so small that the survivorship analysis becomes difficult to interpret, as the error bars, which are seldom shown, may cover the entire graph.

Results can be skewed in many ways. If the implant is difficult to use, as, for example, a threaded cup, it is possible that a master surgeon will produce results unobtainable in the hands of others. Results produced by the designer himself may be better than those produced by his followers because of potential observer bias, not necessarily intentional, and because he has gone through the development process and learning curve and knows how to optimally insert the implant. Patient selection may influence longevity. If, for example, one limits one's practice to patients over 65 years of age with weight under 170 lb, the results are liable to be excellent almost regardless of the implant. This may alter how far back one should search the literature.

Some 20 to 30 years ago, very few young patients were being given the option of total hip replacement, but now many are.

Results from teaching hospitals should be inferior to those produced by a single subspecialized surgeon in private practice, as with the best will in the world, very few residents have either the experience or the eye-hand coordination that they will subsequently develop. The results of those surgeons, doing small numbers of procedures, should also be inferior to those of the expert doing large numbers. None of this should be viewed as a criticism; it is simply a fact of life and everyone is doing his or her best for the patient.

Radiological analysis is also fraught with difficulties. When is "loose" loose? An implant is loose if it has migrated or changed orientation. However, it can restabilize in a new position and remain unchanged for years. Under these circumstances, is it loose? Radiolucent lines show huge intraobserver error. A lucent line in one zone nay mean nothing, but if it is in zone 3, it may be a "wake" phenomenon as the cup moves proximally; therefore it may be of significance. Does a complete lucent line around the acetabular component suggest loosening if it is less than 1 mm thick? Probably not, but if it is more than 2 mm thick, it does imply loosening.

In looking at the results of cemented sockets, I thought it realistic to look at the results in younger patients only. It is only common sense, after all, that an implant will survive longer in the elderly, low-demand patient than it will in a younger high-demand individual. Early reports of cemented total hip replacements in young patients with an average 5- to 10-year follow-up showed 25–70% of hips either radiologically loose or revised. Master surgeons such as Ritter (21) and Ranawat (22) have superior results. Three recent studies in patients under the age of 50 (23) at 18 years showed 41.3% of acetabular components loose or revised. Callaghan (24) at 23.3 years mean follow-up showed 41.7% acetabular components loose or revised. Chiu et al. (25), in a recent study of young, active Chinese patients, showed that at 15 years, 100% of cemented acetabular components used in cases of avascular necrosis were revised or showed evidence of loosening. Their overall group loosening or revision rate was about 30% at 15 years, but the investigators stress that the error bars are very large. The literature suggests that survivorship of cemented sockets is affected by age, body weight, and disease, at least in avascular necrosis.

One has to conclude that most cemented sockets have a finite life expectancy, probably of the order of 15–20 years. As long as the socket has not migrated more than 2 cm, revision is not particularly difficult. Because a loose socket will migrate, it becomes crucial to review patients annually when the socket is 10 years or more out from the index operation. Unfortunately, many patients who turn up faithfully for review for the first 5–10 years or so lose interest at that point. They may retire or move away. They may have increasing difficulties with transportation, and they may become increasingly forgetful. Slow socket migration can be fairly insidious, producing little discomfort in the patient with very low demand.

Every surgeon has to make his own choice, but in my hands patients over age 65 with a primary procedure are cemented unless there is a reason not to. However, the results of revision with cemented sockets are poor. In my hands, the only indication for a cemented socket in a revision is when a cage with a graft is required.

II. THREADED CUPS

The initial threaded cups were the truncated-cone type introduced by Mittlemeier and the truncated ellipsoid designed by Lord. The Mittlemeier prosthesis was an aluminum ceramic; the threads were large and thick and had to be pretapped (Figure 2). A truncated cone had to be reamed, which occasionally necessitated perforation of the acetabular floor, and it had to be inserted much more horizontally than normal. This made it a very unforgiving cup that was technically difficult to insert and had a steep learning curve. Inserted properly, however, the cups have been surprisingly durable (26). The cup of Lord was a truncated ellipsoid with a metal shell and a polyethylene liner. The threads were thin and sharp and could self-tap. Both reaming and insertion were technically easier than with the Mittlemeier, and again early results were good (27).

These cups sparked interest in the rest of the world and several modifications were made for easier insertion. One such was the Anderson cup, which had a hemispherical shape that would allow easier insertion with less bone removal (28).

The cup was a grit blast titanium alloy (Ti6A14V). The thread profile was such that the compressive load fell on the horizontal face. In a pilot study, 2-mm threads were used if the bone was very hard; but after a few cases, it became obvious that deeper threads could be inserted into even very hard eburnated bone. A thread depth of 2.5 mm was therefore chosen as it was felt that deeper threads would require pretapping. The threads were self-tapping with vertical grooves to collect the bone debris generated by cup insertion. Initially the threads were conical, but subsequently spherical threads were developed which theoretically allowed more complete cup seating. A large dome hole was provided to visualize the depth of cup insertion.

After cup seating, a polyethylene liner was inserted. This liner was available for a range of head sizes, primarily 28- and 32-mm inner diameter.

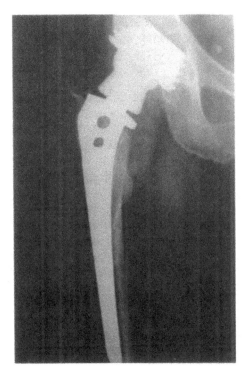

Figure 2 This Mittlemeier truncated cone had to be pretapped in being seated more horizontally than normal.

Neutral, 10-, 15-, and 20-degree offset liners were available, including a constrained socket. The liner was held in placed by a bayonet lock, which allowed the cup, even after reduction, to be dialed around to leave the offset at the position of maximum instability. The plastic liner was then locked in place by inserting screws, which penetrated the outer shell of the cup. These screws were felt to aid initial cup anchorage and perhaps absorb some of the torque forces to which the acetabulum would be subjected.

This locking mechanism was very stable, allowing minimum movement between the liner and the shell and thus generating very little backside wear of the polyethylene. To reduce this further, the inner part of the shell was polished. This mechanism has withstood the test of time and remains in widespread use today in the Arthropor and ZTT cup series (Johnson & Johnson DePuy, Warsaw, Indiana). The supplementary screws were 5 mm in most instances, but with the smallest cup they were 3.5 mm. In general, two screws were used. It was not felt possible to make cups smaller than 45 mm in outer diameter as the liner would then be too thin.

A. Insertion

The acetabulum was reamed with spherical mira reamers, which progressively increased in size until firm anterior and posterior wall contact was made. The subchondral bone plate was usually left intact. The cup was inserted at 45 degrees to the vertical, with 10–15 degrees of anteversion. It was partially seated with hammer blows to make sure that it was well within the acetabulum before screwing began. Initially at T-handled torque wrench with a measuring scale was used and loads of over 600 in./lb could routinely be generated. Initially the inserter locked tightly to the cup; after a few cases, however, this was discontinued, as it was found that if the surgeon did not hold the inserter in exactly the correct alignment, the leverage generated would break the bone threads. A connector was therefore developed which would unlock if more than 5–7 degrees of wobble occurred. A reciprocating wrench was developed later which could generate greater forces. Finally, a pneumatic-powered inserter was developed. The advantage of this was that the surgeon no longer needed to provide power but could concentrate instead on maintaining the appropriate angle. The pneumatic inserter delivered a uniform torque of 1200 in./lb, thus ensuring more than adequate thread seating (28).

If, after generating this torque load, the apex of the cup had not bottomed out in the dome of the acetabulum, bone graft was added through the dome hole. All patients were kept non–weight bearing for 8 weeks after cup insertion to allow development of a periimplant bone plate before service loads were applied (Figure 3).

B. Clinical Experience

The initial results were extremely good and were routinely reported in the literature. This report deals with three separate series. In the first series, the cup was used with a cemented Mittlemeier xenophore stem. Either a cemented cup or a threaded cup was used in a semirandomized fashion. The cemented cup was inserted using multiple subchondral plate perforations, pressure lavage, and cement prepressurization. Age- and sex-matched controls are available for this series. In the second series, the stem used was the Richard's International cemented stem. Due to financial constraints, the threaded cup was reserved for those less than 65 years of age and a cemented cup thereafter, so that age-matched controls are not possible in this series. In both of these series a 32-mm ceramic head was used. The head/neck taper was 14–16.

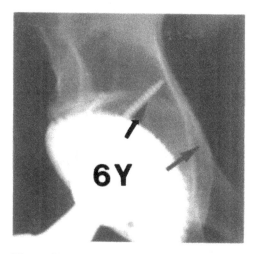

Figure 3 This threaded cup was inserted to be wall-bearing only in this protrusio case. The floor was grafted through the dome hole. At 6 years, the floor has completely reconstituted.

In the third series, the threaded cup was used in patients under the age of 60 with the S-ROM proximally modular stem. A 28-mm cobalt chrome head was used on an 11/13 taper.

As only long-term results are important, only patients with a documented follow-up of more than 7 years were considered. For the purposes of this study, primary cases only were included, as the number of revision cases were too small and other factors such as bulk allograft influenced the outcome. To simplify matters, three endpoints were used—cup revision for aseptic loosening, loose but not revised (i.e., the cup had obviously migrated or changed position), and cup functioning well (Figure 4A and B).

C. Results

1. Series 1

There were 24 threaded cups with a follow up of 7–15 years. Of these, 10 (41.7%) had been revised at an average of 12 years. One was loose but not revised, as the patient died prior to revision. In an age- and sex-matched group of cemented sockets, 1 was loose but not revised. In 130 cemented sockets with a follow up of 7–15 years, 3 (2.3%) had been revised for aseptic loosening and a further 4 (3.1%) were loose but not revised.

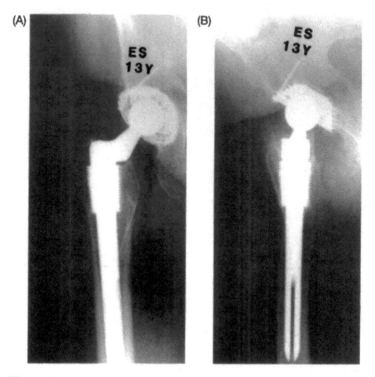

Figure 4 A and B. At 13 years, this threaded cup shows no loosening, no osteo-lysis, and no wear.

2. Series 2

In series 2, there were 40 threaded cups with a follow up of 7–14 years. Of these, 14 (35%) had been revised for aseptic loosening and 1 (2.5%) was loose but not revised. In the remaining 280 cemented sockets in this group, all with a minimum follow up of 7 years, 5 (1.8%) had been revised for aseptic loosening and 4 (1.4%) were loose but not revised. Of interest in this series, 25 ingrowth cups had been used, of which none have as yet required revision.

3. Series 3

In the third series, there were 47 threaded cups with a follow up of 7–15 years. 18 (38.3%) had been revised for aseptic loosening and 5 (10.6%) were loose but not revised.

The long-term results of this particular threaded cup were poor, and this has been a general experience in North America with all threaded cups.

Perhaps if the surface had been rougher, osseointegration might have significantly influenced long-term results. The Anderson cup was modified with this in mind, to produce a very rough surface ("the gripper") and was used extensively in Australia; it remains in use today. A further variant was the partially porous coated cup ("the super cup"), which was widely used in the United States for a time.

In Europe threaded cups seem to enjoy a better reputation. The original Zweymuller cup resembled a truncated cone and was made of polyethylene. Early failures prompted a change to a metal shell with a polyethylene liner. Threaded cups continued to be used principally in the German-speaking world.

One variation of the threaded cup is a remake of the original Peter Ring prosthesis, in which the cup had a long threaded post at the dome. This was introduced into the cancellous bone of the dome of the acetabulum and obtained purchase close to the sacroiliac joint. The results of Ring himself were poor in the long term and he later abandoned this design. The newer version is HA-coated and is conical rather than parallel-sided. Long-term results have yet to be reported.

III. INGROWTH CUPS

The concept of bone ingrowth into porous metal or fibrous metal was pioneered in the early 1970s (29). Ingrowth cups are now the commonest type of cup used in North America. The materials were either a titanium alloy or cobalt chrome alloy and the ingrowth coating is either porous metal beads, fiber metal, or hydroxyapatite. Recently tantalum has been introduced also. Most cups have a detachable (modular) liner of polyethylene. There are several possible variations in design and implantation techniques.

A. Implantation

1. Press Fit or Line to Line

The concept of press fit is that bone is elastic. If a hole is drilled and a larger object forced into that hole, hoop tension is generated. "Line to line" implies that the object inserted into the hole has the same diameter as the hole. Obviously a press fit gives greater initial stability. In general, more than 1 mm of press fit is used in the acetabulum. The surgeon can either calculate this himself or the instruments can be built to provide this press fit. For example, with some systems, if the reamer says an outer diameter of 50 mm and a 50-mm cup is inserted, then the reamer is either 1.5 mm undersized (i.e., 48.5 mm in reality) or the cup is oversized (i.e., 51.5 mm in reality). The advantage of this is that it gives the surgeon one less thing to think about during surgery. A press fit of up to 3 mm is possible but becomes increasingly risky, as the hoop stress on the pelvis is so high that a pelvic fracture, politely called a dissociation, can occur. The greater the degree of press fit, the less likelihood that the cup can be bottomed out (i.e., the more likely it is that the cup will become wall-bearing only). This, of course, is acceptable. The residual gap in the floor can be filled with graft or the cup may migrate a little in the first few weeks to reach a stable position.

B. Visualization Ports

The majority of modular cups have a hole in the dome to enable the floor of the acetabulum to be visualized. Monoblock cups do not have this option. There is some concern that a visualization port may provide a channel for wear debris and the production of osteolysis. This was probably true for the initial, very large visualization ports, but they have since been downsized (Figure 5). As cold flow into this dome hole is possible, one additional design feature employed in some plastic liners is to thicken the polyethylene to insert it into the hole (Figure 6). Whether this is an advantage remains to be seen. Several cups now offer additional features of a "manhole cover" to occlude the hole once the cup has been inserted. This can be done by means of a short screw or a convex metal shell, which can be turned concave by striking it with a curved tool. Not enough time has elapsed as yet to determine whether this is effective in reducing dome-hole osteolysis, but it certainly can do no harm.

C. Supplementary Fixation

1. Pegs and Fins

Some cups have pegs or fins to provide additional fixation. Most require no predrilling and are simply driven into the bone. Usually these are grit blast titanium, which may osseointegrate. The advantage is additional fixation. One disadvantage is that the pegs and fins may impede removal, as they interrupt the path of the curved cup-removal chisel. The main disadvantage, however, is that the bone in the acetabulum may be of variable hardness, especially in the revision situation. If the peg or fin hits very hard bone, it may force the cup into softer bone in another area, thus changing the alignment and preventing full seating. The original PCA cup had "rabbit ears" or tumble locks, which were porous coated and had to be predrilled. Removing these can be somewhat of a challenge.

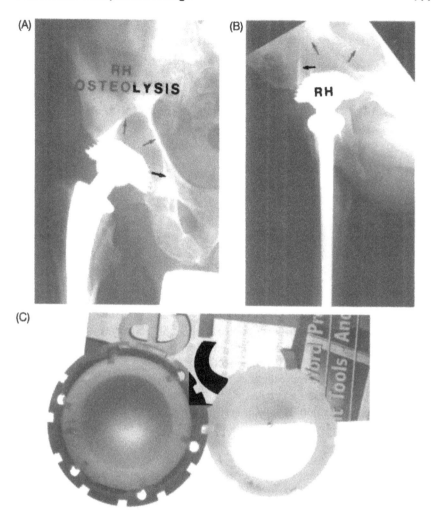

Figure 5 A to C. A very large osteolytic cyst has developed adjacent to the dome hole. The polyethylene liner became so thin that it eventually developed a hole. One can almost read newsprint through the dome of the cup.

2. Screws

Many cups offer dome-screw capacity and a few peripheral screws. The dome screws are usually cancellous (i.e., about 6.5 mm in diameter), with big threads. Fortunately most of the manufacturers see no need to reinvent

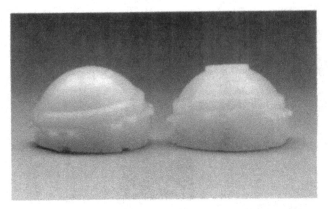

Figure 6 The polyethylene in the dome-hole area has been thickened to help to occlude the hole in the dome of the shell. Long-term data on this modification is not available.

the wheel and most use an Allen key head, which will take either a fixed or multiaxial AO screwdriver. Unfortunately, some manufacturers have propriety screw heads that add nothing to the design and simply make life tedious for the revision surgeon, as recognizing a cup on x-ray is not always easy. Such ill-considered practices should be discouraged. There are other ways to "brand name" a product.

Screws are generally sold as self-tapping, which they are to some extent because they have a cutting flute. However, in the revision situation, where the bone may either be very dense or very thin and eroded, pretapping greatly eases screw insertion.

The holes for the dome screw can be either in the upper part of the cup alone, the so-called "cluster cup," or throughout the whole cup. It has been said that screws are bad, as they prevent settling of the cup, and holes provide another port for osteolysis. If a good press fit is achieved, almost no supplementary fixation with screws is required. If a good press fit cannot be achieved, especially in the revision situation, multiple screws are necessary. The "four-screw sign" indicates that the surgeon who inserted the cup did not trust the press fit—i.e., that the cup was not particularly stable at the time of insertion and therefore multiple screws were used.

My own feeling is that a cluster cup is a cup designed by a committee, being neither fish nor fowl. If there is a good press fit, as in most primary situations, there is no need for dome screws. If there is a poor press fit, as in some revisions, multiple screws are required. It is often remarkable how bad the bone in the dome of the eroded acetabulum is. In watching cups fail, the general pattern is for the upper part of the dome (i.e., zone 1) to act as a fulcrum and the lower part of the cup (i.e., in zone 3) to move generally out to make the cup more vertical. Occasionally the cup moves medially to become more horizontal. The vertical cup in general requires revision a lot sooner than the horizontal cup, which can often, in spite of being obviously loose, survive for a remarkably long period of time.

It is a general principal that less force is required to block movement when it is applied farthest away from the fulcrum. For this reason, in an unstable situation, it is preferable to insert screws through the cup into the ischium and pubis. It is not always possible to do this, or the screws may be very short. However, it is very comforting if this can be achieved. I personally feel, therefore, that two cups are required—one with no dome-screw capacity for a good press fit and one with multiple dome-screw capacity for a poor press fit.

The other advantage of multiple holes is the ability to backfill with graft after cup insertion. If the acetabulum is grafted prior to cup insertion, other than filling the very obvious defects, the cup may rest on graft and not on host bone. Under such circumstances the cup must move through the graft to rest on host bone in the first few weeks. If the distance is small (i.e., a few microns), then this probably does not matter; but if the distance is sizable (i.e., a few millimeters), this is a worrying situation. My own preference, therefore, is to insert the cup first and backfill later. This used to be tedious as packing particulate graft or ceramic particles such as tricalcium phosphate at right angles to the plane of insertion is not easy. The development of reverse-phase gel, such as Dynagraft (GenSci Co. Ltd., Irvine, CA), has greatly simplified this. Normally, when a material is heated, it will turn liquid (i.e., it undergoes a phase change). In a reverse-phase gel, the material is liquid outside the body and can thus be injected via a syringe and a tube. The increased heat of the human body after implantation turns the gel solid.

Holes for dome screws are not entirely innocuous. They potentially allow passage of debris, leading to osteolysis. They can also result in increased polyethylene wear. The polyethylene may cold flow into the holes. If the holes have sharp edges they can act as a shaver at the microscopic level. The edges of the dome holes, therefore, should be rounded. Furthermore, it must be remembered that there is a danger zone in the acetabulum. The upper anterior one-third of the acetabulum has significant vessels deep to it (30). There is supposed to be a characteristic feel as the tap winds up the internal iliac vein, but it is probably better never to experience this feeling. Sometimes screws have to be inserted into this area, but the surgeon should do so only with extreme trepidation.

3. Peripheral Screws

Some cups offer peripheral screw capacity. These vary in size from 5–3.5 mm, depending on the wall thickness of the cup. They may be used additionally to block movement of the liner. They can be either unicortical or, in the revision situation where additional stability is required, bicortical for increased grip. Cups smaller than 45-mm outer diameter cannot accommodate dome screws, as the holes will reduce the volume of porous coating and the cup may then be too weak. Therefore only peripheral screws can be used in very tiny cups (Figure 7).

D. Locking Mechanisms

Some of the initial mechanisms that locked the polyethylene to the shell were not secure and allowed macromotion, leading to backside wear. Fortunately most of these deficiencies have now been corrected, but the revision surgeon must be aware of them. There is little point in inserting a new

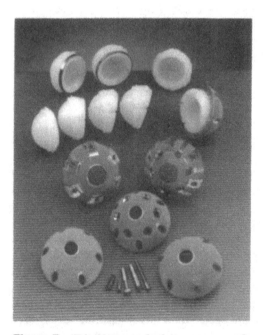

Figure 7 This photograph shows a range of cups. All have peripheral screw capacity and some dome screw capacity also. One has additional spikes. There is also a range of liners varying from neutral to 20 degrees offset. The cups with the metal bands are constrained liners.

polyethylene into a cup with a poor locking mechanism or a locking mechanism that is suspect with reuse (31). It is very embarrassing to have a liner come loose within a short time of revision. If such a cup can be removed easily, it should be. However, if the cup is well ingrown and especially if it crosses the teardrop, then removal is fraught with hazard. The pelvis may break during removal or the cup may come out with the entire medial wall and ischium firmly attached to it.

If the pelvis breaks, it must be plated before a new cup is inserted (Figure 8A and B). I have on a couple of occasions used screws through the cup to stabilize the pelvis, but the patients were uncomfortable for such a long time before the pelvis healed that I would not recommend it. I find anterior plating difficult and of dubious value, so I limit myself to plating the posterior column.

If the cup is across the teardrop and is well fixed, in general it must be cut up to be removed. It is cut with metal cutting burrs like a Mercedes

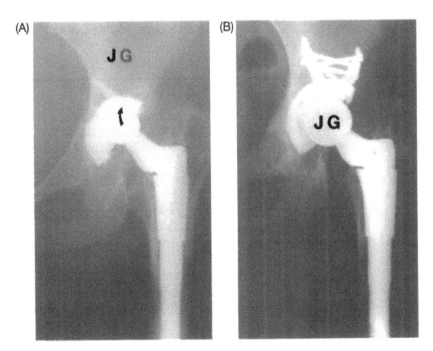

Figure 8 A. This cup was very small with a very thin liner. It was felt that exchange to a bigger cup, which would allow a thicker liner, should be carried out. The cup was only just across the teardrop and it was felt that it could be extracted safely. B. A pelvic fracture occurred. The pelvis was plated with a posterior plate and a newer, larger cup inserted. The fracture healed uneventfully.

emblem into three parts, and each segment is removed separately. Care must be taken to ensure that the burr does not advance too deeply through the metal, as it will also cut the floor. This is a tedious, time-consuming process. In spite of covering the exposed tissue with wet towels, the amount of debris generated as well as tissue contamination is quite extraordinary. Cutting up a titanium cup is bad enough, but anyone who has cut up a chrome cup will never use one again.

To avoid these trials and tribulations, the interior of the metal shell can simply be roughened by the metal-cutting burr and an appropriately sized new liner, not necessarily from the original cup manufacturer, cemented in place with PMMA. This technique is particularly useful for the deeply seated, retroverted, well-ingrown shell, as the usual reason for retroversion is a posterior wall that was deficient to begin with (Figure 9A and B).

Many different locking mechanisms are available. Most are fixed (i.e., removal of the polyethylene liner will damage the liner such that a new liner is required for reinsertion). One system uses a bayonet lock, which allows the liner to be spun into the optimum position after hip reduction, if necessary, before being locked down.

E. Liners

The liners in general are polyethylene. They are usually offered in neutral, or with 10-, 15-, and 20-degree lips or offsets. These offsets provide stability. They are not to be regarded as load-bearing, as the plastic in the offset is unsupported by metal and can deform and break. Offsets of 20 degrees are seldom required and often induce the condition they are supposed to prevent (i.e., dislocation). The 20-degree offset, and to a lesser extent the 15-degree offset, if placed posteriorly, makes the neck of the femoral component strike the plastic lip. At the very least, this increases the volume of wear debris and may produce a click which worries the patient. At worst the contact results in the head being levered out of position.

When a soft and hard material are joined together and subjected to load, the soft material deforms more than the hard—the "Poisson ratio" effect. This means that no matter how good the bond is, some micromotion must occur, thus liberating wear debris. Recognizing the inevitability of micromotion, most manufacturers now polish the inside of the cup to a varying degree to reduce this backside wear.

A polyethylene liner must fill the cup as closely as possible, as it will cold flow into any gaps. Some of the initial cups have large gaps between the polyethylene and metal. Fortunately all companies have now recognized this and have taken steps to rectify it as much as possible.

(A)

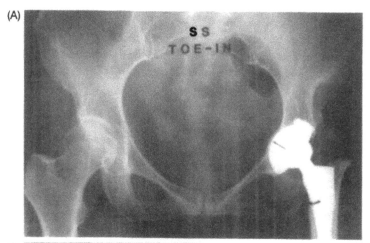

(B)

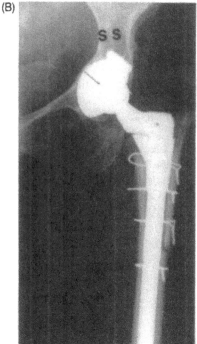

Figure 9 A. This cup has been inserted very deeply and in significant retroversion. To compensate the surgeon inserted the stem in close to 60 degrees of anteversion, resulting in an extremely in-toed gait. The stem arrow shows the absence of the lesser trochanter, a sign of extreme stem anteversion. B. The cup was well fixed, so it was left; the floor was roughened up and a new liner was cemented in place in the corrected version. An extended trochanteric osteotomy was required to remove the well-fixed original stem and to insert a new stem in neutral version.

The optimum minimal thickness of polyethylene is probably about 8 mm. In some situations, however, this cannot be achieved. In a cup with a 40-mm outer diameter, assuming use of a 22-mm head and a wall thickness of metal of 3.5 mm, this will leave a liner thickness of 5.5 mm. Liner wear under such circumstances is assured and may become significant after 7–10 years, especially in young, high-demand patients. Perhaps some of the newer, heavily crosslinked polyethylenes will reduce this, but only time will tell.

Because of what is seen by many as the inevitability of wear of soft/hard bearings, hard/hard bearings have been explored. These can either be metal or ceramic.

The locking mechanism for these hard/hard liners is usually a Morse taper, the liner being the male part of the taper and the shell the female part. The orthopaedic industry has had such a huge success with Morse taper locks with interchangeable heads on femoral components that this is an intuitive step. Taper angles have been refined for this new situation, and clearly there are no theoretical reasons why this should not work. One manufacturer prefers to use polyethylene as part of the locking mechanism, as it theoretically would reduce or attenuate impact. In practice, patients with hard/hard bearings on one side and hard/soft bearings on the other cannot tell the difference.

Ceramic/ceramic bearings are aluminum oxide. There is a theoretical risk of catastrophic failure (32), but this is probably less likely to occur when the ceramic is used as the male part of the taper rather than the female part. When the ceramic is the female part, the thrust of the trunion into it may explode it unless taper tolerances are tightly held. For this reason, a new ceramic head cannot be used on an old taper, as the damage to the taper from the previous head may lead to failure. One would have thought that the likelihood of failure would be less with the reverse situation.

The edge of the ceramic liner is susceptible to chipping from contact with the neck, so that it has to be recessed below the edge of the metal shell, potentially making extraction somewhat difficult. Ceramic/ceramic bearings have a very low wear rate once they "lap in," i.e., grind off the asperities. On extraction, a wear scar can generally be seen, at least with the initial ceramic/ceramic bearings. There is some concern that if the cup changes position after the initial wearing process, the wear may accelerate. The wear debris is in general fairly innocuous and one is struck by how thin and elastic the hip capsule generally is at the time of revision.

Metal/metal bearings are cobalt chrome. The original metal used in the McKee-Farrar and Moore-McBride system were high-carbon cobalt chromes. The metallurgy of the modern cobalt chrome is subtly different and wear testing has suggested that it will produce superior results. As mentioned previously, however the science of wear testing could do with significant improvement.

Metal/metal bearings have to be polar-bearing with a fairly tight tolerance. Wall bearing may result in "stiction/friction" and early failure (Figure 10). The big advantage of metal/metal is that it is not likely to suffer catastrophic failure. Patients can understand that wear is inevitable. Catastrophic failure, however, engenders the suspicion that someone is at fault.

The liner edge is not susceptible to chipping, but care must be taken to ensure that the lip does not contact the neck of the femoral component, as these are generally titanium and therefore subject to wear by the cobalt chrome lip, which is much harder. An enhanced lip liner tends to exacerbate this problem of contact and probably should be avoided except in extremely skilled hands.

There should be no problem removing and reinserting or exchanging metal liners, as they will cause the taper inside the cup to deform enough to obliterate minor discrepancies. Another potential advantage of metal/metal bearings is that the friction seems independent of head size. This should

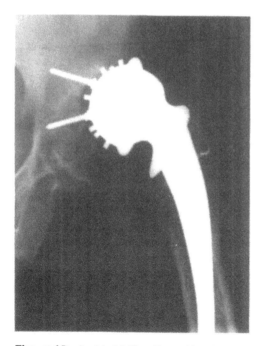

Figure 10 In this McKee-Farrar hip, the head made rim contact, not polar contact. This resulted in bearing freeze and the cup pulled loose.

enable very small heads to be used. If a one-piece or monoblock acetabular component were to be developed, assuming a wall thickness of 5 mm with a 22-mm head, the outer diameter could be as low as 32 mm, which should solve the majority of size problems that plague those who have to take care of very small people, as, for example, patients in Japan.

If the taper angle is correct, there is no theoretical reason why a metal/ceramic or polyethylene liner could not be used with the same shell.

IV. OTHER DESIGN OPTIONS

Several other press-fit or hybrid designs have been introduced and faded from view. The cup of Spotorno remains available. This is a metal cage, the arms of which are not locked. The cage has a rough, spiked outer surface. When the polyethylene liner is driven into the cage, it opens, and the arms are forced into the bone. Little has been written about it, and my only experience with it was that it was very easy to remove. After the plastic was pulled out, the cage could be collapsed in on itself.

A. Modified Cups

Unconventional geometries may be used in cup design to resolve some specific problems. The offset-bore cup designed to allow adequate polyethylene thickness in the cup roof has already been mentioned.

B. Protrusio Acetabulae

A very deep acetabulum can either be developmental or acquired; in revisions, the floor may be missing to varying degrees. Impaction grafting and a cemented socket plus/minus a protrusio ring or wire mesh (Figure 11) or even a "big head" bipolar can be used (33). If an ingrowth cup is to be used, the wall of the acetabulum can be reamed to ensure good contact when the cup is press-fitted and the floor filled up with particulate graft, demineralized bone, or synthetic substitutes such as tricalcium phosphate (Figure 12A to E). The center of rotation can be returned to normal in many instances by these techniques, but they are dependent on reasonably normal walls. If the wall is deficient, the same end can be achieved by using a "deep" or eccentric cup.

If such a cup is used, host bone contact will be made over as large an area as possible, allowing for wall deficiencies. One such cup is the DP+6 (Johnson & Johnson Depuy), which has been thickened in the polar area to allow 6 mm of lateralization of the center of rotation of the hip (34) (Figure

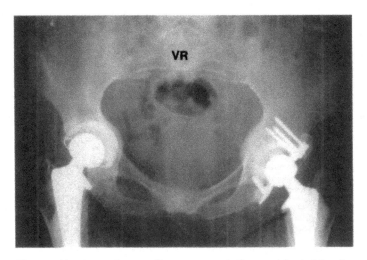

Figure 11 Impaction grafting was carried out on both hips for protrusio. The protrusio ring has given excellent support. On the other side, wire mesh was used. This cup shows lucency in all three zones and is probably loose albeit asymptomatic.

13A and B). If this is not enough, a lateralized liner can also be used. However, there is a limit to how much the liner itself can be made eccentric. If it is much more than 3 mm, a considerable part of the load will fall on the polyethylene unsupported by the metal shell, thus not only overstressing the fixation of the liner to the shell but also producing a significant turning moment on the shell itself, potentially compromising the bone/metal fixation.

A lateralized polyethylene liner can be used with a regular shell. While 3 mm of lateralization may not sound like much, it may increase tissue tension enough to prevent dislocation without lengthening the leg (Figure 14).

V. ROOF DEFECTS

In high-grade acetabular dysplasia, the roof may be deficient. However, in primary total hip replacement, the femoral head is present and autografting is not difficult unless large cysts are present in the head. In the revision situation, however, autograft is generally not available. It is now known that if bulk allografts are to be used, especially if there is less than 50% host bone contact, the graft must be protected with metal, with host bone contact both above and below—i.e., by using something like a Burch-Schneider cage (Figure 15A and B).

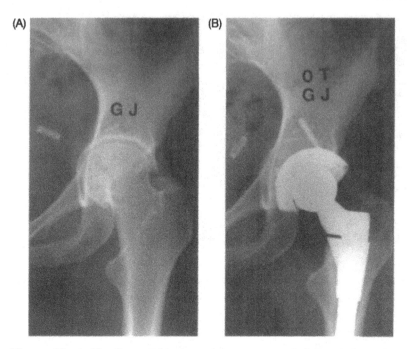

Figure 12   A. The floor of this protrusio case was grafted. B and C. An ingrowth cup has been inserted and is wall-bearing. D and E. Some subsidence was noted within the first few months but the cup has been stable for 3 years. The extent of screw back-out inferiorly indicates the extent of migration of the component.

Alternatives are the high hip center, the jumbo cup, or the oblong socket. In the high-hip-center technique a very small cup is press fitted high on the iliac wing (Figure 16A and B). This, of course, does not restore normal anatomy and the incidence of limp is higher than if the socket is repositioned anatomically, at least in CDH cases (35). In the jumbo-cup technique, the walls are expanded so that a very large cup can be inserted. A press fit may be achieved, or the socket may simply be held in place with multiple screws. If the vertical diameter of the acetabulum is greater than the horizontal diameter, it means that to achieve full contact, the walls must be sacrificed. As the posterior wall is much more important than the anterior wall, reaming must be eccentric, removing more from the front than from the back. However, it is theoretically undesirable to remove any bone that is already in a deficient state.

If the vertical diameter of the acetabulum is 1 cm greater than the horizontal diameter, the metal shell can be made oblong to fill the defect. If

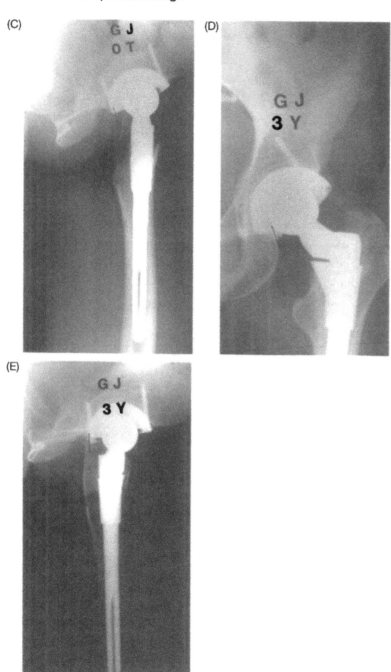

Figure 12 Continued

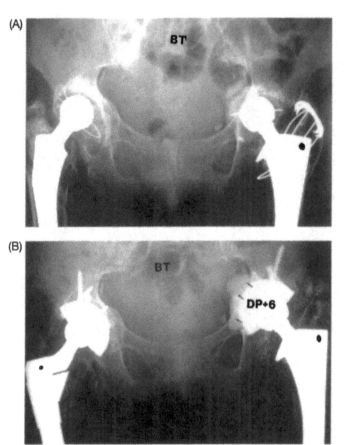

Figure 13   A. Revision of both acetabular components and the cemented stem was required. B. On the right side, a jumbo cup was sufficient to restore the center of rotation. On the left side, a deep cup was used. The hole in the floor of the acetabulum was heavily grafted with tricalcium phosphate.

the liner is seated in the inferior part of the cup, the normal center of hip rotation can be restored. If the back of the cup is vertical, however, the cup has to be inserted vertically in order to make contact with the bony roof. A liner with a 15- to 20-degree lip, therefore, must be used to hold the head in place. This makes the lip load-bearing. As emphasized previously, load bearing is not the function of an extended lip so that polyethylene failure is inevitable in due course (Figure 17A to C).

In designing an oblong socket, therefore, it follows that the cranial part of the socket has to be offset or adducted by 15 to 20 degrees, depending

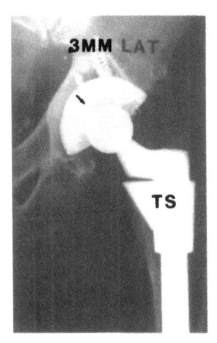

Figure 14 In this case a 3-mm lateralized line has been used to shift the center of rotation laterally thus enhancing the stability of the hip.

on cup length. When stood vertically with respect to the back of the cup, the caudal part bearing the polyethylene liner should make an angle of about 55 degrees to the vertical. If the cranial part of the cup is allowed to protrude from the bony pelvis, this will bring the angle down to the normal 45 degrees.

These cups can be made with varying degrees of eccentricity. The naming system in the cup with which I am familiar measures the distances between the two peaks. At present only two types are available, an E15 and E25, giving 15 and 25 mm of eccentricity respectively. The cup has to be further modified to ensure that it can be inserted in 15 degrees of anteversion. If the upper lobe has the same version as the lower lobe, because there is not the same wall thickness above the true acetabulum, the upper lobe would virtually make no bone contact at all. For this reason, with the E25, it is necessary to retrovert the upper part of the cup (Figure 18A and B). The current design is 15 degrees of retroversion, but this could with advantage be increased to 30 or 40 degrees of retroversion. Cup modifications are in progress.

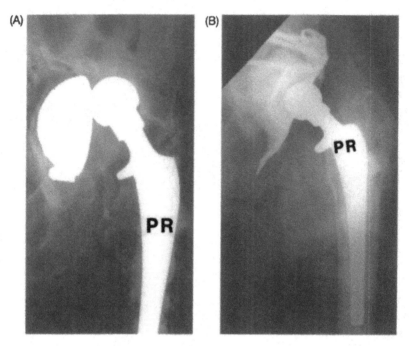

Figure 15 A and B. In this case the defect in the floor was so great that a Burch-Schneider cage has been used with particulate allograft and a cemented cup.

The initial reaming technique is to ream the lower part of the acetabulum to size to determine cup diameter. A hemispherical guide is then inserted into the prereamed lower floor and, holding it firmly seated in the lower part of the acetabulum, the reamer is swung gently vertically, pivoting on the lower guide until bone contact is made. An appropriate amount of bone is removed and the cup is then press-fitted.

While this is appropriate for the odd primary case that requires an oblong socket, I have come to realize that in revision cases the inferior floor is always somewhat eroded, which leaves a wall of bone inferiorly. As this wall potentially prevents the cup from swinging out inferiorly if it loosens, it seems to me rational to preserve this wall. Currently, therefore, I do virtually no reaming and simply grind off the high spots in the floor of the acetabulum. Trials are then used to find an appropriate size and shape and again the superior bone is reamed little if any. The cup is then inserted by hand and driven distally inside the ischial bony ridge using a metal punch and taking care to avoid damage to the locking mechanism. When firm distal floor contact is made, the cup is driven medially to make an appropriate

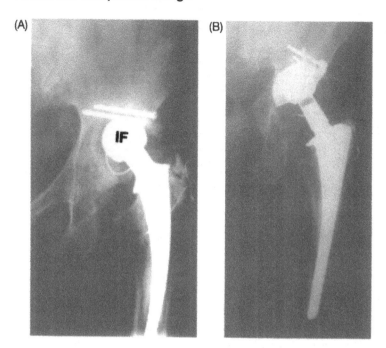

Figure 16 A. This very loose cup has migrated proximally. B. A small cup found reasonable purchase on the top of the defect. Some bone grafting was required. In order to balance leg lengths, a neck extension has been used. The x-ray looks strange but the patient functions well.

angle to the vertical and tapped into the appropriate version. This modification of the technique ensures that virtually no additional bone is removed. As many screws as possible are then inserted unless the press fit is surprisingly good. The remaining bone defects are then backfilled with Dynagraft gel injected through the remaining screw holes.

For the purposes of this chapter, I looked up the results achieved in the last 8 years with this cup. There were 42 cases with a follow-up of 1–8 years. There were 25 cases with E15 and 17 with E25. Three patients died with a follow-up of less than 2 years. Two were primary cases, one a very eroded acetabulum, and one a previous Chiari osteotomy. The femoral heads in these cases were unsuitable for bulk graft. In 14 cases the original diagnosis was CDH, indicating that the problem with the deficient acetabulum was not necessarily solved by autografting during the primary procedure. A total of 27 cases had one total hip replacement, 9 had two and 4 had three or more revisions; 2 were Girdlestones and 1 had a pelvic dissociation. The

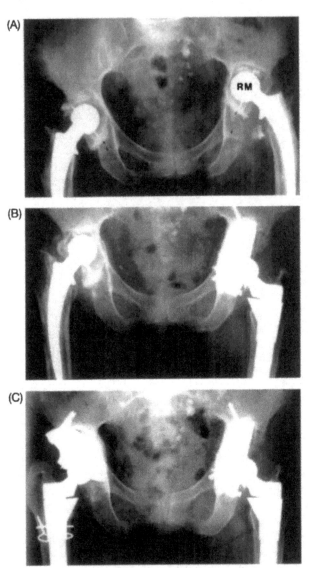

Figure 17 A. Both acetabulae are loose and migrating. B. A custom "bathtub" implant has been used for acetabular revision. In order to gain host bone support superiorly, the cup had to be inserted almost vertically; the head is held in place only by an extended lip liner, an unsatisfactory state of affairs. C. The upper part of the oblong socket on the other side had been adducted to allow the polyethylene-bearing lower part of the cup to be placed at a much better angle.

(A)

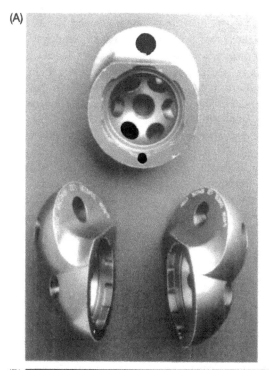

(B)

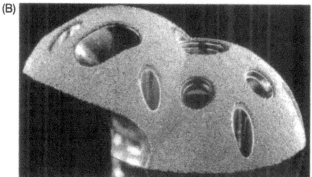

Figure 18   A. The E15 cup is neutral. The top of the E25 trials have been retro-verted so that left and rights are required. B. The degree of adduction of the upper part of the cup is obvious.

original stem was retained in 13 cases, while 4 new cemented stems were used. In 25, a proximally modular noncemented stem was employed. No bulk grafting was required. Autografts were used in 3 cases, morcellized allograft in 5, Dynagraft gel in 6, and tricalcium phosphate in 14. Pain was largely abolished. Limp was absent in 61%, mild (i.e., present with fatigue) in 18%, and severe (i.e., Trendelenburg-positive) in 21%. The Harris hip score was excellent in 51.5%, good in 38.5%, fair in 5%, and poor in 5%. One case, an E25, dislocated and had a stem revision and a constrained socket. The cup later loosened. *Staphylococcus aureus* was cultured, but immediate exchange to a Burch-Schneider cage was carried out. In the pelvic dissociation case, the screws through the cup were used to stabilize the fracture without a supplementary plate. There was an alteration in cup angle in the first year until the fracture healed, but there has been no further migration in the last 4 years. Given that only one case of loosening, possibly septic, occurred in this series, the results are quite acceptable.

Three studies of the oblong socket have been reported. Although no instruments were available, the first study compared oblong sockets favorably with custom cups (36). In the second study, it was found possible to reduce the average vertical displacement from 45.7 to 20.7 mm with 97% cup retention, no progressive migration, and average hip scores of 84% (37). My own results have been equally good (38).

Given these results and the refinement in insertion technique, I have become increasingly confident in this cup and I am therefore expanding its use. The current contraindication for use is an absent posterior column. This requires the use of a Burch-Schneider–type cage plus allograft. A fractured pelvis should first be stabilized with a plate and then the cup used. The cup itself does not give adequate stability in cases of pelvic dissociation.

VI. CAPTURE CUPS—CONSTRAINED SOCKET

Dislocation following total hip replacement, especially revision total hip replacement, remains a problem. The reported results of revision for recurrent dislocation are poor (39,40). For these reasons a constrained socket or capture cup was developed which would fit into a conventional metal shell. It must clearly be stated that there are many drawbacks to the use of a constrained socket. In order to capture the head of the femoral component, a liner must cover more of the head than a hemisphere. This will reduce the range of movement before the neck of the femoral component strikes the lip of the cup (Figure 19). This impingement will tend to release more wear debris and the impact will stress the constraining mechanism, the liner/cup interface, and the cup/bone interface. If redislocation occurs, an open re-

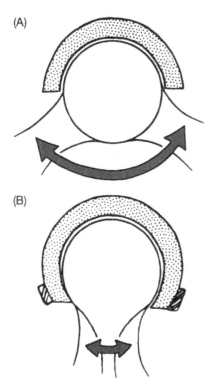

Figure 19 A and B. In order to capture the head, the liner must extend beyond the maximum circumference of the head, thus reducing the range of movement before the neck strikes the edge of the cup.

duction will be required. To limit this, the constrained socket is best used with an 11/13 or 10/12 taper. I have used it with a 14/16 taper but repeated edge contact leading to excessive wear in one case resulted in late redislocation.

The plastic liner is longer than a hemisphere and the mouth of the socket smaller than the size of the femoral head. The mouth is split into gussets to allow expansion of the mouth, thus enabling the head to be snapped in. An additional metal ring is then forced down over the cup to keep the gussets closed. The lever-out resistance is 150 in./lb and the pullout resistance 325 in./lb. The fact that the head can be pulled out of the plastic indicates that these cups are not fully constrained but rather partially constrained. The advantage of this partial constraint is that dislocation will occur in extreme situations rather than avulsion of the metal shell from the bony

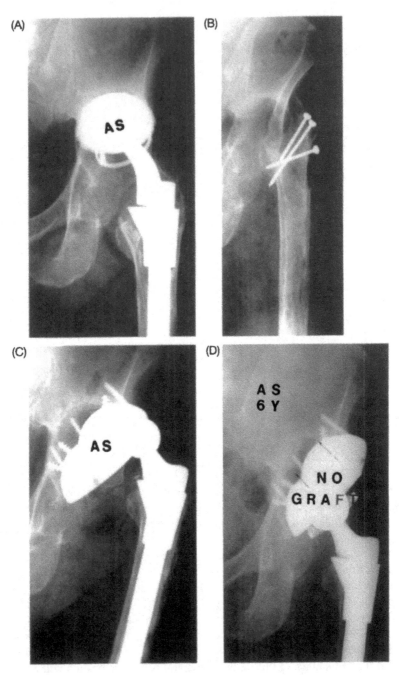

pelvis. It is preferable to use a spherical head with these sockets, as if the head is less than a sphere, the flat area may lead to "plowing" at the extreme range of movement, increasing the likelihood of lever-out. A 32-mm head will give a better range of movement before impingement occurs than a 28-mm head, and a lesser-diameter head should not be used.

The loads on a constrained socket occasioned by impingement may be high. If the initial fixation of the metal shell is poor, as it may be in a complex revision, there is, theoretically, a risk of shell loosening. Under these circumstances, it is probably preferable to use a normal plastic liner. If repeat dislocation occurs, a constrained liner can be substituted once solid bone ingrowth has been achieved (Figure 20A to D). Alternatively, the patient can be protected for a few months with an abduction brace with locks to limit range of motion.

The published results for this cup are quite good (41), but I felt it reasonable to update my own data for this chapter. There were 44 cases with an age range of 47–96 (mean 66) with 28 females and 16 males. Prior operations were one previous total hip replacement in 10, two previous total hip replacements in 24, and third time revision in 6, of which 2 were Girdlestones, 2 were primary cases, 1 was an old polio case, and 1 patient who felt loose for some reason at the time of total hip replacement. Liner exchange only was carried out in 10, cup exchange in 18, and total hip revision in 16. The reason for the use of a constrained socket was recurrent dislocation in 31, nonunion of the trochanter in 5, absent trochanter in 3, avulsed glutei in 1, gluteal polio in 1, leg shortening in 2, loose at revision in 4, massive myositis ossificans excision in 1, and a too-short fully porous-coated fully ingrown stem in 2. The head size was 32 mm in 35 and 28 mm in 9. Three hips were removed for sepsis and one drained, but the patient died at less than 6 months. A femoral component which was too short was eventually revised and constraint was no longer necessary. This left 39 cases for review. The complications included ring dislodgement and redislocation

---

Figure 20 A. This is a multiply revised infected joint with a constrained liner. B. A Girdlestone procedure has been carried out. An extended trochanteric osteotomy was required to remove a well-fixed stem. C. Six months later, an oblong socket has been inserted. No bone graft was used because of the infection. The fixation was tenuous. The abductors were of poor quality and the hip was subsequently dislocated on several occasions. D. Six months after insertion, the oblong socket fixation was felt adequate and a constrained liner was inserted. No further problems have been encountered. Six years later, the acetabular recovery in the absence of bone grafting is quite remarkable.

in 1, original stem loosening requiring revision in 3, nonunion of the greater trochanter in 4, ring dislodgement with no dislocation in 1, and 1 ring fracture in an asymptomatic patient. Limp was absent in a remarkable 69% of cases, mild in 13%, and Trendelenburg-positive in 18%. The Harris hip rating (39 cases) was 31% excellent, 36% good, 23% fair, and 10% poor. The range of motion has been better than expected and blinded observers cannot distinguish patients with a constrained socket from normals. The few patients with constraint in one side and not on the other cannot differentiate.

A major concern with constrained sockets is potential for abuse. They should be used only when there is no alternative. In 10 years with a large revision practice, I have used them in only 45 cases. Better methods of repair of trochanteric nonunion, judicious use of lateralized sockets and stems, and careful repair or reattachment of the glutei will decrease the indications.

The cup should be regarded as an internal splint that will keep the hip in place until soft tissue healing occurs. When used with this thought in mind, the results have been quite acceptable, with a redislocation rate of 2.2%.

REFERENCES

1. Miller J et al. Loosening of arthroplasty components as a result of blood clot interposed between PMMA and bone at the time of surgery. Presentation ORS, Los Vegas, Nevada, 1997.
2. Geiger MH, Keating EM, Ritter MA, et al. Clinical significance of vacuum mixing of bone cement. Clin Orthop 382:258, 2001.
3. Lee AJC et al. Some clinically relevant variables affecting the mechanical behaviour of bone cement. Arch Orthop Traumat Surg 92:1, 1978.
4. Lee AJC, Ling RSM. A device to improve the extrusion of bone cement into the bone of the acetabulum in replacement of the hip joint. J Biomed Eng 9: 1, 1974.
5. Schreiber A et al. Complications after joint replacement—long-term follow up: Clinical findings and biomechanical research. In: Schaldach M, Hohman D, eds. Artificial Hip and Knee Joint Technology. Berlin: Springer-Verlag, 1976.
6. Cameron HU. Cemented acetabulum. In: Cameron HU, ed. Bone Implant Interface. Toronto: Mosby–Year Book, 1994.
7. Linders L, Ivarsson B. Evaluation of biocompatibility of polymers implanted into bone using titanium mosaic on bone cement. Biomaterials 7:17, 1986.
8. Linders L. The reaction of bone to bone cement in animal and humans. In: Older J, ed. Implant Bone Interface. Berlin: Springer-Verlag, 1990.
9. Branemark PI et al. Osseointegrated implants in the treatment of the edentulous jaw. Scand J Plast Reconstr Surg 16:1, 1977.
10. Willert HG. Morphology of implant bone interface in cemented and non-cemented endoprosthesis. In: Oder J, ed. Implant Bone Interface. Berlin: Springer-Verlag, 1990.

11. Fornasier VL. The pathology of prosthetic implants. In: Cameron HU, ed. Bone Implant Interface. Toronto: Mosby–Year Book, 1994.
12. Ericksson, AH. Heat induced injury. Thesis. Gothenburg, Sweden: University of Gothenburg, 1984.
13. Tossing-Larsen S, Franzen H. Cement/interface temperatures in hip arthroplasty. Acta Orthop Scand 62:102, 1991.
14. Cameron HU. Use of a cemented ceramic acetabular component. Can J Surg 35:321, 1991.
15. Moberg, B et al. Early detection of prosthetic hip loosening. Acta Orthop Scand 61:273, 1990.
16. Humphrey PK et al. An investigation into cyclic loading and frequency on the temperature of PMMA bone cement and hip prosthesis. N Engl J Med 203: 167, 1989.
17. Cameron HU, Chiu H. A long-term review of 3 different cemented acetabular components. In press.
18. Ritter M. What's wrong with we've got. Lecture at Current Concepts in Joint Replacement. Orlando, FL, 2000.
19. Livermore J, Illstrup D, Morrey B. Effects of femoral head size in wear of the polyethylene acetabular components. J Bone Joint Surg 72A:518, 1990.
20. Schuller MH, Marti PK. 10 year socket wear in 66 hip arthroplasties—ceramic versus metal heads. Acta Orthop Scand 61:240, 1990.
21. Ritter MA. Cemented acetabulum—clinical considerations. In Cameron HU ed. Bone Implant Interface. Toronto: Mosby–Year Book, 1994.
22. Ranawat C. The all poly cemented cup, back to the future. Lecture at Current Concepts in Joint Replacement. Orlando, FL, 2000.
23. Sullivan PM, MacKenzie JR, Callaghan JJ, et al. Total hip arthroplasty with cement in patients who are less than 50 years old—a 16 to 22 year follow up. J Bone Joint Surg 76A:863, 1994.
24. Callaghan JJ, Forest FE, et al. Charnley total hip arthroplasty in patients less than 50 years old: A 20 to 25 year follow up. J Bone Joint Surg 80A:704, 1998.
25. Chiu KY, Ng TP, Tan WM, et al. Charnley total hip arthroplasty in Chinese patients less than 40 years old. J Arthrop 16:92, 2001
26. Cameron HU, Loehr J, Fornasier VL. Early clinical trials with a ceramic total hip prosthesis. Orthop Rev 12:49, 1983.
27. Cameron HU, Bhimji S. Design rationale and early clinical trials with a hermispherical threaded acetabular component. J Arthrop 4:299, 1988.
28. Cameron HU, McTighe T. Techniques of insertion and results of threaded acetabular components. Surg Rounds Orthop 3:22, 1989.
29. Cameron HU, Pilliar RM, McNab I. Porous vitallium in implant surgery. J Biomed Mater Res 8:283, 1974.
30. Wasslewski RC, Cooperstein LA, Kruger MP, et al. Acetabulum anatomy and transacetabular fixation of screws in total hip arthroplasty. J Bone Joint Surg 72A:501, 1990.
31. Cameron HU. Dissociation of a polyethylene liner from an acetabular cup. Orthop Rev 10:1160, 1993.

32. Cameron HU. Ceramic head failure in total hip replacement. J Arthrop 6:185, 1991.
33. Cameron HU, Jung YB. Acetabular revision with a bipolar prosthesis. Clin Orthop 251:100, 1990.
34. Cameron HU. Modified cups. Orthop Clin North Am 29:277, 1998.
35. Cameron HU, Botsford D, Park YS. Influence of the Crowe rating on the outcome of total hip arthroplasty in congenital hip dysplasia. J Arthrop 11:582, 1996.
36. Sutherland CJ. Treatment of type III acetabular deficiencies in revision total hip arthoplasty without structural bone graft. J Arthrop 11:91, 1996.
37. Deboer DK, Christie MJ. Reconstruction of the deficient acetabulum with an oblong shaped prosthesis. J Arthrop 13:674, 1998.
38. Cameron HU, Smula V. Use of the oblong socket in revision surgery. Acta Chir Orthop Traumat Checkosl 66:8, 1999.
39. Woo RYG, Morrey BF. Dislocation after total hip arthroplasty. J Bone Joint Surg 64A:1295, 1982.
40. Cameron HU, Hunter GA, Welsh RP. Dislocation requiring revision in total hip arthroplasty. Acta Orthop Traumat Surg 95:265, 1979.
41. Cameron HU, Smula V. Review of constrained acetabular components in total hip replacement. Acta Chir Orthop Traumat Checkosl 65:236, 1996.

5
Biological Fixation in Hip Replacement

Noreen J. Hickok and James J. Purtill
Thomas Jefferson University, Philadelphia, Pennsylvania

Michele Marcolongo
Drexel University, Philadelphia, Pennsylvania

Rocky S. Tuan
National Institute of Arthritis and Musculoskeletal Diseases, National Institutes of Health, Bethesda, Maryland

I. HISTORICAL PERSPECTIVE ON BIOLOGICAL FIXATION IN TOTAL HIP ARTHROPLASTY

Since the widespread use of total joint replacement surgery for patients with arthritic conditions of the hip began in the late 1960s, this procedure has been revolutionary in providing pain relief and improvement in function. Hip replacement surgery came into widespread use before its longevity was clearly delineated. When mid- to long-term follow-up became available in the mid-1980s, survivorship analyses revealed implants to be in place and functioning well in 85% (Wroblewski, 1986) to 91% (McCoy et al., 1988) of patients at 15 years.

Excellent results of cemented total hip arthroplasty were not universal, however. Some authors reported high rates of mechanical failure, which raised concern for the long-term survival of these implants. Griffith reported on a series of 547 cemented hip replacements with 8-year follow-up and noted a mechanical failure rate of 2.2% (Griffith et al., 1978). However, 12% of the hip replacements had concerning cement–bone radiolucent lines, which appeared to be progressive. DeLee reported on 141 cemented total hip arthroplasties at 10-year follow-up and noted a 69% rate of radiographic demarcation in the bone–cement interface, with a 9.2% rate of migration of the hip replacement components (DeLee and Charnley, 1976). Gruen reported on a series of 389 total hip replacements with 19.5% rate of radiographic evidence of "mechanical looseness" at an average 3 years of follow-up (Gruen et al., 1979). Beckenbaugh reported a 24% rate of femoral loosening at 4- to 7-year follow-up in 333 Charnley total hip replacements (Beckenbaugh and Ilstrup, 1978). Cotterill reviewed a series of 166 cemented total hip arthroplasties with 6 months' to 11 years' follow-up and noted an incidence of 73% of loosening of the femoral component (Cotterill et al., 1982).

Cemented total hip replacement in young patients raised specific concerns. Salvati noted excellent results in reviewing a series of 100 total hip replacements with 10-year follow-up. However, he noted that 75% of the patients were old and inactive (Salvati et al., 1981). He stated that similar results could not necessarily be expected in young, healthy patients. Marmor reported on 10 cases of early failure (<6 months) in a series of 160 cemented Charnley hip replacements (Marmor, 1976). Loosening of the femoral component was found to be associated with young age and obesity. In a study of patients younger than 30, with a 5-year follow-up, an excessively high rate of loosening (57%) was seen (Chandler et al., 1981). These authors associated premature loosening with a diagnosis of avascular necrosis, an increased level of activity, and weight greater than 180 lb. This series of young patients was thought to represent an "accelerated model of what is occurring in all patients with joint replacements." Carlson noted a 36% rate of lucency at the cement–prosthesis interval (Carlsson and Gentz, 1980). Increased body mass, younger age at the time of surgery, and male sex were associated with this radiographic finding.

Despite excellent clinical results in some series of cemented total hip replacements, concerning radiographic findings and high rates of loosening and failure in other series began to raise concern over the use of polymethylmethacrylate (PMMA) bone cement as a source of fixation for total hip arthroplasty in the mid 1980s. For some hip surgeons, loosening of prostheses fixed with PMMA was felt to indicate a "pathologic response to a foreign material" (Jones and Hungerford, 1987). PMMA was seen as "an imperfect material which undergoes alteration with time and becomes biologically active in a negative sense" (Rothman and Cohn, 1990). "Cement disease," or osteolysis, was later more clearly defined as a biological process of bone destruction secondary to the body's reaction to the microscopic particulate debris formed in the vicinity of total joint replacements.

The concern over the longevity of PMMA-stabilized total hip replacement resulted in a divergence of efforts in an attempt to improve hip arthroplasty. On one hand, refinements were made in cementing technique (the use of a distal cement restrictor, meticulous preparation and drying of the endosteal canal, insertion of doughy bone cement under pressure) that resulted in significant improvement in the rates of survival of cemented femoral components (Harris and Davies, 1988). While improvements were being made in cementing techniques, however, interest also evolved in developing implants and techniques to achieve biological fixation for hip replacement components. Galante stated, "An open pore material into which bone could grow should provide ideal skeletal fixation" (Galante et al., 1971).

The use of porous metallic surfaces as a basis for attachment of implants to bone was studied extensively in canine models. Vitallium implants with a surface coating of sintered beads that formed an openly porous structure were found to bind actively with the surrounding bone with no apparent adverse tissue reaction (Welsh et al., 1971). Metabolically active woven bone was seen in the porous spaces between the sintered beads. Similarly, a sintered titanium fiber composite was found to have bony ingrowth at 2 weeks after implantation, with deep penetration of bone into the composite at 3 weeks. These authors suggested that a porous coating "bonded to a central solid metal core would provide fixation to bone and uniform stress distribution at the implant bone interface" (Galante et al., 1971). Acetabular fixation through bony ingrowth was also demonstrated in a canine model with bony ingrowth to a depth of three layers of the sintered balls (Harris et al., 1983; Hedley et al., 1983). Bony ingrowth was demonstrated using a porous titanium fiber coating on both acetabular and femoral components in a canine model under conditions of in vivo loading (Chen et al., 1983). Active bone remodeling was demonstrated in samples procured at various lengths of time after surgery and was thought to be secondary to the imposed stresses of weight bearing.

Austin Moore first reported on a prosthetic proximal femoral replacement consisting of an uncemented vitallium stem used to replace the proximal femur in a patient with a pathological femur fracture from a giant cell tumor (Moore and Bohlman, 1943). He was encouraged because of the patient's eventual pain-free function as well as the lack of corrosion of the implant, "as it was unaffected by its period of service in the body." He later reported on a prosthesis inserted without cement for patients with femoral neck fractures (Moore, 1957). A tight wedge fit achieved initial stability. Permanent fixation was secured by bone growth into large fenestrations in the prosthesis. This provided pain-free function in the majority of patients.

Hip replacement surgery using femoral components with porous surface was begun in humans in the late 1970s. Engh (Engh, 1983) reported on a series of 26 patients who underwent hip replacement surgery using a modified Moore prosthesis with cobalt chrome sintered bead coating. Excellent clinical performance was noted at 4-year follow-up in a population of young patients at high risk for failure of cemented prostheses.

Judet and Lord (Judet et al., 1978) had a similar experience with cobalt chrome alloy porous-surfaced prostheses. These authors, in their early experience, expressed a "controlled enthusiasm" after observing so few failures in such a large number of cases (Judet et al., 1978; Lord and Bancel, 1983; Lord et al., 1979). Remodeling of bone "provides for long-term anchor of the prosthesis and eliminates the chemical intermediary that leads with time, to loosening of the implant in a significant number of cases" (Lord et al., 1979).

These positive early experiences with biological fixation for total hip arthroplasty have indeed proven to be long-lasting. Many series with 15-year follow-up confirm the long-term stability of this form of fixation (Engh and Culpepper, 1997; McLaughlin and Lee, 1997; Sakalkale et al., 1999). Biological fixation in cementless total hip arthroplasty is an active process with bone remodeling. Many series indicate that once bony ingrowth has been achieved, it is permanent and may provide a biological seal from the deleterious effects of wear-debris generated at the articulation (Emerson et al., 1999).

As biologic fixation has become the standard for many hip arthroplasties, understanding of the biomaterial properties that mediate active bony ingrowth has greatly increased.

II. BONE–IMPLANT INTERACTIONS

Whether a bioactive material surface (calcium phosphate, like hydroxyapatite or bioactive glass) or a biocompatible material surface (e.g., titanium, Ti6Al4V, or a Co Cr Mo alloy) is used, there are certain surface characteristics that can influence osseointegration. These include surface chemistry, surface energy, surface charge, and surface topography or roughness.

The interactions between bone tissue and implant materials have been well investigated throughout the 1980s and 1990s. Many of these investigations relied on implantation of the target material into animal models. Typically, implant materials were inserted transcortically into the weight-bearing limb of an animal. To evaluate the degree of osseointegration between the implant and surrounding bone tissue, either a push-out or pullout test was utilized—i.e., a test that evaluated the interfacial shear strength between the implant and bone tissue at some time after implantation. These data, in conjunction with histological analyses of the same interface, have been central to the identification of fixation mechanisms associated with biomaterials. Unfortunately, while push-out/pullout tests have yielded much useful information, the technique itself can lead to variable results, especially in comparing different studies (Black, 1989). Specifically, the alignment of the specimen to the load application is of critical importance in establishing reliable measurements. Other factors that can affect the outcome of the measured shear strengths include the material and its surface treatment, the animal model, the implantation site, and the implantation time period.

Keeping in mind these differences between studies, there are still useful data for comparison of osseointegration in vivo. For a femoral stem, several variations on the implants of the porous-coated type have been examined. These include hydroxyapatite (HA) coatings of various stoichiometry, crystallinity, and application techniques. After 12 weeks in the canine transcortical model, interfacial bond strengths can approach 20 MPa for both porous-coated titanium and HA-coated, porous-coated Ti (Klein et al., 1994). When similar studies were conducted in the rabbit femur, the bond strengths after 12 weeks were around 6 MPa (Maxian et al., 1993). The fixation surfaces reported in these non-load-bearing studies have led to clinically successful fixation surfaces for femoral hip prostheses.

The objective of many studies was to somehow treat the surface of the biomaterial to enhance osseointegration. This was accomplished by either roughening the surface of a metal to enable bone to lock into the implant material mechanically or by applying a bioactive coating intended to provide attachment through a chemical bond. The chemical bond typically provided a higher interfacial bond strength to bone tissue; but over time, the bonding between the implant material and the bioactive coating in a load-bearing site became the weakest link, with failures resulting in a coating that was attached to bone tissue but not to the substrate implant. A summary of coatings and bond strengths is provided below and in Table 1.

In comparing bioactive coatings on polymers, a wide range of bond strengths were measured. Zimmerman et al. (1993) coated polysulfone with particles of calcium phosphate (95% hydroxyapatite and 5% tetracalcium phosphate). After implantation in the rabbit femoral cortex for 26 weeks, bond strengths of 9.5 MPa for a smooth coating of HA and 11.8 MPa for a rough coating were reported. However, in many instances, the rough coating of HA resulted in failure of the bond between the HA particles and the underlying polymer. Thus, the integrity of the material apparently could have been increased by improving the bond between the surface layer of calcium phosphate and the polymer.

The interfacial bond strengths for various compositions of bioactive glass were determined by Andersson et al. using the rabbit transcortical model in the proximal tibia. They showed bulk bioactive glasses in a range of compositions to display interfacial bond strengths in the range of 16–24 MPa after eight weeks implantation (Andersson et al., 1992).

Table 1 Interfacial Bond Strengths of Representative Coated Biomaterials

Material	Implantation Time	Interfacial Bond Strength (MPa)				Model	Reference
TCP-coated Ti (TCP) HA-coated Ti (HA) Porous	3 months 28 months	TCP 10 31	HA 34 44	Porous Time 9 30		Canine Transcortical Femur	Black, 1989
Alumina Zirconia Stainless steel Sintered dense HA	4 weeks 12 weeks	Alumina 0.1 0.8	Zirconia 0.1 0.9	Stainless steel 0.1 0.5	HA 6.8 12.1	Canine Transcortical Femur	Hayashi et al., 1990
HA plasma-sprayed Ti (porous) Porous Ti	3 weeks 12 weeks	HA coated Ti 7.5 17	Porous-Ti 7.7 18			Canine Transcortical Femur	Cook et al., 1994
Ha-coated triazin Triazin alone Porous coated Ti	7.2 months average (4–8 months)	Ha coated triazin 2.72	Triazin alone 0.14	Porous Ti 3.29		Canine Femoral Hip Components	Maistrelli et al., 1992
PLLA HA/PLLA HA (sandblasted) PLLA (rough)	3 weeks 3 months 6 months	PLLA 0.7 1.8 1.7	HA/PLLA 1.0 5.2 3.3	HA (sand) 2.9 9.8 3.3	PLLA (rough) 1.0 3.3 4.0	Goat Transcortical Femur	Verheyen et al., 1993

Material	Time				Model	Reference
HA coated Ti	4 weeks	HA coated Ti 7.7	HA 7.7	Ti 0.1	Canine Transcortical Femur	Hayashi et al., 1993
Sintered HA	12 weeks	9.7	11.7	0.5		
Uncoated Ti						
HA coated Ti (rough)	4 weeks	HA coated Ti 2.5–3.4	HA coated Ti 1.8–3.0		Rabbit Transcortical Femur	Klein et al., 1994
AHA coated Ti (rough)	12 weeks	3.5–6.2	3.4–6.4			
HA-coated porous CoCr	2 weeks	HA coated CoCr 5.04	Uncoated CoCr 3.11		Canine Transcortical Femur	Cook et al., 1992
Uncoated porous CoCr	12 weeks	15.73	11.1			
	26 weeks	27.06	22.08			
	52 weeks	21.21	18.71			
Bioactive glass fiber/ polysulfone composite	3 weeks	Bioactive glass/PS 6	Polysulfone 4		Rabbit Transcortical Femur	Marcolongo et al., 1998
All polysulfone (PS)	6 weeks	12.4	5.2			
Bulk bioactive glasses: S45P7 S46P0 S55.5P4	8 weeks	S45P7 23.0	S46P0 16.4	S55.5P4 19.4	Rabbit Transcortical Femur	Andersson et al., 1992

Maistrelli et al. (Maistrelli et al., 1992) evaluated the interfacial bond strengths of HA-coated carbon fiber/triazin femoral hip prostheses after a mean 7.2 months of functional implantation. They showed interfacial bond strengths of HA-coated composites (2.72 MPa) to be greater than uncoated composites (0.14 Mpa) and less than a porous-coated Ti prosthesis (3.29 MPa).

Previous work by Marcolongo et al. examined the interfacial bond strength of bioactive glass fiber/polysulfone composites (Marcolongo et al., 1997, 1998). While polysulfone is limited in its fatigue life due to surface crazing associated with the presence of lipids (Trentacosta and Cheban, 1995), the composite showed reasonable bond strength in the static trans-cortical model of a rabbit distal femur. After 6 weeks, the composite had an interfacial bond strength of 12.4 MPa compared with an all-polysulfone control that had a bond strength of 5.2 MPa. In addition, microscopic failure analysis showed that the polysulfone samples failed at the bone–implant interface, while the composite failed away from the interface, indicating that the interfacial bond was not the weakest link in this system (Marcolongo et al., 1998).

More recent work has addressed a material's ability to promote enhanced osseointegration controlling the surface characteristics of the material, thus developing techniques that could potentially be applied to any substrate material. One approach has been to functionalize a surface with a chemistry, energy, and charge so as to encourage the formation of a hydroxyapatite layer on the surface of any biomaterial, with the goal of utilizing this thin layer as the bioactive interface in achieving bone tissue fixation to the substrate (Nishiguchi et al., 2001; Wen et al., 1998). It has been shown that a negative surface charge and hydrophilic surface will encourage this biological response. With the appropriate surface conditions, the attachment proteins will then provide the route for the attachment of cells to the surface through integrin–ligand interactions (McFarland et al., 2000; Qiu et al., 1998).

An alternate approach that has gained much popularity has attempted to facilitate integrin receptor-mediated cell attachment (see Sec. III). It has been shown that a portion of extracellular matrix proteins containing the Arg-Gly-Asp (R-G-D) amino acid sequence on proteins, such as fibronectin, plays a major role in attachment of cells, including stem cells and osteoblasts to a substrate material. Recent materials, rather than using an intermediate hydroxyapatite layer, place this peptide, specifically the R-G-D sequence, directly onto the material surface through the use of a surface chemical treatment. By tethering this sequence to the substrate, enhanced cell attachment can be achieved (Healy et al., 1999; Park et al., 1998; Rezania and Healy, 1999). Critical points to consider are that the bond strength between the peptide and substrate must be at least as strong as that between the peptide and cell, so that there is no weak link in the system. In addition, the length of the tether attaching the sequence, the planar spacing, and the density of the attachment sites will all lead to more or less successful surfaces (Griffith and Lopina, 1998; Maheshravari et al., 2000; Rezania and Healy, 2000). Finally, the R-G-D sequence interacts with integrin receptors on many cell types and thus is not specific for osteoblasts; therefore, some concern arises as to the clinical usage, where fibroblasts are plentiful. However, even with these concerns, more sequences and more tethering techniques are being developed every day, and this approach may be a viable clinical alternative for optimizing the biological fixation of hip prostheses in the near future.

Therefore material development is starting to use knowledge of biological processes to develop more biocompatible materials. However, despite our detailed knowledge of the different material surfaces used for hip prostheses, we still have only limited knowledge of how alterations in surface structure/chemistry affect the cellular and molecular events mediating bony ingrowth.

III. BIOLOGICAL FIXATION

When a prosthesis is introduced, extensive damage to the bone and the marrow occurs. This damage initiates a series of events that form the basis for the biological fixation of the hip implant, with the initial response to the reaming of the bone and implantation of the prosthesis being that of inflammation (Tang and Eaton, 1995).

During the inflammatory response, macrophages and other mediators of cellular inflammation are recruited to the site of injury to initiate a wound-healing response. In addition to the natural consequences of surgery, the composition of the prosthesis plays an important role in determining the duration of this response. The inflammatory response can indeed be the initial response to injury by the biomaterial, with the timing of the response predicated by the composition and topography of the implant (Clark et al., 1976; Hench and Paschall, 1973; Johansson et al., 1998). This wounding response can be a fairly extensive foreign-body reaction, where the prosthesis will be largely encapsulated in a fibrous coating of varying thicknesses.

During the initial stages of the wounding response, degradative enzymes, such as metalloproteinases, are released, causing degradation of cellular debris and extracellular matrix and resulting in degradation of the existing bone lining the insertion site. Small debris is also cleared from the space surrounding the implanted prosthesis by phagocytic ingestion by macrophages. Upon implantation, the prosthesis is first surrounded by a fluid space and becomes coated with abundant serum proteins, such as fibronectin and vitronectin (Overgaard et al., 1998; Santavirta et al., 1992). Fibronectin and vitronectin form key components of the extracellular matrix, and their coating of the prosthesis allows for subsequent stable cellular adhesion to occur (Clubb et al., 1999; Degasne et al., 1999). In fact, the nature and biological activity of the extracellular matrix proteins that are adsorbed to the prosthesis may have profound downstream consequences. Specifically, different cell types preferentially adhere to specific extracellular matrix proteins (Ruoslahti et al., 1994). Thus, the nature and timing of the coating determines if the newly biologically modified prosthesis is hospitable for stable adhesion of cells of the osteoblastic lineage and whether these cells will be able to differentiate and mature on this surface.

The implant plays a critical role in the duration of the inflammatory response and the response of the surrounding tissue (Thomsen and Ericson, 1991). While the chemistry of the prosthesis is important in this process, the surface topography may also contribute to the duration of the inflammatory response. Specifically, some studies suggest that rougher surfaces elicit a more prolonged inflammation than smooth surfaces. This prolonged response would, on the whole, be detrimental to bony ingrowth, as the foreign-body reaction to the prosthesis would favor fibrous encapsulation of the implant (Clubb et al., 1999). On the other hand, the roughened surfaces, whether generated by sandblasting or application of a porous coating, are found to promote greater bony ingrowth and osseointegration, suggesting that the balance between these two responses determines the success of the fixation of the implant (Anselme et al., 2000; Groessner-Schreiber and Tuan, 1992; Lincks et al., 1998). It is clear from many studies that fixation of the implant involves both the fibrous soft tissue interface as well as the bony interface (Boss et al., 1994; De Benedittis et al., 1999; Masuda et al., 1998; Santavirta et al., 1992). These interfaces are formed by cells recruited to the surface of the implant that, under favorable conditions, proliferate to cover the surface. To favor bone ingrowth, the cells must be osteoblastic or undergoing commitment to the osteoblastic lineage.

As in all wound-healing responses, the activated cells involved in this process release cytokines and growth factors; furthermore, degradation of the bony matrix releases additional factors. These factors include interleukins, members of the insulin-like growth factor family, and matrix-bound growth factors, such as those of the transforming growth factor-β family (TGF-β), which includes the bone morphogenetic proteins (BMPs) (Deuel, 1996). These paracrine/autocrine factors and cytokines directly modulate new bone formation, which probably occurs both through stimulation of existing osteoblastic cells resident in the endosteum of the injured bone and through commitment and differentiation of osteogenic precursor cells present in the bone marrow (Pazzaglia et al., 1998; Rahal et al., 1993). Thus, in breaching the bone to insert the prosthesis, wound-healing responses are activated that are critical initiators of the steps necessary for the formation of new bone and the biological fixation of the implant.

In order to model the cellular and molecular parameters that govern ingrowth, we and others have used in vitro model systems. Much of our knowledge of the steps that occur during bone ingrowth is derived from these systems. This chapter first reviews the current state of knowledge of such early events governing bone formation and then surveys the application of this knowledge to understand how implants affect osteoblastic cell maturation.

IV. CELLULAR AND MOLECULAR EVENTS DURING OSTEOBLAST PROLIFERATION AND MATURATION

Regrowth of bone after injury is an integrated response of osteoblasts, osteoclasts, and other cells in the vicinity of bone, such as chondrocytes and hematopoietic cells, to metabolic signals.

Osteoblasts are derived from mesenchymal cells and molecular markers of the progression from osteoprogenitors to mature osteoblasts have been mapped both in vivo and in vitro. The molecular steps governing new bone formation by osteoblast maturation are still being elucidated and are known to be regulated by master transcription factors, specifically the RUNX/cbfa family members (Banerjee et al., 1997; Ducy et al., 1997, 1999; Gao et al., 1996; Karsenty et al., 1999; Komori and Kishimoto, 1998; Komori et al., 1997; Otto et al., 1997), hormones including estrogens, androgens, vitamin D_3, thyroid hormones, parathyroid hormone, and parathyroid hormone-related peptide, and paracrine/autocrine factors that include insulin-like growth factor, TGF-βs, BMPs, and fibroblast growth factor (Centrella et al., 1994). Bone-specific extracellular matrix synthesis is a critical part of the maturation program and alters cell–matrix interactions that, in turn, modify intracellular signaling and gene expression (Centrella et al., 1994; Franceschi, 1999; Karsenty, 2000). Transcription factors required for endochondral bone development include Indian hedgehog (Ihh) and the RUNX/Cbfa family of transcription factors (Ducy et al., 1997; Mundlos et al., 1997; Otto et al., 1997); these factors are also necessary for fracture repair (Ferguson et al., 1999; McCarthy et al., 2000). Notably, transgenic mice that have had their RUNX/Cbfa1 genes inactivated are unable to initiate endochondral formation, with development of the bony elements arrested in the cartilaginous stage (Mundlos et al., 1997; Otto et al., 1997). Transcription factors of the

RUNX/Cbfa family are themselves regulated by known regulators of osteoblastic differentiation and maturation, such as the TGF-βs, BMPs, and protein kinase A signaling pathways. Furthermore, these transcription factors regulate expression of phenotypic markers of osteoblastic maturation, such as osteocalcin and alkaline phosphatase (Karsenty, 1999, 2000). The osteogenic BMPs are necessary for normal skeletal development, with altered levels of expression causing, along with other developmental defects, profound skeletal abnormalities. As an example, mutation of the BMP-5 gene is the cause of the multiple skeletal abnormalities observed in the short-ear mouse (Centrella et al., 1994; Kingsley, 1994a,b; Kingsley et al., 1992).

Finally, the role of cell–extracellular matrix interactions is critical for normal bone development. This is illustrated by some of the less severe forms of osteogenesis imperfecta. In these cases, due to gene mutations, secretion of collagen type I is decreased. The resulting bone is fragile and immature (Fedarko et al., 1995a,b), suggesting that a complex sensing system exists in which gene expression is tightly coupled to interactions with and secretion of the extracellular matrix. This coupling determines the maturation state of the osteoblast and thus the degree of matrix mineralization. This is particularly important in terms of the biological fixation of total joint arthroplasty, as the surface of the implant must support the initial osteoblast–extracellular matrix interactions to optimize the subsequent downstream biological events.

The proliferative osteoblast, which is responsible for ultimately filling much of the surface that becomes osseointegrated, has been referred to as a "sophisticated fibroblast," (Karsenty, 1999), as its morphology and, with notable exceptions, gene expression profile resemble those of the fibroblast. Characteristics of the proliferative osteoblast include synthesis of extracellular matrix proteins such as collagen type I, the most abundant protein in mineralized bone, osteopontin, thrombospondin, and fibronectin (Owen et al., 1990), normal regulation of housekeeping and cell cycle proteins, and active DNA synthesis (Smith et al., 1995). Differential regulation of *fos* and *jun* transcription factor family members during maturation suggest that maturation-dependent regulation of AP-1-responsive genes may be important (McCabe et al., 1995).

The osteoblast deposits a matrix that, through remodeling, matures and becomes suitable for mineralization. The maturing osteoblasts organize within nodules and express the extracellular matrix proteins collagen type I, fibronectin, and some vitronectin. These maturing osteoblastic cells express a full complement of extracellular matrix receptors (integrins) and show increased alkaline phosphatase activity such that inorganic pyrophosphate is being actively metabolized for later mineralization. Finally, the mature osteoblastic cells show increased matrix calcium incorporation. During the temporal progression of this maturation process, collagen type I and fibronectin synthesis become suppressed, while synthesis of osteopontin, osteocalcin, and bone sialoprotein are increased, as is the synthesis of proteins important for the structure of the bony matrix involved in normal bone turnover, e.g., gelatinase and tissue inhibitor of metalloproteases (TIMP) (Giachelli and Steitz, 2000; Meikle et al., 1992; Owen et al., 1990).

Throughout osteoblastic differentiation and maturation, the RUNX/cbfa family of transcription factors play critical roles in determining osteoblastic cell phenotype (Ducy et al., 1997; Gori et al., 1999). Activity of these transcription factors is actively regulated via feedback mechanisms throughout this process. For instance, interruption of interactions between collagen type I and its integrin receptor $\alpha 2\beta 1$ abrogates activation of cbfa1 and suppresses osteocalcin synthesis. These data suggest at least one mechanism for interdependence of osteoblastic maturation and extracellular matrix composition (Xiao et al., 1998). In addition, activity of members of the RUNX/cbfa transcription family are suppressed or increased by the TGF-β pathway and increased by the BMP-2 pathway (Lee et al., 1999; Li et al., 1998). Pathways that can be activated through cell–extracellular matrix interactions have been shown to alter RUNX/cbfa activity. Specifically, cbfa1 activity is suppressed (Tintu et al., 1999) or increased (Selvamurugan et al., 2000) by the PKA pathway and is increased by MAP kinase pathways (Xiao et al., 2000). Some of the reported differences in the direction and magnitude of the response to a particular stimulus may be dependent on the cell line used and the maturational state of the osteoblastic cells. Thus, the effects of ablation of cbfa1 in vivo are profound, and these factors regulate and are regulated by known regulators of osteoblastic maturation.

V. MODELS OF OSTEOBLASTIC CELLULAR BEHAVIOR

In order to investigate how bony ingrowth occurs, we and others have used in vitro models to study osteoblastic differentiation, maturation, and mineralization. These models have used primary cells, cell lines, or generic cells, such as the fibroblast, to model cellular behavior on prostheses (Bundy et al., 1993; Cannas et al., 1988; Goldring et al., 1989; Horbett and Schway, 1978; Kononen et al., 1992; Meyle et al., 1991; Naji and Harmand, 1990).

The cells that are most likely to recapitulate the key biochemical sequences initiated upon bone being placed in proximity with the prosthesis are primary human osteoblastic cells. These cells are grown as outgrowths of explants of minced, protease-digested trabecular bone obtained as surgical waste during hip arthroplasty ((Robey and Termine, 1985), as modified by Sinha et al. (1994). Within 10–14 days of plating, cells are apparent growing from the bone chips, with cultures reaching confluence at 3–4 weeks. Relatively immature cells migrate out of the bone chips and, interestingly, these cells maintain some pluripotency, as they can differentiate into osteoblastic, chondrocytic, or adipogenic cells, depending on the culture conditions (Noth et al., 2001). Under osteogenic conditions—including dense cell-cell contact and supplementation with ascorbic acid—the cells grown from the bone chips express alkaline phosphatase and osteocalcin, hallmarks of the maturing osteoblast. The osteoblastic cells derived from bone chips have been well characterized; they faithfully recapitulate the proliferation-to-mineralization sequence of the maturing osteoblast, with normal hormone responsiveness and expression of phenotypic maturation markers (e.g., collagen type I, alkaline phosphatase, osteopontin, and osteocalcin) (Sinha et al., 1994). Because these are primary cultures from explants, several drawbacks to these cells are present, including donor-to-donor variability in the magnitude of responses to various agents and the relative paucity of cells. Specifically, while the numbers of cells obtained from a single hip are certainly sufficient to perform most experiments, the cells are used at the first to second passage after 3–6 weeks of culturing. This is therefore a work-intensive, limited method of obtaining cells.

Alternate cell sources include immortalized cell lines and primary cultures of osteoblastic cells from nonhuman sources, where tissue is not limiting. Osteosarcoma cell lines, such as the ROS and SaOS cell lines, show an accelerated expression of maturation and mineralization markers while retaining their proliferative capability. Because of the genetic lesions that are present in these cell lines, their use must be strictly validated by comparison with normal cells. Osteosarcoma cell lines have been used to great effect in testing cellular adhesion and osteoblastic cell response, such as alkaline phosphatase induction, to many different biomaterial surfaces. Primary osteoblastic cells have been established from other species, i.e., chicken, rat, mouse, and rabbit. Like the osteosarcoma lines, osteoblastic cells from different species have been used to elucidate markers of osteoblastic differentiation and osteoblastic cell response to a variety of biomaterials, with the caveat that some biochemical responses can be more critical in one species than in another. Like primary human osteoblastic cells, mesenchymal stem cells (MSCs), albeit a younger population, can model osteoblastic interactions with prostheses. The MSCs are available as a source of cells that can be expanded many times to yield a plentiful supply. Upon culturing in the appropriate osteogenic medium, these MSCs are rich cellular sources of osteoblastic cells and are very promising for use in tissue engineering applications requiring supplemental bone formation.

Finally, over the years, fibroblasts have been used to model the cellular/biomaterial interface. While these studies have defined many parameters important for cellular interactions with prostheses, fibrous growth often competes with bony ingrowth. This competition draws into question the wisdom of optimizing fibroblastic interactions with the prosthesis biomaterials. Equally important, fibroblasts do not synthesize the same repertoire of extracellular matrix proteins as osteoblasts, and as the biomaterial surface actively influences the expression of extracellular matrix proteins and thus their availability for initiating cell-extracellular matrix interactions, observations on fibroblasts are not a basis to predict the outcome of osteoblastic-specific interactions (Auf'mkolk et al., 1985; Bellows et al., 1986; Bobyn and Engh, 1984; Bobyn et al., 1980). Based on these considerations, osteoblastic cells, preferably human, remain the preferred model.

VI. FIRST STEPS IN BIOLOGICAL FIXATION OF IMPLANTS—CELLULAR ADHESION

The ingrowth of bone into implants, a direct result of osseointegration, occurs when mature living bone interacts directly with the prosthetic component without intervening soft or fibrous tissue (Branemark et al., 1977). During the surgical implantation of the prosthesis, the implant is press-fitted into a cavity, bringing it into close contact with the bone and thereby facilitating any interactions between osteoblasts and the implant interface. In our in vitro model systems, this close approximation between bone and implant occurs when bone chips and/or osteoblasts settle onto the implant surface. As a first step, the surface of the biomaterial must have interacted with the soluble extracellular matrix (ECM) proteins in a way to facilitate osteoblast adhesion and maturation. This is especially important, as our data suggest that this biocoated surface actively influences the repertoire of ECM proteins synthesized by the cell (Shah et al., 1999b; Sinha et al., 1994; Sinha and Tuan, 1996a), thus affecting both the initial adhesion of the osteoblast to the surface and the later synthesis and organization of ECM proteins important for osteoblast maturation. This influence of the ECM on the cellular fate is achieved by intracellular signaling initiated by clustering of integrins—the cell surface receptors that interact with the ECM.

Initial cellular adhesion to the surface of the implant may or may not involve integrins but certainly does involve charge interactions between the biomaterial surface and cell surface–charged components, such as glycoproteins and sialoproteins. On the metal alloys, both integrin-independent and -dependent initial cellular adhesion has been reported. These differences in the reported dependencies are probably both a function of the cell type used in the experiment as well as the method used to interrupt adhesion. Whether this initial adhesion is dependent on integrins, *stable* adhesion and

subsequent proliferation and differentiation are determined by the engage-
ment of integrin receptors with the ECM.

We and others have attempted to understand how prosthetic features
that contribute to stable fixation affect osteoblastic cell adhesion, morphology, and maturation. In a series of experiments, osteoblastic cells were used
to investigate the role of roughness while holding material chemistry constant as well as the role of the chemistry of the material with roughness
being constant. Specifically, in order to dissect the contributions of biomaterial topography and chemistry on osteoblastic cell proliferation, we have
examined three surfaces: (1) polished smooth, (2) roughened by sandblasting, and (3) sinter-coated porous surfaces. Using these three roughnesses,
we examined two different chemistries, i.e., CoCrMo or Ti6Al4V, two alloys
commonly used for orthopedic prostheses. Importantly, these three surfaces
have been custom-fabricated (courtesy of Biomet, Inc., Warsaw, IN, and
Zimmer, Inc., Warsaw, IN) to yield composition and topography parameters
similar to those found in orthopedic prostheses used for arthroplasty. These
surfaces are passivated in nitric acid and sterilized with ultraviolet light prior
to use. By scanning electron microscopy, the smooth surfaces display randomly spaced, narrow, parallel grooves of different depths; the sandblasted
rough surfaces display unevenly spaced pits of variable size ($\sim 3-100$ μm);
porous surfaces appear globular with large peaks and valleys (pore size,
$100-300$ μm), with a fine structure similar to that of roughened surfaces.

In our early experiments, we tested the effects of a rough or porous
Ti6Al4V surface on proliferation and maturation of embryonic chicken osteoblastic cells. Effects of material were assessed as a function of extracellular matrix synthesis, morphology, matrix organization, and incorporation
of calcium into the maturing matrix. Our observations of these cultures suggested that both materials supported osteoblastic cell adhesion, spreading,
and maintenance of a normal osteoblastic morphology. Importantly, osteoblastic maturation correlated with these parameters and was supported on
these materials. In particular, the topography of the Ti6Al4V surface actively
influenced the degree of maturation and matrix mineralization of the cultured
osteoblasts, which were enhanced as a function of the roughness of the
substrate (Groessner-Schreiber et al., 1991; Groessner-Schreiber and Tuan,
1992). From these observations, we hypothesized that initial cell adhesion
leading to a normal osteoblastic morphology represented an important first
step in the establishment of the intimate association between bone and metal
at the interface that ultimately results in osseointegration.

As a first step in the testing of this hypothesis, a fluorescent dye cell
adhesion assay was developed and optimized for use with osteoblastic cells
plated on metallic surfaces (Sinha et al., 1994), as it was not possible to
count the cells directly on the opaque surfaces of the metal alloys. Osteo-

blasts adhered to both polished Ti6Al4V and rough Ti6Al4V at all times tested, with cells plated on rough Ti having a slight adhesive advantage over cells plated on smooth Ti6Al4V. We then tested the effect of substrate composition on the adhesion kinetics of normal human osteoblastic cells. Osteoblastic cells on Ti6Al4V alloys adhered in greater numbers than those plated on CoCrMo alloys, suggesting that osteoblastic cells on the Ti6Al4V alloys had an adhesive advantage over cells on CoCrMo (Shah et al., 1999b). These studies suggest that surface chemistry in part determined the nature of the ECM proteins adsorbed and thus influenced the relative health and function of the cell with respect to its proliferation and maturation (Figure 1).

Again, in order for the prosthesis to be stably integrated, cellular migration onto the surface must occur, as must cellular proliferation to fill the available surface area. These functions are coordinately regulated by integrins and by kinases that interact with the cytoskeleton and the clustered integrins at the focal contact. Integrins are the major transmembrane receptors that mediate stable adhesion and—with activation of signalling proteins like the small ras-like kinases, rho, rac, and cdc42—mediate cell spreading, projection of cell extensions, and migration.

VII. MOLECULAR BASIS FOR CELL ADHESION

Many studies have addressed the role of cell–matrix interactions in signaling from the ECM to control cellular proliferation, differentiation, or apoptosis. A major synthetic activity of the osteoblast is to produce a bone-specific extracellular matrix consisting primarily of collagen type I, fibronectin, vitronectin, osteocalcin, osteopontin, osteonectin, and bone sialoprotein. Osteoblasts, as they mature, will remodel this matrix into mineralized bone; this matrix remodeling event is itself an important factor in osteoblastic maturation (Stein et al., 2000). The composition of the extracellular matrix regulates osteoblastic cell function; specifically, interaction of osteoblasts with the extracellular matrix through integrins may determine the maturation sequence that occurs (Owen et al., 1990). Plating of osteoblastic cells on collagen type I increases early adhesion and accelerates their maturation (Owen et al., 1990). In contrast, when less collagen type I is present in the extracellular matrix, as is characteristic of some of the less severe forms of osteogenesis imperfecta, osteoblast maturation is retarded, causing an immature, fragile bone (Fedarko et al., 1995a,b) Taken together, these studies suggest that the composition of the ECM, specifically that adsorbed to the prosthesis biomaterial, plays an active, dynamic role in determining osteoblast maturation. Stable osteoblastic cell adhesion has been shown by us and

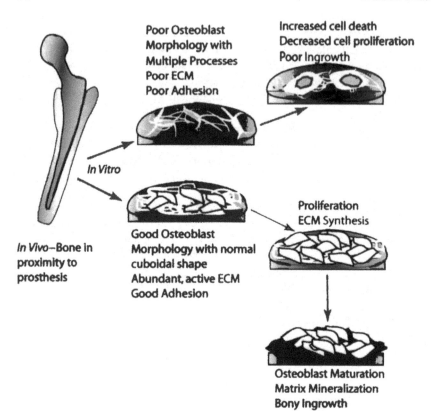

Figure 1 In vivo to in vitro model systems. In the hip prosthesis, the bone would be in close approximation to the prosthesis through press-fitting. In the in vitro system, this proximity is achieved by allowing osteoblastic cells to settle onto biomaterial surfaces. On surfaces suitable for osteoblastic proliferation and maturation, cells will deposit an extracellular matrix (ECM), proliferate, and mature to produce a bony matrix that interacts with the biomaterial (bottom pathway). In situations where the interactions of the cells with the biomaterial are poor, probably due to a less than optimal coating with serum ECM components, cellular morphology is elongated with multiple processes. This poor ECM composition and cellular morphology leads to decreased cellular functions associated with maturing osteoblastic cells and, in extreme cases, cellular death (top pathway).

by others to be dependent on the interactions of the ECM with integrins— cell surface receptors that, upon binding to a specific ECM protein, coordinate cellular spreading and stimulate intracellular signaling pathways (Gronowicz and McCarthy, 1996; Moursi et al., 1996, 1997; Shah et al., 1999a,b)

Integrins are membrane-spanning heterodimeric proteins that are made up of α and β subunits. The C-terminus of integrins is necessary for formation of focal contacts or ECM contacts which are clusters of membrane and cytosolic proteins involved in intracellular signaling and in organization of the actin stress fiber network. The N-terminus of integrins is responsible for ligand binding which, in many cases, involves interaction with an R-G-D amino acid motif in the ECM protein. An important activity of integrins that also resides in the N-terminus is their ability to reorganize the ECM as they migrate to cluster to form the focal adhesion contact (Ruoslahti, 1991). This ability to organize the ECM has been shown to be extremely important in integrin interactions with fibronectin. We have shown that fibronectin and vitronectin, abundant serum proteins, are extensively organized by osteoblastic cells during adhesion to a roughened, sandblasted Ti6Al4V surface identical to that used in hip prostheses (Shah et al., 1999a). This organization of the fibronectin matrix is consistent with data from Damsky's group, which examined rabbit coastal osteoblastic cells on tissue culture polystyrene. Her group has shown that osteoblastic cells, through the activity of integrin $\alpha5\beta1$, organize the fibronectin matrix within 15 min of plating to initiate signaling pathways necessary for osteoblastic cell maturation. Furthermore, when integrin $\alpha5\beta1$ is mutated such that it is still able to bind to fibronectin but is not able to organize the matrix, osteoblastic cells that express these mutant integrins undergo cell death (Moursi et al., 1996, 1997). They have also shown that fibronectin serves as a survival and maturation signal for osteoblastic cells (Globus et al., 1998). These studies emphasize the importance of both the binding and the organizing ability of the integrins in both initial osteoblast–ECM interactions and in osteoblastic maturation (Globus et al., 1998; Moursi et al., 1996, 1997). The results from Damsky's group and from others thus underline the critical role of the initial adhesion of serum ECM proteins to the biomaterial surface and the importance of the components of this ECM, specifically fibronectin and collagen type I, in determining the maturation program of the osteoblastic cell in vitro and bone in vivo.

The molecular recognition sequences for integrins have been mapped, and, in most cases, consist of an R-G-D amino acid motif, although integrins that interact with laminin and collagen type I and II, to name a few, use other amino acid sequences for recognition. For instance, the $\alpha2\beta1$ integrin that binds to collagen type I and to a lesser extent, collagen type II recognizes a (F/Y)Y(F/G)DLR amino acid motif and this binding is dependent on the native three-dimensional structure of this motif. Similarly, the other major integrin receptor for collagen, $\alpha 1 \beta 1$, recognizes an R-X-X-X-D amino acid motif, where X is any amino acid. More than 15α and 8β integrin subunits have been described, and different combinations of these yield integrins with different specificities; the majority of the specificity appears to be contributed by the α subunit (Ruoslahti, 1996).

For any specific α-β combination of integrin subunits, generally more than one ECM protein can bind; conversely, most ECM proteins can interact with more than one combination of integrin α and β subunits. For instance, the $\alpha V\beta 3$ integrin receptor binds not only fibrinogen, but fibronectin, vitronectin, von Willebrand factor, thrombospondin, and osteopontin; whereas fibronectin can bind to $\alpha 3\beta 1$, $\alpha 4\beta 1$, $\alpha 5\beta 1$, $\alpha IIb\beta 3$, and $\alpha V\beta 3$ integrins. The integrin dimer with which any ECM protein interacts will be determined by (1) the integrins expressed by that cell type, (2) the abundance of the different expressed integrins with respect to each other, and (3) the affinities of these expressed integrins for the particular ECM proteins. Importantly, ECM proteins can interact with more than one integrin subclass in any particular cell type, with the ultimate fate of the cell dependent on the different signaling pathways initiated (Ruoslahti et al., 1994; Ruoslahti and Reed, 1994). In human osteoblastic cells, we and others have found expression of the $\alpha 1$, $\alpha 2$, $\alpha 3$, $\alpha 4$, $\alpha 5$, αV, $\beta 1$, and $\beta 3$ integrins, with relative amounts of these integrins dependent on the substrate surface (Clover et al., 1992; Sinha and Tuan, 1996b).

VIII. EFFECTS OF PLATING SUBSTRATE ON FOCAL CONTACT DISTRIBUTION AND CYTOSKELETAL ORGANIZATION

Based on studies of other cell types, it has been suggested that cell attachment and cell spreading need not be coupled, with cell spreading necessary for the initiation of intracellular signaling events that are regulated through the cell adhesion site, the focal contact (Frisch et al., 1996). The signaling pathways that are initiated are dependent on the integrin-ECM identity. In order to assess the degree of cell spreading, the focal contact distribution, the cytoskeletal organization that is directly influenced by focal contact distribution, and the topography of the substrate, we imaged osteoblastic cells by means of confocal laser scanning microscopy (CLSM). A laser beam can be focused onto a plane of finite width, thereby making it possible to optically section the osteoblastic cell as it interacts with the biomaterial surface.

Using CLSM, we collected data on cell size, shape, and the three-dimensional relationship of the osteoblastic cells to the substrate. Furthermore, through use of multiple fluorescent labels, we related cell spreading with focal contact distribution, actin cytoskeletal organization, and surface topography to begin to understand the mechanistic basis for specific interactions of osteoblastic cells with different surfaces, in this case, sand-blasted, roughened Ti6Al4V or CoCrMo.

When the osteoblastic cell stably adheres to Ti6Al4V or CoCrMo, it does so through establishment of focal adhesion contacts. Integrins cluster to form the focal contact and this initiates the assembly of a macromolecular complex that includes signaling molecules such as the focal adhesion kinase $p125^{FAK}$, proto-oncogenes such as *src* and *ras*, and proteins important for tethering the actin cytoskeleton to the focal contact, such as vinculin and talin (Schaller and Parsons, 1994). In Figure 2, such cell anchoring via focal contacts and cytoskeletal architecture is shown. Focal contacts are visible throughout the cells with an enrichment at cell edges. These focal contacts serve as tethering points for the array of actin stress fibers that provide mechanical strength to the cell.

When osteoblastic cells were examined on these substrates, several characteristic differences were noted. Consistently, osteoblastic cells plated on Ti6Al4V had smaller cell areas, more focal contacts, were more elongated, and had a greater percentage of their membranes devoted to focal contacts than osteoblasts plated on CoCrMo. That osteoblasts were more elongated but had a smaller cell area on Ti6Al4V could be explained when the three-dimensional relationship of the osteoblastic cells relative to the sandblasted, roughened surfaces was examined.

The three-dimensional relationship of osteoblastic cells to the metal surfaces was determined by computer-aided three-dimensional reconstruction after CLSM. Cells were immunostained for the focal contact protein vinculin, stained for the actin cytoskeleton, and the topography of the metal surface visualized by reflectance. Osteoblastic cells adhered to the two metal surfaces quite differently, with focal contacts apparent at all membrane to surface contact points (Figure 3). On the rough Ti6Al4V surface, osteoblastic cells appeared to conform to the topography of the surface (Figure 3A). Focal contacts were distributed along the contours of the surface, with actin stress fibers following the contour of the surface (Figure 3E). On roughened CoCrMo, osteoblastic cells spanned the topographic valleys found in the surface (Figure 3B and D). The cells extended multiple processes to achieve its stable adhesion, explaining its larger cell area and irregular cell shape (Figure 3F). In contrast to what we observed on roughened Ti6Al4V, osteoblastic cells on roughened CoCrMo exhibited parallel actin filaments only

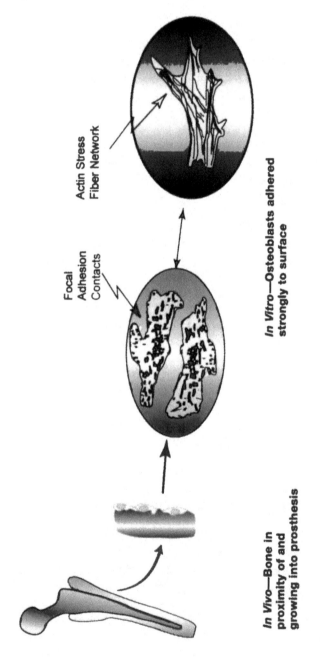

In Vivo—Bone in
proximity of and
growing into prosthesis

Focal
Adhesion
Contacts

Actin Stress
Fiber Network

In Vitro—Osteoblasts adhered
strongly to surface

Figure 2 Bony ingrowth—in vivo to in vitro. As the bone grows into the prosthesis, individual cells coat the crevasses and peaks epitomized in the roughened and porous coatings. The cellular events that underlie this conforming of the cell to the undulating surface of the implant have to do with the establishment of focal adhesion contacts, which are close contacts mediated by cell surface receptors that bind to the extracellular matrix coating the prosthesis. These focal adhesion contacts provide anchoring points for the actin stress fiber network that gives the cells their ability to adhere in the face of mechanical stress.

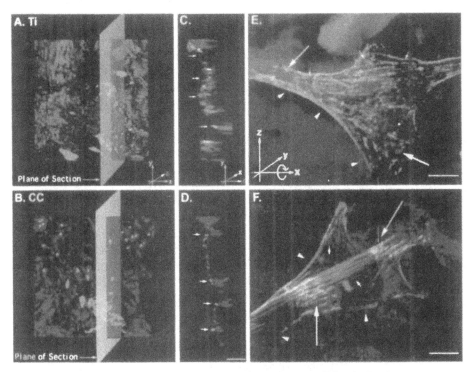

Figure 3 Three-dimensional relationship of osteoblastic cell focal adhesion contacts, cytoskeletal organization, and substrate surface as reconstructed by confocal laser scanning microscopy. Panels A to D. Osteoblasts immunostained for the focal contact protein vinculin (green) and the biomaterial surface as detected by reflectance (red or blue) were optically sectioned by confocal laser scanning microscopy (CLSM) followed by computer-aided three-dimensional reconstruction of the osteoblast-Ti6Al4V (Ti) or osteoblast CoCrMo (CC) interface. Optical sectioning (see plane of section) along the indicated y-z axis shows focal contacts following contours of the surface on Ti while remaining localized to relative topographical peaks on CC. Arrows indicate corresponding points of focal contacts and surface reflectance. Magnification: Bar = 25 μm. Panels E and F. Three-dimensional images of osteoblastic cells stained for the focal contact protein vinculin (blue in E, green in F) as well as stained with a dye that detects filamentous actin (green in E, red in F), were gathered using CLSM. In addition to the two biochemical markers, substrate topography was simultaneously recorded using reflectance (red for Ti6Al4V surface in E; blue for CoCrMo surface in F). The resulting images were stacked and rotated by 90 degrees along the x axis for Ti6Al4V (E) or 45 degrees for CoCrMo (F). Close approximation of the actin, vinculin, and substrate signals is indicated by yellow or white. Black regions of the substrate are located out of the plane of the section and thus represent areas either above or below the section. On Ti6Al4V (E), the osteoblasts can be seen following the contour of the surface (arrowheads), while on CoCrMo (F), the osteoblasts appear to span topographic valleys (arrowheads). On both surfaces, focal contact formation appears to be localized to membrane to surface contact points (long arrows) with no focal contact formation occurring along the dorsal membrane of the cells (short arrows). Magnification: Bar = 25 μm. (From *Bone* 24:499–506, 1999.)

in the cellular extensions that spanned valleys (arrows, Figure 3E), and focal contacts were present in the cellular extensions only where they resided on the relative topographical peaks. No focal adhesion contacts were visualized on the dorsal membrane, as would be expected due to lack of contact with any substrate.

These results, taken together, strongly indicate that biomaterial composition significantly affects focal contact formation and ordering of actin microfilament systems in adherent osteoblasts. Importantly, these findings offer a molecular explanation for our early observations that osteoblastic cells adhere in greater numbers on Ti6Al4V than on CoCrMo. Such differences in other cellular systems have important downstream consequences on activation of proteins and on gene expression. It is interesting to speculate that similar cellular events could take place in vivo upon placement of the metallic implant into bony sites, and that these events would govern or guide subsequent events as bone tissue responds to the presence of the biomaterial. To what extent these findings are reproduced during early stages of osseointegration remain to be investigated in vivo.

IX. OSTEOGENIC FACTORS

The ability of a number of growth factors to stimulate new bone growth in cases where inadequate bone formation is present has been tested. In addition to facilitating healing of nonunions and segmental defects, these osteogenic factors have been tested as means to enhance bone ingrowth into screws, plates, and prostheses.

The most potent osteoactive factors identified belong to the TGF-β gene superfamily, which includes the TGF-βs, BMPs, dpp, activins, gdfs, and inhibins. Because the cellular signaling pathways that are critical for new bone formation are still being elucidated, the cellular basis for the osteogenic effects of these factors are still being explored, although important effects are known. Specifically, TGF-βs and BMPs regulate genes that are critical for ECM deposition, and remodeling. Furthermore, they modulate intracellular signaling pathways, transcription factor activity, and gene expression to yield altered expression of proteins important for osteoblastic cell proliferation and maturation.

All members of the TGF-β superfamily are secreted proteins that are active as homodimers or, in combinations with other family members, as heterodimers (Massague et al., 1994). TGFβ1, in vitro, enhances osteoblast adhesion, presumably through increased expression of proteins involved in ECM deposition, cell-ECM interactions and ECM remodeling. For example,

TGF-β1 increases levels of fibronectin, integrins, collagens, osteonectin, tissue inhibitors of metalloproteinases (TIMPs), and osteopontin. In addition, TGF-β affects cell spreading and cell shape as it alters the distribution of focal adhesion contacts, and increases actin stress fiber formation, structures that will bear the mechanical stress of the cells. Finally, although in vitro TGF-β1 increases osteoblastic maturation as indicated by increased alkaline phosphatase activity, it inhibits matrix maturation and mineralization. In keeping with this, osteocalcin and metalloproteinase expression are suppressed (Breen et al., 1994).

The potent osteogenic factor BMP-2, like TGF-β, enhances osteoblast adhesion and actin stress fiber formation. Consistent with its effects on adhesion, BMP-2 increases cell size, promotes a more ordered distribution of focal adhesion contacts, and increases numbers of cells with well-formed actin stress fiber networks. Unlike TGF-β, BMP-2 not only increases alkaline phosphatase activity but also accelerates the temporal expression of the characteristic osteoblastic maturation markers. Two of these, osteocalcin and calcium incorporation into matrix (Shah et al., 1999a), are increased, consistent with a role in both osteoblastic maturation and matrix mineralization for the BMPs. BMPs play critical roles in new bone formation, fracture repair and embryonic bone development (Centrella et al., 1994). BMP injection distal to bone supports ectopic bone formation; TGF-β or BMP injection proximal to bone results in increased bone mass (Centrella et al., 1994).

Members of the TGF-β superfamily are synthesized as precursors with a signal peptide for secretion and a pro-domain that determines the active structure. When TGF-β is cleaved, the pro-domain remains associated with the 110-140 amino acid TGF-β signaling molecule; this inactive complex is the so-called latent form of TGF-β (Massague et al., 1994). The latent form of TGF-β can be stored in the mineralized matrix and its release by osteoclasts may induce osteoclast apoptosis (Hughes et al., 1994). BMPs are also synthesized as precursors and, after secretion, can associate with the mineralized matrix (Zhu et al., 1999).

Members of the TGF-β superfamily bind to two membrane-spanning cell surface receptors that associate as tetramers. Two BMP receptor-I's (BMPR-I) are present in osteoblastic cells and can mediate BMP signaling. The BMPR-IB has been associated with differentiation of osteoblastic cells whereas the BMPR-IA has been associated with suppression of the osteoblastic phenotype, driving the cells toward the adipocytic lineage (Chen et al., 1998). Other studies suggest that BMPR-IB and -IA are functionally equivalent (Fujii et al., 1999).

The activated receptors initiate intracellular signaling through activation of cytoplasmic proteins called Smads. These Smads, after phosphorylation and coassociation with the common Smad4, translocate to the nucleus. Once in the nucleus, they interact with other transcription factors to modulate gene expression. Interestingly, members of the TGF-β superfamily, including the BMPs also activate intracellular signaling pathways that are initiated by formation of the focal contact and/or by calcium fluxes. These other pathways have been shown to interact with the Smad pathways to produce the biological effects of the TGF-β family member. Such integration of pathways, as shown for the BMPs in Figure 4, suggests how cell specific gene regulation occurs in response to the different osteogenic factors.

X. OSTEOGENIC FACTORS AND ENHANCEMENT OF BONE INGROWTH

We and others have asked if treatment with osteogenic factors could enhance bony ingrowth (Cole et al., 1997; Shah et al., 1999a,b; Sinha et al., 1994; Sinha and Tuan, 1996a; Sumner et al., 1995, 2001). Specifically, both the Ti6Al4V and CoCrMo surfaces showed relatively good adhesion of osteoblasts; however, from in vivo studies, it is known that the extent of actual bony ingrowth is only a fraction of the available implant surface (Bellows et al., 1986; Bobyn and Engh, 1984; Goldring et al., 1989). Therefore, these agents are good candidates to enhance osteoblastic interactions with prostheses. We have examined this question, in vitro, using normal human osteoblastic cells plated on the Ti6Al4V alloys.

When osteoblastic cells were pretreated with BMP-2 and allowed to adhere to roughened, sandblasted Ti6Al4V, several differences were noted between the control cultures and cultures treated with BMP-2. Notably, numbers of adherent cells were greater at times less than 24 h after BMP-2 treatment. By 24 h, when all cells had had a chance to settle and spread, differences in numbers of adherent cells were no longer significant. Other morphological changes in cell shape, focal contact number, and actin stress fiber organization were apparent. In control cells, focal adhesion contacts appeared throughout the cells, including the cellular processes, suggesting that all of these areas were being used for cell contact to the substrate. In BMP-2–treated cells, focal contacts were large and concentrated in the cell body. Unlike in control cells, BMP-2–treated cells showed very few focal contacts in cellular processes that appeared to be mostly used to establish cell-cell contact to enhance communication between cells, important functions for the mature osteoblast or osteocyte. This cell-cell communication was more apparent several weeks after treatment, where control cultures mineralized in discrete foci. In contrast, BMP-2–treated cultures showed

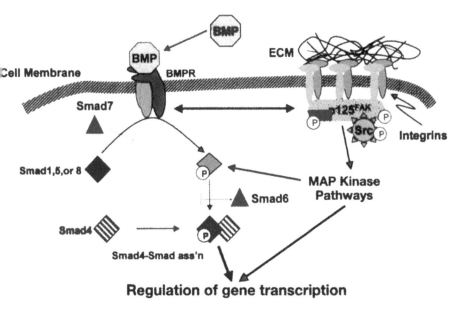

Regulation of gene transcription

Figure 4   Cartoon of BMP signaling as integrated with cellular adhesion. When BMP interacts with its receptor, the intracellular proteins that mediate BMP signaling, Smad 1, 5, or 8, are phosphorylated and associate with the common Smad, Smad 4. This Smad/Smad 4 complex is translocated to the nucleus, where, after interaction with transcription factor partners, gene transcription events are modified. These activation steps initiated by binding of BMP to the BMP receptors (BMPR) can be blocked by the inhibitory Smads, Smad 6 and Smad 7. Concurrent with Smad activation, integrin receptor activation, clustering and formation of focal adhesion contacts occur, mobilizing the MAP kinase pathways that can be initiated by these events. Whether direct signaling occurs between the two types of pathways is still uncertain, but accumulating knowledge suggests that it does. Activation of the MAP kinase pathways can then alter the phosphorylation state of the Smads, as well as causing altered gene transcription events. We propose that integration of these signaling pathways are largely responsible for the cell type–specific responses to TGF-β and BMPs.

extensive mineralization, both in foci and in between foci, where cells appeared to be recruited. Overall, this morphological picture of the effects of BMP-2 treatment on osteoblastic cell growth emphasizes the proposed role for BMP-2 in enhancing bony ingrowth.

Finally, as described in the previous Sec. IX, osteoblasts on Ti6Al4V synthesized and secreted a complex extracellular matrix that interacted with cellular receptors to initiate signaling pathways. BMP-2 altered organization

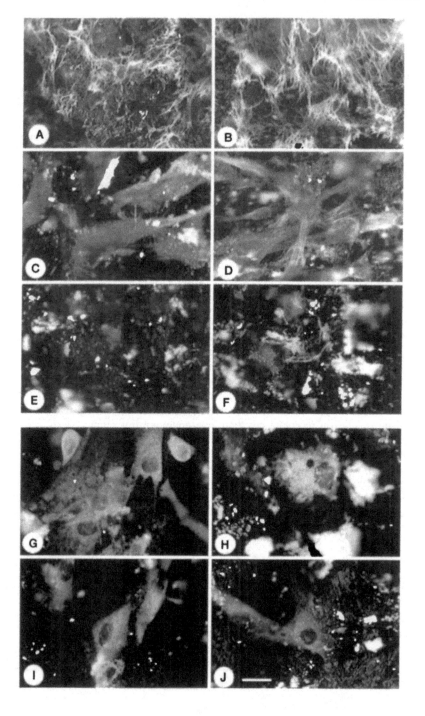

and expression of the extracellular matrix proteins (Figure 5) as well as expression of their cognate integrin receptors and activation of intracellular signaling pathways (Shah et al., 1999a).

Observations such as these from many in vitro studies suggest that osteogenic factors, including the BMPs, enhance bone healing and formation by having direct effects on gene expression and, importantly, altering cellular pathways initiated early in cellular adhesion. The effects observed on the metal alloys are consistent with known in vivo effects of these agents, i.e., accelerated maturation and recruitment of cells to the mature osteoblastic phenotype. The actual cellular mechanisms are similar to that observed in the normal, maturing osteoblast, but at an accelerated rate. Thus, by studying the in vitro systems, we and others have gained a better understanding of the cellular processes that lead to new bone growth and osseointegration. The nature of the initial adhesion appears to determine subsequent maturation steps. Thus the prosthetic surface must support not only cellular adhesion but also do so in a way that leads to a normal osteoblastic morphology. The maturational steps leading to new bone formation and osseointegration thus become the natural consequences of this initiating event and suggests additional criteria for judging prospective prosthetic surfaces.

XI. FUTURE DIRECTIONS

The integrity of the bone–biomaterial interface is the keystone of long-term biological fixation of the implant. Optimization of the integrity of the interface should enhance bony ingrowth as well as reduce the opportunistic infiltration and harboring of wear debris particles derived, for example, from

---

Figure 5 Effects of BMP-2 pretreatment on organization of the osteoblastic cell extracellular matrix on rough Ti6Al4V. Normal human trabecular osteoblastic cells were pretreated with 10 ng/mL BMP-2 for 12 hr, and plated on rough Ti6Al4V. After 12 hr, cells were fixed and stained for fibronectin (A,B), vitronectin (C,D), collagen type I (E,F), osteopontin (G,H) or osteonectin (I,J). In all panels, treatment with BMP-2 (B,D,F,H,J) caused a more extensive organization of the extracellular matrix than in the control cultures (A,D,E,G,I). Note, that at 12 hr after plating, the fibronectin (A,B) and vitronectin (C,D) matrices are the most abundant and more extensively organized, whereas collagen type I is barely detectable, with some fibril-like structures apparent in (F). Both osteocalcin and osteopontin, at these early times, give positive signals but appear to be confined within the cellular area (G–J). Magnification: Bar = 25 μM. (From *Biol. Cell.* 91:131–142, 1999.)

the polyethylene liner material, known to contribute to subsequent aseptic osteolysis. Understanding the scientific basis of bone–implant interaction is therefore crucial to developing a rational design of implants that have optimal mechanical and biological characteristics.

Some of the major issues to be considered for the future include the following:

Determining the physical and chemical attributes of biomaterial surface that positively or negatively influence bone cell biology. Parameters to consider include surface chemistry and energy and topography in terms of micro- and macrotexture.

Characterizing the initial cellular responses that are predictive parameters for long-term, effective maturation of osteoblasts that will lead to functional tissue remodeling and integration into the biomaterial surface.

Identifying the bioactive factors and/or matrix molecules, both natural or synthetic, that stimulate such osseointegrative cellular responses.

Designing regulated and effective delivery systems for such factors to the bone–implant interface.

Applying contemporary material manufacturing processes to produce, in a consistent, reproducible, and cost-effective fashion, implant devices with the desired surface characteristics.

Designing a meaningful functional testing regimen that encompasses both in vitro and animal models and logically leads to clinical trials.

While the progress in biological fixation of hip implants has been impressive, the design and application of new technologies that can address these challenges promises development of new, multifunctional, long-lived prostheses.

XII. ACKNOWLEDGMENT

The authors gratefully acknowledge past and present members of the Jefferson Orthopaedic Research Laboratory in contributing to various aspects of the work summarized in this review and the NIH and the Orthopaedic Research and Education Foundation for funding support.

REFERENCES

Andersson, O. H., Liu, G., Kangasniemi, K., and Juhanoja, J. (1992). Evaluation of the acceptance of glass in bone. Mater. Med. 3, 145–150.

Anselme, K., Linez, P., Bigerelle, M., Le Maguer, D., Le Maguer, A., Hardouin, P., Hildebrand, H. F., Iost, A., and Leroy, J. M. (2000). The relative influence of the topography and chemistry of TiAl6V4 surfaces on osteoblastic cell behaviour. Biomaterials 21, 1567–1577.

Auf'mkolk, B., Hauschler, P. V., and Schwartz, E. R. (1985). Characterization of human bone cells in culture. Calcif. Tiss. Int. 37, 228–235.

Banerjee, C., McCabe, L. R., Choi, J. Y., Hiebert, S. W., Stein, J. L., Stein, G. S., and Lian, J. B. (1997). Runt homology domain proteins in osteoblast differentiation: AML3/CBFA1 is a major component of a bone-specific complex. J. Cell. Biochem. 66, 1–8.

Beckenbaugh, R. D., and Ilstrup, D. M. (1978). Total hip arthroplasty. J. Bone Joint Surg. 60A, 306–313.

Bellows, C. G., Aubin, J. E., Heersche, J. N. M., and Artosz, M. E. (1986). Mineralized bone nodules formed in vitro from enzymatically released rat calvarial cell populations. Calcif. Tiss. Int. 38, 143–154.

Black, J. (1989). "Push-out" tests. J. Biomed. Mater. Res. 23, 1243–1245.

Bobyn, J. D., and Engh, C. A. (1984). Human histology of the bone-porous metal implant interface. Orthopaedics 7, 1410–1422.

Bobyn, J. D., Pilliar, R. M., Cameron, H. U., and Weatherly, G. C. (1980). The optimum pore size for the fixation of porous-surface metal implants by the ingrowth of bone. Clin. Orthop. Rel. Res. 150, 263–270.

Boss, J. H., Shajrawi, I., and Mendes, D. G. (1994). The nature of the bone-implant interface. The lessons learned from implant retrieval and analysis in man and experimental animal. Med. Prog. Technol. 20, 119–142.

Branemark, P. I., Hansoon, B. O., Adell, R., Breine, U., Lindstrom, J., Hallan, O., and Oham, A. (1977). Osseointegrated implants in the treatment of the edentulous jaw. Scand. J. Plast. Reconstr. Surg. 16, 1–132.

Breen, E. C., Ignotz, R. A., McCabe, L., Stein, J. L., Stein, G. S., and Lian, J. B. (1994). TGFβ alters growth and differentiation related gene expression in proliferating osteoblasts in vitro, preventing development of the mature bone phenotype. J. Cell. Physiol. 160, 323–335.

Bundy, K., Rahn, B., Gerber, H., Schlegel, U., Peter, R., and Geret, V. (1993). Cell and tissue adhesion to orthopaedic biomaterials. Trans. Orthop. Res. Soc. 18, 513.

Cannas, M., Denicolai, F., Webb, L. X., and Gristina, A. G. (1988). Bioimplant surfaces: binding of fibronectin and fibroblast adhesion. J. Orthop. Res. 6, 58–62.

Carlsson, A. S., and Gentz, C. F. (1980). Mechanical loosening of the femoral head prosthesis in the Charnley total hip arthroplasty. Clin. Orthop. Rel. Res. 147, 262–270.

Centrella, M., Horowitz, M. C., Wozney, J. M., and McCarthy, T. L. (1994). Transforming growth factor-β gene family members and bone. Endocr. Rev. 15, 27–39.

Chandler, H. P., Reineck, F. T., Wixson, R. L., and McCarthy, J. C. (1981). Total hip replacement in patients younger than thirty years old. A five-year follow-up study. J. Bone Joint Surg. 63A, 1426–1434.

Chen, D., Ji, X., Harris, M. A., Feng, J. Q., Karsenty, G., Celeste, A. J., Rosen, V., Mundy, G. R., and Harris, S. E. (1998). Differential roles for bone morphogenetic protein (BMP) receptor type IB and IA in differentiation and specification of mesenchymal precursor cells to osteoblast and adipocyte lineages. J. Cell. Biol. 142, 295–305.

Chen, P. Q., Turner, T. M., Ronnigen, H., Galante, J., Urban, R., and Rostoker, W. (1983). A canine cementless total hip prosthesis model. Clin. Orthop. Rel. Res. 176, 24–33.

Clark, A. E., Hench, L. L., and Paschall, H. A. (1976). The influence of surface chemistry on implant interface histology: a theoretical basis for implant materials selection. J. Biomed. Mater. Res. 10, 161–174.

Clover, J., Doods, R. A., and Gowen, M. (1992). Integrin expression by human osteoblasts and osteoclasts in situ and in culture. J. Cell. Sci. 103, 267–271.

Clubb, F. J., Jr., Clapper, D. L., Deferrari, D. A., Hu, S. P., Seare, W. J., Jr., Capek, P. P., Armstrong, J., McGee, M. G., Billings, L. A., Fuqua, J. M., Jr. et al. (1999). Surface texturing and coating of biomaterial implants: effects on tissue integration and fibrosis. ASAIO J. 45, 281–287.

Cole, B. J., Bostrom, M. P., Pritchard, T. L., Sumner, D. R., Tomin, E., Lane, J. M., and Weiland, A. J. (1997). Use of bone morphogenetic protein 2 on ectopic porous coated implants in the rat. Clin. Orthop. Rel. Res. 345, 219–228.

Cook, S. D., Thomas, K. A., Dalton, J. E., Volkman, T. K., Whitecloud, T. S. III, and Kay, J. F. (1992). Hydroxylapatite coating of porous implants improves bone ingrowth and interface attachment strength. J. Biomed. Mater. Res. 26, 989–1001.

Cook, S. D., Thomas, K. A., Kay, J. F., and Jarcho, M. (1988). Hydroxylapatite-coated porous titanium for use as an orthopaedic biologic attachment system. Clin. Orthop. Rel. Res. 230, 303–312.

Cotterill, P., Hunter, G. A., and Tile, M. (1982). A radiographic analysis of 166 Charnley-Müller total hip arthroplasties. Clin. Orthop. Rel. Res. 120–126.

De Benedittis, A., Mattioli-Belmonte, M., Krajewski, A., Fini, M., Ravaglioli, A., Giardino, R., and Biagini, G. (1999). In vitro and in vivo assessment of bone-implant interface: a comparative study. Int. J. Artif. Organs 22, 516–521.

Degasne, I., Basle, M. F., Demais, V., Hure, G., Lesourd, M., Grolleau, B., Mercier, L., and Chappard, D. (1999). Effects of roughness, fibronectin and vitronectin on attachment, spreading, and proliferation of human osteoblast-like cells (Saos-2) on titanium surfaces. Calcif. Tiss. Int. 64, 499–507.

DeLee, J. G., and Charnley, J. (1976). Radiological demarcation of cemented sockets in total hip replacement. Clin. Orthop. Rel. Res. 121, 20–32.

Deuel, T. F. (1996). Growth factors. In Principles of Tissue Engineering, (eds. R. P. Lanza, R. Langer, and W. L. Chick), pp. 133–149. Austin, TX: R.G. Landes Co., and Academic Press.

Ducy, P., Starbuck, M., Priemel, M., Shen, J., Pinero, G., Geoffroy, V., Amling, M., and Karsenty, G. (1999). A Cbfa1-dependent genetic pathway controls bone formation beyond embryonic development. Genes Dev. 13, 1025–1036.

Ducy, P., Zhang, R., Geoffroy, V., Ridall, A. L., and Karsenty, G. (1997). Osf2/Cbfa1: a transcriptional activator of osteoblast differentiation. Cell 89, 747–754.

Emerson, R. H., Sanders, S. B., Head, W. C., and Higgins, L. (1999). Effect of circumferential plasma-spray porous coating on the rate of femoral osteolysis after total hip arthroplasty. J. Bone Joint Surg. 81A, 1291–1298.

Engh, C. A. (1983). Hip arthroplasty with a Moore prosthesis with porous coating. A five-year study. Clin. Orthop. Rel. Res. 176, 52–66.

Engh, C. A., and Culpepper, W. J. (1997). Long-term results of use of the anatomic medullary locking prosthesis in total hip arthroplasty. J. Bone Joint Surg. 79A, 177–184.

Fedarko, N. S., D'Avis, P., Frazier, C. R., Burrill, M. J., Fergusson, V., Tayback, M., Sponseller, P. D., and Shapiro, J. S. (1995a). Cell proliferation of human fibroblasts and osteoblasts in osteogenesis imperfecta: influence of age. J. Bone Miner. Res. 10, 1705–1712.

Fedarko, N. S., Robey, P. G., and Vetter, U. K. (1995b). Extracellular matrix stoichiometry in osteoblasts from patients with osteogenesis imperfecta. J. Bone Miner. Res. 10, 1122–1129.

Ferguson, C., Alpern, E., Miclau, T., and Helms, J. A. (1999). Does adult fracture repair recapitulate embryonic skeletal formation? Mech. Dev. 87, 57–66.

Franceschi, R. T. (1999). The developmental control of osteoblast-specific gene expression: role of specific transcription factors and the extracellular matrix environment. Crit. Rev. Oral Biol. Med. 10, 40–57.

Frisch, S. M., Vuori, K., Ruoslahti, E., and Chan-Hui, P. Y. (1996). Control of adhesion-dependent cell survival by focal adhesion kinase. J. Cell. Biol. 134, 793–799.

Fujii, M., Takeda, K., Imamura, T., Aoki, H., Sampath, T. K., Enomoto, S., Kawabata, M., Kato, M., Ichijo, H., and Miyazono, K. (1999). Roles of bone morphogenetic protein type I receptors and Smad proteins in osteoblast and chondroblast differentiation. Mol. Biol. Cell 10, 3801–3813.

Galante, J., Rostoker, W., Lueck, R., and Ray, R. D. (1971). Sintered fiber metal composites as a basis for attachment of implants to bone. J. Bone Joint Surg. 53A, 101–114.

Gao, T. J., Lindholm, T. S., Kommonen, B., Ragni, P., Paronzini, A., Lindholm, T. C., Jamsa, T., and Jalovaara, P. (1996). Enhanced healing of segmental tibial defects in sheep by a composite bone substitute composed of tricalcium phosphate cylinder, bone morphogenetic protein, and type IV collagen. J. Biomed. Mater. Res. 32, 505–512.

Giachelli, C. M., and Steitz, S. (2000). Osteopontin: a versitile regulator of inflammation and biomineralization. Matrix Biol. 19, 615–622.

Globus, R. K., Doty, S. B., Lull, J. C., Holmuhamedov, E., Humphries, M. J., and Damsky, C. H. (1998). Fibronectin is a survival factor for differentiated osteoblasts. J. Cell. Sci. 111, 1385–1393.

Goldring, S. R., Flannery, M. S., Petrison, K. K., Evins, A. E., Jasty, M. J., and Goldring, M. B. (1989). In vitro model for characterization of the biochemical and cellular responses to orthopaedic implant materials. Trans. Orthop. Res. Soc. 13, 495.

Gori, F., Thomas, T., Hicok, K. C., Spelsberg, T. C., and Riggs, B. L. (1999). Differentiation of human marrow stromal precursor cells: bone morphogenetic protein-2 increases OSF2/CBFA1, enhances osteoblast commitment, and inhibits late adipocyte maturation. J. Bone Miner. Res. 14, 1522–1535.

Griffith, L. G., and Lopina, S. (1998). Microdistribution of substratum bound ligands affect cell function: hepatocyte spreading on PEO-tethered galactose. Biomaterials 19, 979–986.

Griffith, M. J., Seidenstein, M. K., Williams, D., and Charnley, J. (1978). Eight year results of Charnley arthroplasties of the hip with special reference to the behavior of cement. Clin. Orthop. Rel. Res. 137, 24–36.

Groessner-Schreiber, B., Kreitzer, D., and Tuan, R. S. (1991). Bone cell response to hydroxyapatite-coated titanium surfaces in vitro. Semin. Arthrop. 2, 260–267.

Groessner-Schreiber, B., and Tuan, R. S. (1992). Enhanced extracellular matrix production and mineralization by calvarial osteoblasts cultured on titanium surfaces in vitro. J. Cell Sci. 101, 209–217.

Gronowicz, G., and McCarthy, M. B. (1996). Response of human osteoblasts to implant materials: integrin-mediated adhesion. J. Orthop. Res. 14, 878–887.

Gruen, T. A., McNeice, G. M., and Amstutz, H. C. (1979). "Modes of failure" of cemented stem-type femoral components: a radiographic analysis of loosening. Clin. Orthop. Rel. Res. 141, 17–27.

Harris, W. H., and Davies, J. P. (1988). Modern use of modern cement for total hip replacement. Orthop. Clin. North Am. 19, 581–589.

Harris, W. H., White, R. E., McCarthy, J. C., Walker, P. S., and Weinberg, E. H. (1983). Bony ingrowth fixation of the acetabular component in canine hip joint arthroplasty. Clin. Orthop. Rel. Res. 176, 7–11.

Hayashi, K., Inadome, T., Mashima, T., and Sugioka, Y. (1993). Comparison of bone-implant interface shear strength of solid hydroxyapatite and hydroxyapatite-coated titanium implants. J. Biomed. Mater. Res. 27, 557–563.

Hayashi, K., Inadome, T., Tsumura, H., Mahima, T., and Sugiokaa, Y. (1990). Bone-implant interface mechanics of in vivo bio-inert ceramics. Biomaterials 14, 1173–1179.

Healy, K. E., Rezania, A., and Stile, R. A. (1999). Designing biomaterials to direct biological responses. Ann. N.Y. Acad. Sci. 875, 24–35.

Hedley, A. K., Kabo, M., Kim, W., Coster, I., and Amstutz, H. C. (1983). Bony ingrowth fixation of newly designed acetabular components in a canine model. Clin. Orthop. Rel. Res. 176, 12–23.

Hench, L. L., and Paschall, H. A. (1973). Direct chemical bond of bioactive glass-ceramic materials to bone and muscle. J. Biomed. Mater. Res. Symp. 4, 25–42.

Horbett, T. A., and Schway, M. B. (1978). Correlation between mouse 3T3 cell spreading and serum fibronectin adsorption on glass and hydroxyethylmethacrylate copolymers. J. Biomed. Mater. Res. 22, 763–793.

Hughes, D. E., Wright, K. R., Mundy, G. R., and Boyce, B. R. (1994). TGFβ1 induces osteoclast apoptosis in vitro (Abstract). J. Bone Miner. Res. 10 (Suppl. 1), 71.

Johansson, C. B., Han, C. H., Wennerberg, A., and Albrektsson, T. (1998). A quantitative comparison of machined commercially pure titanium and titanium-aluminum-vanadium implants in rabbit bone. Int. J. Oral Maxillofac. Impl. 13, 315–321.

Jones, L. C., and Hungerford, D. S. (1987). Cement disease. Clin. Orthop. Rel. Res. 225, 192–206.

Judet, R., Siguier, M., Brumpt, B., and Judet, T. (1978). A noncemented total hip prosthesis. Clin. Orthop. Rel. Res. 137, 76–84.

Karsenty, G. (1999). The genetic transformation of bone biology. Genes Dev. 13, 3037–3051.

Karsenty, G. (2000). Bone formation and factors affecting this process. Matrix Biol. 19, 85–89.

Karsenty, G., Ducy, P., Starbuck, M., Priemel, M., Shen, J., Geoffroy, V., and Amling, M. (1999). Cbfa1 as a regulator of osteoblast differentiation and function. Bone 25, 107–108.

Kingsley, D. M. (1994a). The TGF-beta superfamily: new members, new receptors, and new genetic tests of function in different organisms. Genes Dev. 8, 133–146.

Kingsley, D. M. (1994b). What do BMPs do in mammals? Clues from the mouse short-ear mutation. Trends Genet. 10, 16–21.

Kingsley, D. M., Bland, A. E., Grubber, J. M., Marker, P. C., Russell, L. B., Copeland, N. G., and Jenkins, N. A. (1992). The mouse short ear skeletal morphogenesis locus is associated with defects in a bone morphogenetic member of the TGF beta superfamily. Cell 71, 399–410.

Klein, C. P., Patka, P., Wolke, J. G., de Blieck-Hogervorst, J. M., and de Groot, K. (1994). Long-term in vivo study of plasma-sprayed coatings on titanium alloys of tetracalcium phosphate, hydroxyapatite and alpha-tricalcium phosphate. Biomaterials 15, 146–50.

Komori, T., and Kishimoto, T. (1998). Cbfa1 in bone development. Curr. Opin. Genet. Dev. 8, 494–499.

Komori, T., Yagi, H., Nomura, S., Yamaguchi, A., Sasaki, K., Deguchi, K., Shimizu, Y., T., B. R., Gao, Y.-H., Inada, M. et al. (1997). Targeted disruption of Cbfa1 results in a complete lack of bone formation owing to maturational arrest of osteoblasts. Cell 89, 755–764.

Kononen, M., Hormia, M., Kivilahti, J., Hautaniemi, J., and Thesloff, I. (1992). Effect of surface processing on the attachment, orientation, and proliferation of human gingival fibroblasts on titanium. J. Biomed. Mater. Res. 36, 1325–1341.

Lee, M. H., Javed, A., Kim, H. J., Shin, H. I., Gutierrez, S., Choi, J. Y., Rosen, V., Stein, J. L., van Wijnen, A. J., Stein, G. S. et al. (1999). Transient upregulation of CBFA1 in response to bone morphogenetic protein-2 and transforming growth factor beta1 in C2C12 myogenic cells coincides with suppression of the myogenic phenotype but is not sufficient for osteoblast differentiation. J. Cell. Biochem. 73, 114–25.

Li, J. M., Tsuji, K., Komori, T., Miyazono, K., Wrana, J. L., Ito, Y., Nifuji, A., and Noda, M. (1998). Smad2 overexpression enhances smad4 gene expression and suppresses cbfa1 gene expression in osteoblastic osteosarcoma ROS17/2,8 cells and primary rat calvaria cells. J. Biol. Chem. 273, 31009–31015.

Lincks, J., Boyan, B. D., Blanchard, C. R., Lohmann, C. H., Liu, Y., Cochran, D. L., Dean, D. D., and Schwartz, Z. (1998). Response of MG63 osteoblast-like cells to titanium and titanium alloy is dependent on surface roughness and composition. Biomaterials 19, 2219–2232.

Lord, G., and Bancel, P. (1983). The madreporic cementless total hip arthroplasty. New experimental data and a seven-year clinical follow-up study. Clin. Orthop. Rel. Res. 176, 67–76.

Lord, G. A., Hardy, J. R., and Kummer, F. J. (1979). An uncemented total hip replacement: experimental study and review of 300 madreporique arthroplasties. Clin. Orthop. Rel. Res. 141, 2–16.

Maheshravari, G., G., B., Lauffenburger, D. A., Wells, A., and Griffith, L. G. (2000). Cell adhesion and motility depend on nanoscale RGD clustering. J. Cell. Sci. 113, 1677–1686.

Maistrelli, G., Mahomed, N., Garbuz, D., Fornasier, V., Harrington, I., and Binnington, A. (1992). Hydroxyapatite coating on a carbon composite hip implant in dogs. J. Bone Joint Surg. 74B, 452–456.

Marcolongo, M., Ducheyne, P., and Garino, J. (1998). Bioactive glass fiber polymeric composites bond to bone tissue. J. Biomed. Mater. Res. 39, 161–170.

Marcolongo, M., Ducheyne, P., and Lacourse, W. (1997). Surface reaction layer formation in vitro on a bioactive glass fiber/polymeric composite. J. Biomed. Mater. Res. 37, 440–448.

Marmor, L. (1976). Femoral loosening in total hip replacement. Clin. Orthop. Rel. Res. 121, 116–119.

Massague, J., Attisano, L., and Wrana, J. L. (1994). The TGF-β family and its composite receptors. Trends Cell. Biol. 4, 172–178.

Masuda, T., Yliheikkila, P. K., Felton, D. A., and Cooper, L. F. (1998). Generalizations regarding the process and phenomenon of osseointegration. Part I. In vivo studies. Int. J. Oral Maxillofac. Impl. 13, 17–29.

Maxian, S. H., Zawadsky, J. P., and Dunn, M. G. (1993). Mechanical and histological evaluation of amorphous calcium phosphate and poorly crystallized hydroxyapatite coating on titanium implants. J. Biomed. Mater. Res. 27, 717–728.

McCabe, L. R., Kockx, M., Lian, J., Stein, J., and Stein, G. (1995). Selective expression of fos- and jun-related genes during osteoblast proliferation and differentiation. Exp. Cell. Res. 218, 255–262.

McCarthy, T. L., Ji, C., Chen, Y., Kim, K. K., Imagawa, M., Ito, Y., and Centrella, M. (2000). Runt domain factor (Runx)-dependent effects on CCAAT/ enhancer-binding protein delta expression and activity in osteoblasts. J. Biol. Chem. 275, 21746–21753.

McCoy, T. H., Salvati, E. A., Ranawat, C. S., and Wilson, P. D. (1988). A fifteen-year follow-up study of one hundred Charnley low-friction arthroplasties. Orthop. Clin. North Am. 19, 467–476.

McFarland, C. P., Thomsa, C. H., DeFillipis, C., Steele, J. G., and Healy, K. E. (2000). Protein adsorption and cell attachment to patterned surfaces. Biomed. Mater. Res. 49, 200–210.

McLaughlin, J. R., and Lee, K. R. (1997). Total hip arthroplasty with an uncemented femoral component. Excellent results at ten-year follow-up. J. Bone Joint Surg. 79B, 900–907.

Meikle, M. C., Bord, S., Hembry, R. M., Compston, J., Croucher, P. I., and Reynolds, J. J. (1992). Human osteoblasts in culture synthesize collagenase and other matrix metalloproteinases in response to osteotropic hormones and cytokines. J. Cell. Sci. 101, 1093–1099.

Meyle, J., von Recum, A. F., Gibbesch, B., Huttemann, W., Schlagenhauf, U., and Schulte, W. (1991). Fibroblasts shape conformation to surface micromorphology. J. Appl. Biomater. 2, 273–276.

Moore, A. T. (1957). The self-locking metal hip prosthesis. J. Bone Joint Surg. 39A, 811.

Moore, A. T., and Bohlman, H. R. (1943). Metal hip joint. A case report. J. Bone Joint Surg. 25, 688.

Moursi, A. M., Damsky, C. H., Lull, J., Zimmerman, D., Doty, S. B., Aota, S., and Globus, R. K. (1996). Fibronectin regulates calvarial osteoblast differentiation. J. Cell. Sci. 109, 1369–1380.

Moursi, A. M., Globus, R. K., and Damsky, C. H. (1997). Interactions between integrin receptors and fibronectin are required for calvarial osteoblast differentiation in vitro. J. Cell. Sci. 110, 2187–2196.

Mundlos, S., Otto, F., Mundlos, C., Mulliken, J. B., Aylsworth, A. S., Albright, S., Lindhout, D., Cole, W. G., Henn, W., Knoll, J. H., et al. (1997). Mutations involving the transcription factor CBFA1 cause cleidocranial dysplasia Cell 89, 773–779.

Naji, A., and Harmand, M. (1990). Study of the effect of the surface state on the cytocompatibility of a Co-Cr alloy using human osteoblasts and fibroblasts. J. Biomed. Mater. Res. 24, 861–877.

Nishiguchi, S., Kato, H., Neo, M., Oka, M., Kim, H. M., Kokubo, T., and Manamuru, T. (2001). Alkali- and heat-treated porous titanium for orthopaedic implants. J. Biomed. Mater. Res. 54, 198–208.

Noth, U., Osyczka, A. M., Tuli, R., Hickok, N. J., Danielson, K. G., and Tuan, R. S. (2001). Trabecular bone-derived human mesenchymal stem cells. J. Bone Miner. Res. Submitted.

Otto, F., Thornell, A. P., Crompton, T., Denzel, A., Gilmour, K. C., Rosewell, I. R., Stamp, G. W., Beddington, R. S., Mundlos, S., Olsen, B. R. et al. (1997). Cbfa1, a candidate gene for cleidocranial dysplasia syndrome, is essential for osteoblast differentiation and bone development. Cell 89, 765–771.

Overgaard, L., Danielsen, N., and Bjursten, L. M. (1998). Anti-inflammatory properties of titanium in the joint environment. An experimental study in rats. J. Bone Joint Surg. 80B, 888–893.

Owen, T. A., Aronow, M., Shalhoub, V., Barone, L. M., Wilming, L., Tassinari, M. S., Kennedy, M. B., Pockwinse, S., Lian, J. B., and Stein, G. S. (1990). Progressive development of the rat osteoblast phenotype in vitro: reciprocal relationships in expression of genes associated with osteoblast proliferation and differentiation during formation of the bone extracellular matrix. J. Cell. Physiol. 143, 420–430.

Park, A., Wu, B., and Griffith, L. (1998). Integration of surface modification and 3D fabrication techniques to prepare patterned poly (L-lactide) substrates allowing regionally selective cell adhesion. J. Biomater. Sci. Polym. Ed. 9, 89–110.

Pazzaglia, U. E., Brossa, F., Zatti, G., Chiesa, R., and Andrini, L. (1998). The relevance of hydroxyapatite and spongious titanium coatings in fixation of cementless stems. An experimental comparative study in rat femur employing histological and microangiographic techniques. Arch. Orthop. Trauma Surg. 117, 279–285.

Qiu, Q., Sayer, M., Kawaja, M., Shen, X., and Davies, J. E. (1998). Attachment, morphology and protein expression of rat marrow stromal cells cultured on charged substrate surfaces. J. Biomed. Mater. Res. 42, 117–127.

Rahal, M. D., Branemark, P. I., and Osmond, D. G. (1993). Response of bone marrow to titanium implants: osseointegration and the establishment of a bone marrow-titanium interface in mice. Intl. J. Oral Maxillofac. Imp. 8, 573–579.

Rezania, A., and Healy, K. E. (1999). Integrin subunits responsible for adhesion of human osteoblast-like cells to biomimetic peptide surfaces. J. Orthop. Res. 17, 615–623.

Rezania, A., and Healy, K. E. (2000). The effect of peptide surface density on mineralization of a matrix deposited by osteogenic cells. J. Biomed. Mater. Res. 52, 595–600.

Robey, P. G., and Termine, J. D. (1985). Human bone cells in vitro. Calcif. Tissue Int. 37, 453–460.

Rothman, R. H., and Cohn, J. C. (1990). Cemented versus cementless total hip arthroplasty. A critical review. Clin. Orthop. Rel. Res. 254, 153–169.

Ruoslahti, E. (1991). Integrins. J. Clin. Invest. 87, 1–5.

Ruoslahti, E. (1996). RGD and other recognition sequences for integrins. Annu. Rev. Cell Dev. Biol. 1996, 697–715.

Ruoslahti, E., Noble, N. A., Kagami, S., and Border, W. A. (1994). Integrins. Kidney Int. 44, S17–S22.

Ruoslahti, E., and Reed, J. C. (1994). Anchorage dependence, integrins, and apoptosis. Cell 77, 477–478.

Sakalkale, D. P., Eng, K., Hozack, W. J., and Rothman, R. H. (1999). Minimum 10-year results of a tapered cementless hip replacement. Clin. Orthop. Rel. Res. 362, 138–144.

Salvati, E. A., Wilson, P. D., Jolley, M. N., Vakili, F., Aglietti, P., and Brown, G. C. (1981). A ten-year follow-up study of our first one hundred consecutive Charnley total hip replacements. J. Bone Joint Surg. 63A, 753–767.

Santavirta, S., Gristina, A., and Konttinen, Y. T. (1992). Cemented versus cementless hip arthroplasty. A review of prosthetic biocompatibility. Acta Orthop. Scand. 63, 225–232.

Schaller, M. D., and Parsons, J. T. (1994). Focal adhesion kinase and associated proteins. Curr. Opin. Cell Biol. 6, 705–710.

Selvamurugan, N., Pulumati, M. R., Tyson, D. R., and Partridge, N. C. (2000). Parathyroid hormone regulation of the rat collagenase-3 promoter by protein kinase A–dependent transactivation of core binding factor $\alpha 1$. J. Biol. Chem. 275, 5037–5042.

Shah, A. K., Lazatin, J., Sinha, R. K., Lennox, T., Hickok, N. J., and Tuan, R. S. (1999a). Mechanism of BMP-2 stimulated adhesion of osteoblastic cells to titanium alloy. Biol. Cell 91, 131–142.

Shah, A. K., Sinha, R. K., Hickok, N. J., and Tuan, R. S. (1999b). High-resolution morphometric analysis of human osteoblastic cell adhesion on clinically relevant orthopedic alloys. Bone 24, 499–506.

Sinha, R. K., Morris, F., Shah, S. A., and Tuan, R. S. (1994). Surface composition of orthopaedic implant metals regulates cell attachment spreading, and cytoskeletal organization of primary human osteoblasts in vitro. Clin. Orthop. 305, 258–272.

Sinha, R. K., and Tuan, R. S. (1996a). In vitro analysis of the bone-implant interface. Semin. Arthrop. (Classics) 7, 47–57.

Sinha, R. K., and Tuan, R. S. (1996b). Regulation of human osteoblast integrin expression by othopedic implant materials. Bone 18, 451–457.

Smith, E., Frenkel, B., Schlegel, R., Giordano, A., Lian, J. B., Stein, J. L., and Stein, G. S. (1995). Expression of cell cycle regulatory factors in differentiating osteoblasts: postproliferative up-regulation of cyclins B and E. Cancer Res. 55, 5019–5024.

Stein, G. S., Lian, J. B., Stein, J. L., and van Wijnen, A. J. (2000). Bone tissue specific transcriptional control: options for targeting gene therapy to the skeleton. Cancer 88, 2899–2902.

Sumner, D. R., Turner, T. M., Purchio, A. F., Gombotz, W. R., Urban, R. M., and Galante, J. O. (1995). Enhancement of bone ingrowth by transforming growth factor-beta. J. Bone Joint Surg. 77A, 1135–1147.

Sumner, D. R., Turner, T. M., Urban, R. M., Leven, R. M., Hawkins, M., Nichols, E. H., and McPherson, J. M. (2001). Locally derived rhTGF-β2 enhances bone ingrowth and bone regeneration at local and remote sites of skeletal injury. J. Orthop. Res. 19, 85–94.

Tang, L., and Eaton, J. W. (1995). Inflammatory responses to biomaterials. Am. J. Clin. Pathol. 103, 466–471.

Thomsen, P., and Ericson, L. E. (1991). Inflammatory Cell Response to Bone Implant Surfaces. In The Bone-Biomaterial Interface, (ed. J. E. Davies), pp. 153–164. Buffalo, NY: University of Toronto Press.

Tintu, Y., Parhami, F., Le, V., Karsenty, G., and Demer, L. L. (1999). Inhibition of osteoblast-specific transcription factor Cbfa1 by the cAMP pathway in osteoblastic cells: Ubiquitin/proteasome dependent regulation. J. Biol. Chem. 274, 28875–28879.

Trentacosta, J. D., and Cheban, J. C. (1995). Lipid sensitivity of polyaryl-etherketones and polysulfone. Proc. Orthop. Res. Soc. 41, 783.

Verheyen, C. C., de Wijn, J. R., van Blitterswijk, C. A., de Groot, K., and Rozing, P. M. (1993). Hydroxylapatite/poly(L-lactide) composites: an animal study on push-out strengths and interface histology. J. Biomed. Mater. Res. 27, 433–444.

Welsh, R. P., Pilliar, R. M., and Macnab, I. (1971). Surgical implants. The role of surface porosity in fixation to bone and acrylic. J. Bone Joint Surg. 53A, 963–977.

Wen, H. B., de Wijn, J. R., Cui, F. Z., and DeGroot, K. (1998). Preparation of bioactive Ti6Al4V surfaces by a simple method. Biomaterials 19, 215–221.

Wroblewski, B. M. (1986). 15–21 year results of the Charnley low-friction arthroplasty. Clin. Orthop. Rel. Res. 211, 30–35.

Xiao, G., Jiang, D., Thomas, P., Benson, M. D., Guan, K., Karsenty, G., and Franceschi, R. T. (2000). MAPK pathways active and phosphorylate the osteoblast-specific transcription factor, Cbfa1. J. Biol. Chem. 275, 4453–4459.

Xiao, Z. S., Thomas, R., Hinson, T. K., and Quarles, L. D. (1998). Genomic structure and isoform expression of the mouse, rat and human Cbfa1/Osf2 transcription factor. Gene 214, 187–197.

Zhu, Y., Organesian, A., Keene, D. R., and Sandell, L. J. (1999). Type IIA procollagen containing the cysteine-rich amino propeptide is deposited in the extracellular matrix of prechondrogenic tissue and binds to TGF-β1 and BMP-2. J. Cell Biol. 144, 1069–1080.

Zimmerman, M., Boone, P., Scalzo, H., and Parsons, J. (1993). A mechanical and histological analysis of the bonding of bone to hydroxylapatite/polymer composite coatings. In Composite Materials for Implant Application in the Human Body: Characterization and Testing. In ASTM STP, vol. 1178 (eds. R. J., and. L. Gilbertson), pp. 145–155. Philadelphia: American Society for Testing and Materials.

6

Osteolysis in Total Hip Arthroplasty: Biological and Clinical Aspects

Gun-Il Im,* Rajiv K. Sethi, Harry E. Rubash, and Arun S. Shanbhag
Massachusetts General Hospital and Harvard Medical School, Boston, Massachusetts

I. PATHOPHYSIOLOGY

A. Historical Background and Pathophysiology

Osteolysis is the bone loss that results from biological processes occurring at the metal-bone or cement-bone interface. Clinical manifestations of osteolysis range from the appearance of new radiolucent lines around previously well-fixed implants, which progress slowly and eventually result in mechanical instability, to the rapid formation of either focal or expansile lesions. The term *aseptic loosening* was previously used to define the linear dissecting processes and *osteolysis* to define the lytic bone loss. These terms are now considered to describe different manifestations of the same biological phenomenon, resulting in both aseptic loosening and osteolysis (1).

   Aseptic loosening of prosthetic components has been observed since the inception of joint replacement in the early 1960s. Charnley first recognized this process when the polytetrafluoroethylene (PTFE) acetabular components he used required revision within 1 to 3 years (2–4). After switching to polyethylene cups, Charnley saw a dramatic decrease in the amount of wear debris generated and consequently the need for revision surgery. In those cases that did require revision, he found granulomatous tissues laden with inflammatory cells surrounding the implant at the cement–bone inter-

---

**Current affiliation*: Hallym University Hospital, Chunchon, South Korea.

face. He believed that those findings suggested of infection even when bacteriological evidence did not exist (3,5). Harris and associates reported extensive localized bone resorption in four femoral components that did not have gross loosening or infection and suggested a benign, noninflammatory adverse tissue response (6).

Based on extensive histopathological analysis, Willert and Semlitsch (7) proposed that aseptic loosening resulted from excess wear debris within macrophages of the periprosthetic tissue. They suggested that wear debris was biologically active and induced a macrophage response in the tissue surrounding the implant. Their views were supported by Mirra et al. (8), who found sheets of macrophages in a fibrous stroma intermingled with multinucleated giant cells, polymethylmethacrylate (PMMA) particles, and metallic wear debris. Goldring et al. (9) demonstrated that these interfacial membranes were capable of producing collagenase and prostaglandin E_2 (PGE_2), a powerful stimulator of bone resorption in vivo. Numerous investigators have shown that the cellular activity within this membrane produces a variety of cytokines, enzymes, prostaglandins, and other mediators that stimulate osteoclastic bone resorption and fibrous tissue formation (10,11). Goodman et al. reported that tissues around loose total hip replacements released significantly higher levels of PGE_2 than tissues around stable components. Kim et al. analyzed a spectrum of cytokines and osteolytic mediators [stromelysin, interleukin (IL)-1α, IL-1β, IL-6, tumor necrosis factor (TNF)-α, and PGE_2] and reported that few differences existed between tissues from failed cemented and uncemented hip components, implying similar mechanisms of aseptic loosening (12). The presence of an ultrahigh-molecular-weight polyethylene (UHMWPE) component was associated with higher levels of inflammatory mediators such as collagenase and IL-1β (13). Shanbhag et al. compared the levels of several pro- and anti-inflammatory cytokines and mediators and suggested that the periprosthetic tissues may represent a biochemically imbalanced situation (11) wherein the mediators initiating and maintaining the inflammatory processes are no longer regulated by anti-inflammatory mediators due to a constant stimulation of the phagocytic cells by wear debris (11).

Jiranek et al. (14) used in situ hybridization to detect the source of cytokines from loose acetabular components. They detected IL-1β protein bound to both macrophages and fibroblasts, but the messenger RNA for IL-1β was detected only within macrophages. Furthermore, using RNA isolation techniques and the quantitative polymerase chain reaction, Glant et al. have shown that cells of interfacial membranes have a high latent capacity to express the gene coding for IL-1 in response to a change in the microenvironment (15).

During the early days of total joint arthroplasty, prosthetic fixation was accomplished through cementing techniques and osteolysis was associated with fragmentation of the cement mantle. Many investigators thus hypothesized that PMMA wear debris was the cause of osteolysis and aseptic loosening, leading to the term *cement disease* (16). Therefore, improvements in cementing techniques and development of uncemented fixation were emphasized as a means to reduce the incidence of aseptic loosening (17,18). Even with these improvements and the introduction of uncemented total hip arthroplasty, the problems of osteolysis and aseptic loosening have persisted. This has led clinicians and researchers to propose that wear debris from other sources, such as UHMWPE and metal, as potential causes of osteolysis and subsequent aseptic loosening (19,20).

B.   Generation of Wear Debris

While wear debris can arise from several sources around total hip components, the predominant wear debris identified in osteolytic lesions, representing 70–95% of the debris burden is particulate UHMWPE (21,22). From the articulating surface of the UHMWPE acetabular liner, UHMWPE debris present around failed uncemented femoral components are predominantly spheroids ranging from 0.1 to 2.0 μm in size, with interconnecting fibrils (21,22) (Figure 1). Wear also occurs at the nonarticulating surface of the

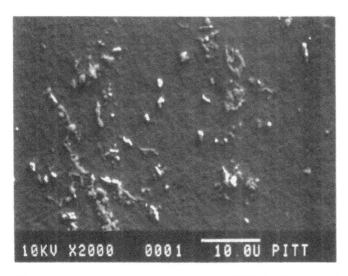

Figure 1   Scanning electromicrograph of UHMWPE (ultrahigh-molecular-weight polyethylene) particles isolated from failed total hip arthroplasties.

UHMWPE acetabular liner, and unfilled screw holes in the metal backing of the acetabular component can become repositories of wear debris (19,23). Unfilled screw holes provide access for wear debris to migrate to the area behind the ingrowth cup, resulting in pelvic osteolysis (24,25). Metal screws that had been used to provide initial cup stability can become a source of fretting and corrosion, causing metal debris. Another important source of metallic debris is fretting corrosion at the modular head and neck junction of the femoral component. Metallic wear debris represents a minor fraction of the debris burden and typically results from abrasion of the stem against bone or cement polishing and lapping treatments of the implant (21,22,26). Around joint replacements, debris can also be generated from unusual sources such as from degradation of the hydroxyapatite coatings (27), fragmentation of cables used for trochanteric fixation (28), as well as residuals from the grit blasting and polishing of the components (29).

C. Particle Dynamics

Wear-debris particles generated within the joint space are phagocytosed by inflammatory cells associated with the joint capsule. Smaller particles (<7 μm) are generally retained within macrophages, while foreign-body giant cells surround larger nonphagocytosable particles. Depending on the biocompatibility and toxicity of the debris material, there is a variable amount of cellular necrosis and associated infiltration by inflammatory cells.

Wear debris is cleared from the joint space by macrophage phagocytosis and transported via the lymphatic system to the reticuloendothelial system (7,30). If the amount of wear debris generated exceeds the capacity of the cells to clear it, granulation tissue is formed at the periprosthetic interface, which compromises bony anchors and results in implant loosening (7,20). Willert et al. and later Schmalzried et al. suggested the concept of the "effective joint space" to indicate that debris generated at the articulation can be carried to all periprosthetic regions by the joint fluid (7,20,30). It has also been suggested that the flow pattern of the wear debris is determined by the degree of access to the interfaces (31–33). Dispersion of particles along the interface is believed to result in linear osteolysis, whereas accumulation in discrete areas is thought to lead to focal osteolysis, which in turn may be associated with stable and loose components (34,35).

D. In Vitro and In Vivo Models for Osteolysis

Because the periprosthetic tissues usually contain a variety of sizes and compositions of particulate debris, it was not possible to determine which of the debris species is primarily involved in stimulating the macrophages to release the mediators. Macrophages cultured with particles in vitro have thus been used as model systems for studying the sequence of events occurring in the process of osteolysis.

Using similarly sized CoCr-alloy and Ti-alloy particles, Haynes et al. (36) studied their ability to stimulate rat peritoneal macrophages to release inflammatory mediators. They found that while CoCr-alloy particles were very toxic and caused cell death, Ti-alloy particles were less toxic and induced the synthesis and release of significant levels of numerous inflammatory mediators such as PGE_2, IL-1, IL-6, and TNF-α. Shanbhag et al. (37) studied the stimulatory capabilities of titanium-aluminum-vanadium (TiAlV), commercially pure titanium (CpTi), and UHMWPE particles retrieved from interfacial tissues, and UHMWPE particles fabricated in the laboratory in clinically similar sizes. TiAlV and CpTi particles were found to be the most stimulatory in eliciting PGE_2, IL-1α, IL-1β, and IL-6 from monocytes. Recent studies have documented that when macrophages are stimulated with wear particles, they can also synthesize and release nitric oxide (NO), in addition to the more traditional mediators and cytokines (38). Because NO is a biologically ubiquitous free radical with many physiological roles, its release may add an extra tier of complexity in understanding the consequences of macrophage–particle interactions. In addition to macrophages, fibroblasts have been investigated as important contributors to periprosthetic bone loss. Maloney et al. reported that a low concentration of Ti and Ti-alloy particles stimulate fibroblast proliferation (39). Yao et al. reported that Ti particles can directly stimulate fibroblasts to produce high levels of collagenase and stromelysin (at both mRNA and protein levels), which can degrade the organic components of bone. In addition, Ti-stimulated fibroblasts release de novo synthesized factor(s) that suppress collagen synthesis in osteoblast cells (40). Collectively, different types of cells within the periprosthetic granulomatous tissues produce various cellular mediators with both autocrine and paracrine function. The autocrine-paracrine effect may result in the activation of macrophages and osteoclasts to resorb adjacent bone (41).

In vivo studies are required to understand the biocompatibility of bulk and particulate materials and the overall effect of these cytokines and mediators released in response to wear debris. Cohen (42) looked at the subcutaneous tissue response in rabbits to different forms and sizes of commonly used CoCr alloy and stainless steel particles. He reported that larger particles (between 5 and 40 μm) provoked very little inflammatory response and mainly took the form of a fibrous tissue encapsulation. On the other hand, finer particles were severely inflammatory and usually associated with tissue necrosis, acute inflammation, and extensive fibrosis. Numerous other studies have confirmed this aspect of host response (43–46).

The enhanced biological response to finer particles was more recently demonstrated by Goodman et al.(45,47,48). Using a tibial defect in a rabbit model, they demonstrated that particulate debris of either PMMA or UHMWPE can elicit the formation of inflammatory granulomatous tissue in an osseous cavity. The particles evoked an intense fibrohistiocytic and giant cell response that was similar to that surrounding loose implants (45,47,48). On the other hand, bulk forms of these biomaterials were surrounded by only a thin fibrous membrane (47,49). Using a subcutaneous rat air-pouch model, Gelb et al. (50) also demonstrated that smaller, irregularly shaped particles allowed for significantly greater amounts of inflammatory mediators such as TNF-α and neutral metalloproteinase. These studies are in agreement with in vitro macrophage models used to study the biological nature of particles of different sizes and compositions (46,51,52).

Spector et al. (53) used a canine model to study the periprosthetic response to implanted PMMA particles. A femoral component was placed in an overreamed dog femur along with PMMA particles. Twelve weeks after surgery, radiolucent lines characteristic of implant loosening were observed at the bone–cement interface and a fibrous tissue lining was observed at the interface when the femora were harvested. Dowd et al. (54) developed a canine model for uncemented total hip arthroplasty. A fiber metal–coated porous TiAlV femoral component articulated against an UHMWPE acetabular liner with a fiber mesh–backed metal shell. Particulate Ti-alloy, CoCr-alloy, or high-density polyethylene was placed at the bone–implant interface. At 12 weeks after surgery, granulomatous tissue was observed at the bone–implant interface: it contained fibroblasts, macrophages, and foreign-body giant cells with intra- and extracellular particulate wear debris. Histologically, it resembled tissues retrieved from clinically loosened arthroplasty components (11). When these membranous tissues were placed in organ culture, they released significant levels of inflammatory cytokines and mediators (54). The study was further enhanced by using UHMWPE particles in clinically similar sizes and shapes and extending the postoperative period to 24 weeks. The pattern of bone loss observed radiographically and associated periosteal reaction was similar to that observed in the clinical setting following total joint arthroplasty (55) (Figure 2).

E.   Other Mechanisms Inducing Osteolysis

While the biological response to wear debris is a widely studied mechanism of implant loosening, there are other possible scenarios that can also lead to implant loosening. Mechanical factors may play an important role. For example, motion of the prosthesis can affect the cellular makeup around the prostheses in two ways: First, by directly activating macrophages to produce

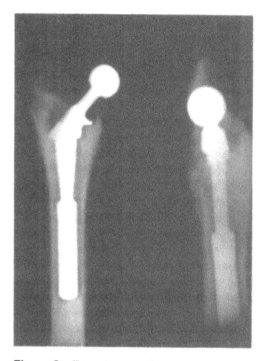

Figure 2 Extensive osteolysis induced with UHMWPE particles in dog model.

cytokines and metalloproteinases thus initiating the inflammatory cascade, and second, by creating conditions that promote mechanical wear and corrosion, thus yielding both metallic and polymeric debris in addition to metal ions, which activate the inflammatory process. Other mechanical factors have also been implicated as causes of aseptic loosening. Some have suggested that the surgical procedure itself may initiate the loosening process (8,56–58). Drilling, reaming, thermal effects of polymerization, and toxicity of the PMMA bone cement monomer can cause necrosis of osseous tissue surrounding implants (59,60). The necrotic tissue is replaced by fibrous tissue, preventing interdigitation of the cement. An initially successful fixation can also fail as the result of fatigue or shock loading (61). The motion of the loosened implant then increases the number and severity of fractures along the interface and stimulates an inflammatory tissue reaction to the particulate PMMA debris in cemented implants. In addition, a combination of high axial loading and poor implant design can also fracture the cement mantle, leading to an adverse foreign-body tissue reaction (61). Adaptive remodeling around the femoral stems also can lead to increased motion at the implant–cement and cement–bone interfaces, leading to cement fatigue and loss of fixation.

Because prosthetic components are constantly exposed to the biological environment, including serum proteins and inflammatory cells involved in the host's response to foreign antigens, it is possible that the host's immune response may be involved in aseptic loosening. Evans et al. (62) were among the first to suggest that an immune response to metal ions released from components may initiate the loosening process. Using an epicutaneous patch test, they found that 9 of 14 patients with loose metal-on-metal total hip implants were sensitive to one or more components of the alloy. In contrast, none of the 24 patients with well-fixed components were sensitive. These investigators postulated that some patients could become sensitized to the cobalt (Co), chromium (Cr), or nickel (Ni) ions released in the local tissues. The subsequent delayed-type IV hypersensitivity reaction could cause obliterative changes in blood vessels of the bone adjacent to the implant, leading to bone death. Since avascular bone is extremely susceptible to fatigue, bony anchors stabilizing the cement mantle are replaced by fibrous tissue at the bone–cement interface, leading to a loose component.

In many subsequent studies of patients with loose metal-on-metal or metal-on-polymer hip implants, delayed hypersensitivity to metal was not associated with aseptic loosening (63–65). Other investigators examined retrieved interfacial tissues from failed cemented and uncemented implants (66–68). Using antibodies to surface receptors for various cell types, they frequently observed T cells and activated macrophages in addition to an absence of B cells or plasma cells. It can be seen from the evidence presented above that there is controversy regarding the role of the immune response in aseptic loosening or osteolysis.

II. INCIDENCE

The incidence of osteolysis in hip replacement is most easily described in terms of the components and their mode of fixation. For cemented cups, the incidence of focal osteolysis has been reported from 0 to 19%, with loss of fixation occurring at rates between 0 and 44% at 8 to 10 years (1). The best result on polyethylene cups implanted using first-generation cementing techniques is from Salvati and associates. At 10 years, two of the patients (3.7%) demonstrated linear osteolysis at the cement–bone interface, leading to component loosening; no patient had expansile osteolysis. Others have reported loosening rates due to linear osteolysis of 11 to 23% for first-generation cemented polyethylene cups after a minimum of 10 years (61,69). Mac-Kenzie et al. reported the results of all-polyethylene cups implanted with second-generation cementing technique in patients with developmental dysplasia or chronic dislocation of the hip. They found focal osteolysis in 7 of 37 patients (19%), and in 16 of 59 patients (27%); linear osteolysis resulted in loosening after an average of 192 months. Second-generation cementing techniques did not show any improvement in a study by Mulroy and Harris (70), with linear osteolysis leading to loosening in 44% of patients a minimum of 14 years after implantation (71).

Acetabular components inserted without cement have shown better results at 5 to 7 years than those implanted with cement. Maloney and colleagues have shown that osteolysis developed in 22% of hip replacements in patients younger than 50 years of age at the time of their index operation after 81 month follow-up of Harris-Galante-I cementless acetabular components. For patients older than 50 years of age at the time of surgery only 7.8% (8 hips) had developed osteolysis of the pelvis (72). For the PCA cup (Howmedica, East Rutherford, NJ), rates of focal osteolysis have been higher, ranging from 1% at 4 years to 36% after more than 5 years (1). Other variables, such as younger age of patients, higher activity levels, and 32-mm heads have been implicated in the high rates of osteolysis. In addition, shedding of the porous coating can accelerate third-body wear. Engh et al. (73,74) reported focal osteolysis in 20% of their patients and loosening in 4% after follow-up of 84–102 months with nonmodular AML (Anatomic Medullary Locking, Warsaw, IN) cups with 32-mm heads.

Threaded cups such as T-TAP (Biomet, Warsaw, IN) have also produced high rates of osteolysis (59 of 68 patients, or 87%) and osteolysis-associated loosening (26 of 68, or 38%) after only 6 years (75). Similarly, 95 of 378 (25%) threaded Mecring (Mecron, Berlin, Germany) cups were found to be radiographically loose only 4.5 years after implantation (76). Although initially quite stable, screw-in cups apparently cause a high concentration of local stress and possibly pressure necrosis. Brujin et al. also suggested that such stress causes bone resorption, decreased stability, increased micromotion, and greater access of wear particles to the metal–bone interface, resulting in rapidly progressive osteolysis. Due to their unusually high rate of failure, threaded acetabular cups are no longer used in the United States (76).

While femoral components inserted with the first-generation cementing techniques loosened at rates between 11 and 30% at 10 years (1), those inserted using second- or third-generation cementing techniques have enjoyed excellent results in terms of osteolysis, loosening, and revision rates. Several authors have reported the long-term incidence of focal osteolysis to be less than 8%, even in difficult reconstructions (1). Intermediate- to long-term rates of loosening associated with osteolysis have increased from 1.5 or 3 to 7% at latest follow-up (1). In a recent study by Clohisy et al. of 86

primary hybrid total hip replacements performed with insertion of the acetabular component without cement and a precoated femoral component with
cement, with an average ten year follow-up, 7 hips had osteolytic areas
located in the proximal aspect of the most proximal zones of Gruen et al.
and 5 had small osteolytic lesions in more distal areas (77). Smith and
colleagues have reported a 10- to 13-year follow-up study with the insertion
of a hemispherical porous-coated acetabular component inserted without cement and the use of screws and a femoral component inserted with second-
generation cementing technique. They found that pelvic osteolysis developed
in 1 hip (2%), femoral osteolysis in 8 hips (15%), and distal femoral osteolysis in 3 hips (6%) (78).

The incidence of osteolysis in femurs with first-generation uncemented
stems is also quite high. The HGP prosthesis was associated with focal
osteolysis rates of 13–52% over short to intermediate follow-up periods (1)
(Figure 3). The incidence of loosening of these components has been between 8 and 32%. With the PCA stem (1), the incidence of osteolysis was

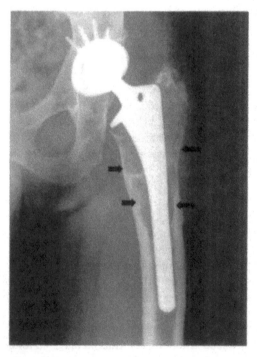

Figure 3 Radiograph demonstrating severe osteolysis extending to diaphysis (arrow) after THA with a HGP stem.

also quite high (13–25%) at 50–84 month follow-up. Although studies suggested high rates (32–34%) of osteolysis with the AML stem (73,74), these lesions were also confined to zones 1 and 7, were quite small, and did not result in loosening. Kim and colleagues have recently shown with 11.3 year follow-up of the AML prosthesis, that 38% of their hips had acetabular and femoral osteolysis and 17% had femoral osteolysis only (79). Hellman and associates followed for 119 months 76 hips with porous-coated Omnifit femoral and acetabular components. They reported that 36% had femoral osteolysis (80).

Newer-generation of uncemented stems do not have adequate follow-up, as the first-generation stems do. Therefore direct comparisons are not possible at this time. Nevertheless, favorable results and fewer incidents of osteolysis are being reported so far. Sakalkale et al. reviewed 71 total hip arthroplasties with a cementless, wedge-fit, cobalt chrome femoral component (Taperloc stem, Biomet, Warsaw, IN) at a minimum 10-year follow-up (mean, 11.5 years). Despite the high incidence of acetabular osteolysis, no osteolysis was seen on the femoral side distal to the lesser trochanter (81). McLaughlin et al. also reported results with the Taperloc femoral component in younger patients (mean, 37 years; range, 20–50 years; and follow-up 10.2 years). In 100 total hip arthroplasties, 2 femoral components were revised for reasons other than aseptic loosening or osteolysis. In the 98 total hip arthroplasties, femoral cortical osteolysis occurred in 7 (7%) hips; major lysis was present in only 1 (1%) (82). Emerson et al. evaluated the follow-up results of the Mallory-Head (Biomet, Warsaw, IN) femoral component with circumferential plasma-spray porous coating. When the 90 hips had been followed for 7.5 years; 9 of 90 hips (10%) were found to have femoral osteolysis. Osteolysis remote from the joint space (distal to zones 1 and 7) was found in none of those 9 stems (83). Christie et al. reported results of the S-ROM (Joint Medical Products, Stamford, CT) modular femoral stem without cement in a series of 175 hips with complete clinical and radiographic data. The average age of the patients was 59 (range 22–93) years. The duration of clinical follow-up averaged 5.3 years. Periprosthetic osteolytic lesions were present around 8 stems (5%), being localized within the greater trochanter or the proximal-medial portion of the femoral neck. No osteolytic lesions were evident distal to the stem–sleeve junction (84). Sinha followed up 124 hips with Multilock stem (Zimmer, Warsaw, IN) for 5 to 9 years. There were no cases of femoral diaphyseal osteolysis, even though 33 (27%) stems had minor osteolysis in zone 1 or 7 (Sinha and Rubash, unpublished report).

Metal-on-metal and ceramic-on-ceramic articulations have been developed in an attempt to decrease wear and are currently in use by orthopaedic surgeons. Dorr and associates reported midterm results from Metasul metal-on-metal articulation in 56 patients (56 hips). After a follow-up period of 5.2 years (range, 4–6.8 years), no hip had radiographic evidence of acetabular osteolysis and two hips had calcar resorption, but there was no other radiographic evidence of focal osteolysis (85). While these results are promising, a longer period of follow-up is needed, because the incidence of osteolysis usually goes up after 5 years of implantation (1). Ceramic-on-ceramic articulations also has the potential to generate wear particles, thus predisposing patients to osteolysis. Yoon and associates reported that femoral osteolysis developed in 23 hips (22%) from103 of early design after mean follow-up period of 92 months (86). More advanced designs of ceramic-on-ceramic total hip arthroplasties have been developed and used in Europe and Asia since 1995. Their long-term results are not currently available. Bizot and associates reported the results from 234 consecutive alumina-on-alumina hip replacements, using a press-fit metal-backed socket, performed on 214 patients. At the median follow-up of 7.8 years, radiographic data were documented for 134 patients (143 hips). Three sockets (2%) had a complete and nonprogressive radiolucent line less than 1 mm thick, one stem (0.7%) had lucencies involving five zones, and two stems (1.4%) had isolated femoral osteolysis. Neither component migration nor acetabular osteolysis were detected (87).

III. CLINICAL MANIFESTATION

A. Cemented THA

Aseptic loosening was first identified around cemented components and subsequently was defined as the development of a radiolucent line around a previously well-fixed prosthesis (1). The natural history of this linear radiolucency at the bone-cement interface with cemented components is important (61). When the zone of radiolucency is wider than 2 mm or becomes circumferential, the prosthesis is considered to be at risk for loosening (88). The radiolucency appears to progress from the intra-articular margin of the interface until it extends circumferentially. On the other hand, focal osteolysis may present as a circumferential periprosthetic endosteal scalloping of bone at the cement–bone interface. Such focal areas of bone loss possibly are more accessible to particulate debris or have a higher concentration of it, but they appear to exhibit similar biological activity (89).

1. Cemented Acetabular Component

With cemented acetabular components, joint fluid and wear particles tend to deposit at the cement–bone interface. The soft tissue membrane created by the inflammatory response to wear particles proceeds along the cement–bone interface, often leading to its damage. As the interfacial disruption progresses to the acetabular dome, fixation can be lost. Radiographically, the osteolytic pattern is usually linear, with the radiolucency occurring at the cement–bone interface. The component tends to migrate into the radiolucent areas in the superior and medial aspects of the acetabulum and may obliterate the radiolucent line. However, a distinct zone will be seen in the inferior aspects of the socket. Bone loss can be extensive, especially if the disease has been long standing and untreated (1) (Figure 4).

2. Cemented Femoral Component

In hip replacements with a cemented femoral component, the path of least resistance for joint fluid migration on the femoral side is alongside the cement–metal or the cement–bone interface. Linear and focal or expansile lesions all have been noted with both the stable and unstable stems (34,74,90–92). Several authors have demonstrated the possibility for a pathway to form at the stem–cement interface (34,92). The formation of such a passage may be a predisposing factor for the focal lytic lesions that tend to develop around the distal aspect of an otherwise well-fixed cemented femoral component. Fluid and particles are driven along the interface by the relatively high intra-articular pressures generated during normal gait, which may reach the cement–bone interface via defects in the cement mantle (92).

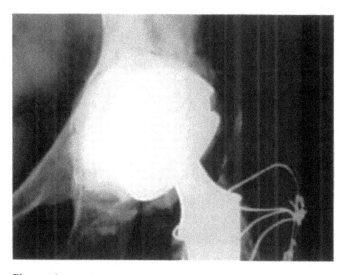

Figure 4 Acetabular osteolysis in a cemented cup.

The resulting biological reaction can lead to focal osteolysis in the presence of a well-fixed cemented stem (1) (Figure 5).

Particles with biological reactivity can also migrate along the cement–bone interface of femoral components. However, in the absence of cement fracture or debonding at the cement–metal interface, the femoral component usually does not loosen for years, probably because of the restricted surface area for access to the femoral canal and the large surface area of fixation (33,93). The 2–3 cm of disruption of the proximal cement–bone interface due to linear osteolysis (i.e., membrane formation) will not significantly compromise the femoral component's stability, whereas 2–3 cm of disruption at the cement–bone interface in the acetabular socket is likely to have a significant effect on implant stability. With modern cementing technique, osteolysis around the proximal femur is rarely the primary cause of loosening (70,71). However, with stem debonding or cement fracture, cement debris is produced. With prolonged access to the cement–bone interface, the

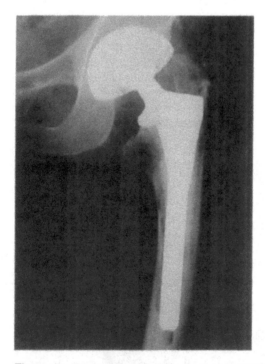

Figure 5 Femoral osteolysis in a cemented THA. Both linear and focal radiolucency (arrow) can be observed.

debris can promote the development of osteolysis as a secondary phenomenon.

A complete radiolucency at the cement–bone interface suggests probable loosening, whereas 50–99% radiolucency suggests possible loosening.
Prudent interpretation of the radiolucent line is critical in determining
whether the radiographic picture is suggestive of linear osteolysis or remodeling (94).

B. Cementless THA

1. The Cementless Acetabular Component

The pattern of osteolysis around a cementless socket often depends on
whether bone ingrowth has occurred. If the socket is stabilized by bone
ingrowth, the path of least resistance is via areas that do not have bone
ingrowth or via screw holes, which allow particles to migrate into the trabecular bone of the ilium, ischium, and pubis. This results in a distinct
pattern of osteolysis in ingrown cups. High particle loads in these areas may
be more likely to result in rapidly growing, expansive lesions with indirect
margins, leading to osteolysis and progressive bone loss. Loosening often
does not result until bone loss is extensive; thus implant failure may be
acute and catastrophic, with the patient remaining clinically asymptomatic
until the component has loosened (Figure 6). The second pattern of acetabular osteolysis is a slowly growing radiolucency that has sclerotic osseous
margins (1). This pattern of osteolysis is quite similar to that seen with
cemented sockets results in progressive, indolent bone loss with subsequent
clinical loosening. These linear radiolucent lines may also be seen in an
uncemented implant that has not stabilized and is loose (aseptic). An important caveat is that radiographs consistently underestimate the size of osteolytic lesions. The combination of iliac oblique views is helpful in evaluating the size of a lesion, since the radiographic appearance is dependent
on the mode of fixation (95).

The patterns of osteolysis around uncemented cups depend on the cup
design. In a 7-year follow-up study (74) on one-piece metal-backed AML
sintered-bead porous-coated cups, 14 (20%) had radiolucent lines in at least
one zone, most commonly zone 3. No component had circumferential linear
osteolysis. One or more periarticular focal lesions occurred in 18% of the
cups. Two cups (3%) also had osteolytic areas remote from the joint. Studies
on PCA cups reported an equal incidence of focal osteolysis in all three
zones (96,97). Reports have noted the occurrence of nonprogressive radiolucent lines around HG-I cups, with few focal osteolytic areas noted at 7 to
11 years of follow-up (97,98).

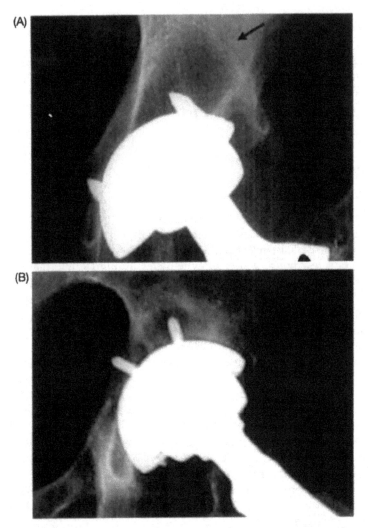

Figure 6 Radiographs showing osteolysis of cementless acetabular component
with marked wear of polyethylene liner (A) and around screws (B).

Regardless of the cup type, both linear and expansile osteolysis has
been noted about the fixation screws (67,75). With the HG cups after 5 years,
the use of screws for internal fixation showed one lesion in 83 cups
(1.2%)(100); no osteolysis was identified in the same cup fixed without
screws in 122 hips (101). Soto and colleagues showed, with HG cups and

a mean follow-up period of 87 months, that 22 (24%) hips had periacetabular osteolysis; 16 of these (73%) were associated with screws (102). Clohisy and colleagues have reported a recent 10-year follow-up study with 188 hips that had HG cups with screw fixation. Osteolytic lesions were noted in 9 hips (5%). Two of these hips had osteolytic lesions, located in zone 1, associated with the acetabular screw (103).

2. Cementless Femoral Components

The pattern of osteolysis with cementless stems also depends on whether bone ingrowth has occurred. In the case of cementless stems, the implant design is a major factor in the location of osteolytic lesions. With patch-porous-coated implants, synovial fluid flows along the smooth portion of the stem into the diaphysis of the femur. Thus, these types of stems are vulnerable to diaphyseal osteolysis, as demonstrated in studies in which partially porous-coated cylinders were implanted into the distal femur of rabbits (32). Polyethylene particles then were injected into the joint, and the femora were harvested several weeks after surgery. Histological analysis demonstrated that the bone-ingrowth areas were relative barriers to the ingress of joint fluid and polyethylene debris. In contrast, a periprosthetic cavity with a membrane formed around the smooth portion of the stem. Polarized light microscopy demonstrated that this soft tissue membrane contained abundant polyethylene particles, and similar findings have been noted in studies examining patch-porous-coated stems that were implanted in humans (34, 35,104,105).

With circumferential porous-coated stems such as the AML or the PCA, focal osteolytic lesions occur most commonly in the proximal aspect of the femur (Figure 7). Occasionally, these lesions have presented as spontaneous fractures of the greater and lesser trochanter (106). With AML femoral components, periarticular lesions occurring in zones 1 and 7 are primarily reported, with minimal clinical significance (greater and lesser trochanters, respectively) (73,74). Osteolysis around the PCA stem also occurred in zones 1, 7, or both in some studies (95,107), and in zones 1, 2, 3, and 7 in another study (106). A 5- to 9-year prospective study of the PCA stem showed 2.8% rate of endosteal osteolysis (108).

In contrast, diaphyseal expansile osteolysis is much more common in patch-porous coated implants such as the original Harris-Galante porous-coated stem, the Anatomic Porous Replacement (APR-I, Intermedics Orthopedics, Austin, TX) stem, and the initial S-ROM (Joint Medical Products, Stamford, CT) implant, which had a seam that allowed joint fluid to reach the diaphysis (1,109–111). The consequence of osteolysis in these cases is progressive diaphyseal bone loss. Loosening can occur when significant sup-

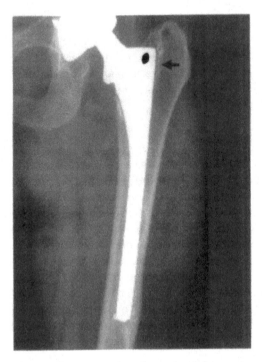

Figure 7 Osteolysis of proximal femur (zone I) in a well-fixed cementless stem.

port for the implant is lost along the smooth and porous portions of the stem. Because loads are then transferred across a small area of bone ingrowth, stress fractures of the ingrown area leading to implant loosening can occur and has been reported (112,113). Thus, it is possible for the surgeon to predict the location, appearance, and prevalence of osteolysis as a function of the implant design.

If bone ingrowth does not occur in a porous-coated cementless stem, a fibrous interface can develop. Radiographically, a sclerotic line adjacent to the fibrous tissue often indicates the presence of a partial barrier restricting the entry of particulate matter to the endosteal zone of the femur, and linear osteolysis in what is described as a "windshield wiper" pattern is seen (1). Progressive loss of diaphyseal bone may occur, which can lead to expansion of the endosteal canal. These patients often present with pain that progressively worsens, leading to revision surgery (114).

IV. SURGICAL TREATMENT OF OSTEOLYSIS

While the pathophysiology of osteolysis has been well understood, its treatment and prevention remain challenging. A longer follow-up is required to further evaluate the efficacy of new treatment and preventive measures (115–118).

The finding of osteolysis must be discussed with patients, and close follow-up is necessary. Besides, the factors causing the development of lesions should be explored with each individual patient. A decision for management can be made after the patient's mechanisms of osteolysis have been studied. Symptoms, location, and the likelihood of progression of the lesions; the amount of bone loss; and the status of fixation of the components must be considered. The surgical procedure must eliminate the osteolytic lesion and the particle generators (the sources of increased wear). Potential particle generators include worn or loose polyethylene liners, scored or burnished femoral heads, titanium (Ti) femoral heads, and fractured cement, among others. Surgery would address removal of granulomatous material when appropriate, filling of the defects with a graft material, and the possible exchange of components, depending on the extent of damage. Attention to normal anatomy and wide exposure help the surgeon to restore the appropriate biomechanical relationships.

A. Femoral Osteolysis

Linear osteolysis around cemented stems is often circumferential, involving all Gruen femoral zones, and can lead to implant loosening if left untreated. Radiographic examination at 3- to 6-month intervals is a reasonable approach until the patient becomes symptomatic or progressive lysis is observed. Although data are not available to indicate when observation should be abandoned in favor of surgery, operative intervention is instituted if structural stability is likely to be threatened or when clinical symptoms are significant. Conditions that may threaten stability include loss of the proximal femoral cortical bone—including the calcar—and large osteolytic lesions that may lead to periprosthetic fracture, such as those at the tip of the stem (119,120).

If the component is loose, it usually needs to be replaced, particularly to prevent further bone resorption. However, if the component is well fixed (as with cementless implants), substantial bone loss can result from injudicious removal. In such cases, curettage and grafting of the lytic lesion and retention of the stem, with exchange of the polyethylene liner, may be appropriate (115–118).

There are two principles in the effective treatment of femoral osteolysis. First, the sources of the particles must be identified and removed. Second, the interfacial bone loss must be treated. Removal of loose components and the appropriate grafting of bony defects are often required. The issue of removing a well-fixed cementless stem with focal osteolysis should be addressed on an individual case basis using the guidelines listed below.

Rubash et al., advocating revision of all loose stems, have proposed an algorithm for the management of femoral osteolysis (Figure 8) (117). Cemented stems are considered to be definitely loose by evidence of migration or subsidence of the component, stem debonding, stem fracture or bending, or cement fracture (121). A circumferential radiolucency at the bone–cement interface suggests probable loosening (121). For cementless components, migration and subsidence are most indicative of a loose stem. Additional signs of instability include cortical or cancellous hypertrophy at the stem tip, distal pedestal formation, shedding of the porous coating, and radiolucent lines along the porous coating (122,123).

Surgery is often indicated for well-fixed stems when there is evidence of progression of osteolysis on serial radiographs. Other factors to be considered include the size and location of the lesion as well as patient age, activity, and medical status. For stems with focal and cavitary osteolysis in zones 1 and 7, the lytic lesions may be grafted, although this has not been done regularly. In addition, the particle generators should be removed. For progressive diaphyseal osteolysis in a distal area, the stem often requires

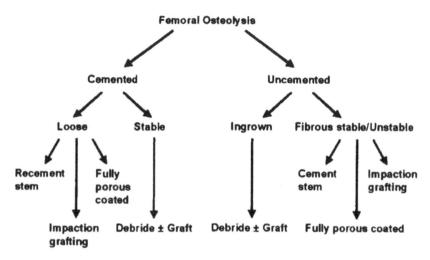

Figure 8 Treatment algorithm for femoral osteolysis. (From Ref. 138.)

revision. For small focal lesions or linear osteolysis, we recommend revision for physiologically young patients and observation for elderly and less active patients.

The location, extent, and type of porous coating must also be considered for uncemented stems. For proximal focal osteolysis, if the component is porous-coated circumferentially, the lesion can be packed with particulate graft and the particle generators exchanged. A non–circumferentially coated component may be retained in elderly, sedentary patients, with removal of the particle generators and grafting of the lesions when appropriate. This approach should be used with young, active patients only if the stem is well fixed and there is no evidence of distal osteolysis. However, if the stem is also a particle generator (e.g., monoblock titanium or extensive fretting of the modular taper), it should be revised as well. For osteolysis distal to zones 1 and 7, the femoral stem and polyethylene liner should usually be changed. Because distal osteolysis is usually progressive with noncircumferentially coated stems, even if they are well fixed, revision of the stem should be strongly considered. Cavitary lesions distal to the stem tip present a high risk of periprosthetic fracture and also should be revised with a stem that bypasses the lesion. Distal osteolysis in extensively coated stems has not been reported; therefore its appearance may imply loosening of the stem.

Bourne and Rorabeck classified femoral osteolysis into four types and suggested possible treatment modalities in accordance with this classification (120). A type 1 defect has intact cancellous bone and cortical tube and well-preserved cancelous bone. Any primary stem, cemented or uncemented, can be used. The type 2 defect has deficient cancellous bone and and an intact cortical tube. Treament options include extensively porous-coated prostheses, and less favorably proximal porous-coated prostheses or cemented prostheses. Impaction allografting with cemented prostheses can be an option for the younger patient (<65 years of age) with a patulous femoral canal (greater than 20 mm). A type 3 defect has deficient cancellous bone and cortical tube. Treatment options are essentially similar to type 2, but distal fixation with a scratch fit of 4–6 cm is more difficult to obtain and cortical strut allograft is needed in many cases. Type 4 has absent cancellous bone and cortical tube, and is the least common type. As a diaphyseal scratch fit is not possible, a proximal femoral allograft or tumor prosthesis is the remaining option.

During the surgical procedure, wide exposure is necessary for complete visualization of defects of the femoral canal. Extensive subperiosteal elevation of the overlying musculature may be required to fully assess the femoral cortex and lytic lesions. An extended osteotomy of the femur may be necessary, particularly in cases of a distally ingrown stems. The osteolytic membrane should be entirely removed, followed by curettage and preparation of of the canal, thus creating an appropriate bed of host bone for either a cemented or an uncemented stem. All structural defects should be reinforced with cortical femoral struts or intact distal femoral allografts. Once cortical support has been re-established, the endosteal cavities can be packed with particulate allograft. Then, the neutral axis of the femur must be identified so that the revision stem can be placed in proper alignment. This is readily accomplished by passing a beaded guide wire into the cancellous bone proximal to the knee. This step also confirms the absence of cortical perforations. Finally, the particle generators must be addressed. Titanium heads, which are associated with higher rates of polyethylene wear, should be replaced with CoCr heads. Similarly, femoral head of appropriate size can be mated with new polyethylene liners. Also, monoblock stems with extensive scoring of the head generally should be replaced, although advanced patient age, decreased activity, and poor medical status may be reasons to consider retaining otherwise well-fixed components (124) (Figure 9).

B.   Acetabular Osteolysis

The algorithm by Rubash et al. (124) provides a systematic approach to the treatment of acetabular osteolysis (Figure 10). For cemented cups, the first step is to evaluate implant stability. Linear or focal osteolysis in two or three acetabular zones has been associated with 71 and 94% incidences of loosening of the component, respectively (125). A loose-cemented component must be revised, preferably with porous-coated shell. Bone stock deficiencies must be treated with appropriate grafting. If the cup is not loose, the degree of wear should be evaluated. Worn cups with eccentricity of the femoral head should be replaced. Recent advancements, including crosslinked polyethylene, may make possible the use of 32-mm heads or ones with an even larger diameter.

Uncemented cups have been classified into three separate groups. The type I cup is stable with discrete focal osteolysis, including zones 1 and 3, and it is occasionally adjacent to screws. The component usually can be retained, and particulate graft can be packed into the defect if readily accessible. In addition, the polyethylene liner in modular cups can be replaced as long as the locking mechanism is intact. For nonmodular metal-backed cups, periodic observation of osteolysis may be appropriate, although early revision is recommended when progression of the osteolysis has been documented. Type II components are also stable by virtue of bone ingrowth, but the function of the cup is compromised. For example, the locking mechanism of a modular cup may be damaged, there may be extensive wear of the shell, or the shell may be malpositioned. In these cases, the entire com-

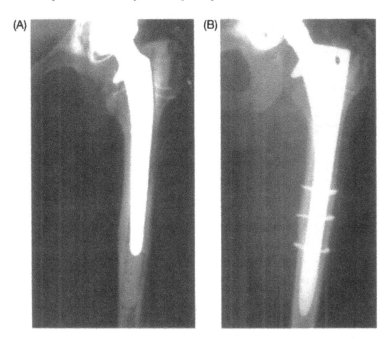

Figure 9 Osteolysis and loosening of a cemented femoral component. Revision was done with an extensively porous coated stem.

ponent is often removed, defects are filled with the appropriate graft, and a new cup is reimplanted without cement. As an alternative, a new polyethylene (often cross-linked) cup can be cemented into a well-fixed metal shell. Type III cups are unstable and have migrated into the osteolytic lesion, necessitating exchange. Cavitary acetabular defects with adequate rim integrity can be packed with particulate allograft. Structural rim deficiencies may require bulk allograft for support.

Two recent studies currently available show that liner exchange and debridement of granulomatous tissue with or without bone graft is effective; revision of a well-fixed uncemented acetabular component is not necessary in the treament of pelvic osteolysis (126,127).

Paprosky and associates developed and recently revised a classification system of acetabular osteolysis based on the integrity of the acetabular rim and its ability to support an implanted component. For classification, the appearance of an osteolytic lesion is first documented in order to confirm that the lesion is in fact a new one and not a radiolucency that was either in the same location either preoperatively or postoperatively. Once confirmed

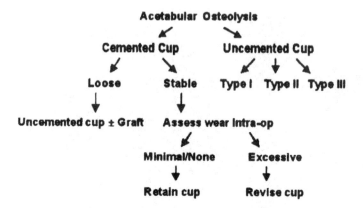

Treatment algorithm for acetabular osteolysis

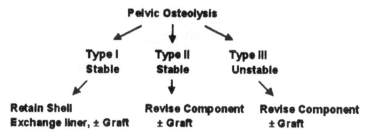

Treatment algorithm for pelvic osteolysis in uncemented cup

Figure 10 Treatment algorithm for acetabular osteolysis. (From Ref. 138.)

to be a definite lesion, its size should be measured and standardized by doing a standing x-ray of the anteroposterior pelvis. Category I lesions have retroacetabular lesions with sizes of 2.4 by 1.7 cm. There is no confluence of lesion. These lesions can be treated with polyethylene exchange with or without graft. They should be observed for 6 months and operated on if progression is documented. Category II lesions are larger and usually represent a confluence of lesions. Because they are thought to be already progressive lesions, they should be operated on within a 3- to 6-month period without further documentation. As fixation is not compromised, they can be treated in the same manner as category I lesions. Category III lesions have fusiform osteolysis superiorly and inferiorly but Kohler's line is intact. There is severe periacetabular osteolysis, and fixation of the cup is only through the medial wall. These cups should not be exchanged, because the only useful medial bone is destroyed during the removal process. They should be operated on within 3 months and peripherally packed with bone graft. Category IV lesions represent a possible compromise of fixation with severe posterior column involvement and larger ischial lesion. The intervention must be immediate, since fixation of the shell is precarious and the shell must be exchanged in order to prevent further bone loss (128).

During the surgical procedure, the appropriate extraction device for each manufacturer's cup should be available in order to remove the polyethylene liner without damaging the locking mechanism, which must be examined to determine whether it is functional. If the shell must be removed, the entire acetabular rim must be accessible. The cup is then separated from the underlying cement mantle or bone bed. Specially shaped osteotomes or gouges are needed to facilitate this step. Occasionally, the component must be broken into pieces for removal because the underlying bond with cement or bone cannot be broken. During component removal, care must be taken not to breach the medial wall, which compromises structural support and threatens intrapelvic contents. Generally, the cup cannot be removed until it is released hemispherically past the widest diameter from the underlying bone or cement (127).

In cases where there is a large amount of intrapelvic cement or when the cup is directly applied to the quadrilateral plate, forceful extraction can rupture underlying bone or vessels. When this is of concern, a computed tomography (CT) scan and/or contrast venogram will identify the anatomic relationships between pelvic structures and components. If the cement is adherent to pelvic vessels or when there is no room to pass an osteotome, an intrapelvic surgical approach can be used to dissect the vessels from cement or implants (129). After removal of the cement, all osteolytic membrane must be curetted, especially within anchor or screw holes. The appropriate grafting technique is used to address the bony defects. Structural grafts should be oriented so the trabeculae are aligned to withstand axial compressive forces across the hip joint (130).

To prepare the acetabulum for a porous-ingrowth cup, the acetabular bed is reamed hemispherically to preserve as much host bone as possible and to maximize the area of bone contact. Subchondral or sclerotic bone is the strongest bone for initial stability and should not be breached. The cup should be placed as near the anatomic position as possible (Figure 11). Screw fixation is often required to secure the cup. In some situations, a polyethylene cup may need to be cemented, such as when allograft comprises greater than 60% of the contact area between component and structural bone, or when the pelvic bed has been previously irradiated (130,131).

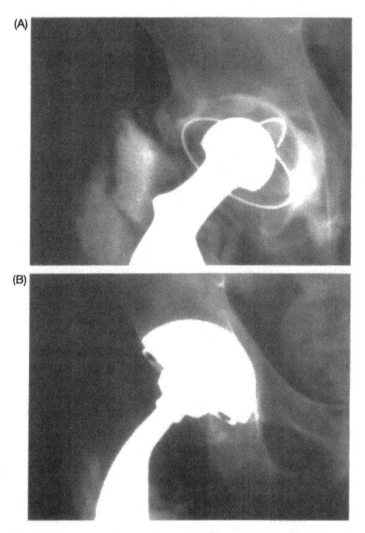

Figure 11   Acetabular osteolysis with bone loss. Revision was done with a ce-mentless acetabular component.

C. Nonsurgical Treatments

As alternatives to surgical intervention, investigators have looked to modi-fying the host response to debris by using nonsteroidal anti-inflammatory drugs to inactivate the inflammatory mediators (53,132). Since TNF-α is a key mediator of the inflammatory process in rheumatoid arthritis as well as in peri-implant bone loss, several investigators have attempted to attenuate particle-induced bone loss by targeting TNF-α (133,134). Schwarz et al. demonstrated that when macrophages are challenged with titanium particles, gene expression of TNF-α and activation of NF-κB precedes the gene expression of other cytokines (133). Schwarz et al. studied the response to titanium particles in the calvariae of genetically modified mice. Mice genetically deficient in TNF-α showed little inflammatory response or bone resorption when titanium particles were introduced over their calvaria, whereas mice that genetically over-produce TNF-α had exaggerated inflammatory response (133). Childs et al. studied the effect of TNF-α inhibitor Etanercept (Wyeth-Ayerst Pharmaceuticals), in a mouse model. When mice were treated with Etanercept at the time of osteolysis induction, bone resorption and osteoclast numbers were reduced to background levels in both normal and human TNF-α transgenic mice (134). Gene transfer techniques can also be used to neutralize proinflammatory mediators with interleukin-1 receptor antagonist protein or anti-inflammatory cytokines (135).

In particle-induced inflammation and bone loss, the final effector cell is the osteoclast. Since bisphosphonates inhibit osteoclastic activity and have been used clinically to prevent and treat osteoporosis, this class of drugs also provides a logical choice (136). Shanbhag et al. demonstrated that in a canine model of total hip arthroplasty, oral bisphosphonate therapy can prevent wear debris–induced bone loss (137). Continuous administration of alendronate effectively inhibited bone lysis for the 24-week duration of the study. To evaluate if such a drug therapy will be effective in treating peri-implant bone loss, multicenter clinical trials of oral alendronate treatment are now under way.

D. Future Directions

Long-term results of the management and treatment approaches proposed here, which are being employed at many centers, will be available. Improved models of osteolysis will enable more detailed study of particular treatment methods such as improved grafting materials and techniques, pharmacologic intervention, or immunologic modulation. In addition, the use of nonmodular femoral stems and the development of crosslinked polyethylene, ceramic, or highly polished metal-on-metal articulations will decrease the generation of wear debris. Various biological treatments will also be available to modulate peri-implant bone loss. With these advances, it is now possible to expect joint replacements to last more than 20 years.

REFERENCES

1. Sinha RK, Shanbhag AS, Maloney WJ, Hasselman CT, Rubash HE. Osteolysis: cause and effect. Instr Course Lect 47:307–320, 1998.
2. Charnley J. Arthroplasty of the hip. Lancet 1129–1132, 1961.
3. Charnley J, Follacci FM, Hammond BT. The long-term reaction of bone to self-curing acrylic cement. J Bone Joint Surg 50-B:822–829, 1968.
4. Wroblewski BM. Charnley low-friction arthroplasty, Review of past, present status and prospects for the future. Clin Orthop 210:37–42, 1986.
5. Charnley J. The bonding of prostheses to bone by cement. J Bone Joint Surg 46-B:518–529, 1964.
6. Harris WH, Schiller AL, Scholler JM, Friberg RA, Scott R. Extensive localized bone resorption in the femur following total hip replacement. J Bone Joint Surg 58A:612–618, 1976.
7. Willert HG, Semlitsch M. Reactions of the articular capsule to wear products of artificial joint prostheses. J Biomed Mater Res 11:157–164, 1977.
8. Mirra JM, Amstutz HC, Matos M, Gold R. The pathology of the joint tissues and its clinical relevance in prosthesis failure. Clin Orthop 117:221–240, 1976.
9. Goldring SR, Schiller AL, Roelke M, Rourke CM, O'Neill DA, Harris WH. The synovial-like membrane at the bone-cement interface in loose total hip replacements and its proposed role in bone lysis. J Bone Joint Surg 65A:575–584, 1983.
10. Dorr LD, Bloebaum R, Emmanual J, Meldrum R. Histologic, biochemical and ion analysis of tissue and fluids retrieved during total hip arthroplasty. Clin Orthop 261:82–95, 1990.
11. Shanbhag AS, Jacobs JJ, Black J, Galante JO, Glant TT. Cellular mediators secreted by interfacial membranes obtained at revision total hip arthroplasty. J Arthrop 10:498–506, 1995.
12. Kim KJ, Rubash HE, Wilson SC, D'Antonio JA, McClain EJ. A histological and biochemical comparison of the interface tissues in cementless and cemented hip prosthesis. Clin Orthop 287:142–152, 1993.
13. Kim KJ, Chiba J, Rubash HE. In vivo and in vitro analysis of membranes from hip prostheses inserted without cement. J Bone Joint Surg 76-A:172–180, 1994.
14. Jiranek WA, Machado M, Jasty MJ, Jevsevar D, Wolfe HJ, Goldring SR, Goldberg MJ, Harris WH. Production of cytokines around loosened cemented acetabular components. Analysis with immunohistochemical techniques and in situ hybridization. J Bone Joint Surg 75-A:863–879, 1993.
15. Glant TT, Valyon M, Mikecz K, Cole A, Jacobs JJ, Yao J, Kuettner KE. Discoordinate expression of IL-1α and IL-1β in interfacial membranes of failed joint prostheses. Agents Actions, Special Conference Issue 41:C172-C173, 1994.
16. Jones LC, Hungerford DS. Cement disease. Clin Orthop 225:192–206, 1987.
17. Park JB, Von Recum AF, Gratzick GE. Pre-coated orthopedic implants with bone cement. Biomat, Med Dev Art Org 7:41–53, 1979.

18. Rubash HE, Harris WH. Revision of nonseptic, loose, cemented femoral components using modern cementing techniques. J Arthrop 3:241–248, 1988.

19. Huk OL, Bansal M, Betts F, Rimnac CM, Lieberman JR, Huo MH, Salvati EA. Polyethylene and metal debris generated by non-articulating surfaces of modular acetabular components. J Bone Joint Surg 76-B:568–574, 1994.

20. Schmalzried TP, Jasty MJ, Harris WH. Periprosthetic bone loss in total hip arthroplasty. J Bone Joint Surg 74-A:849–863, 1992.

21. Maloney WJ, Smith RL, Schmalzried TP, Chiba J, Huene D, Rubash HE. Isolation and characterization of wear particles generated in patients who have had failure of a hip arthroplasty without cement. J Bone Joint Surg 77-A: 1301–1310, 1995

22. Shanbhag AS, Jacobs JJ, Glant TT, Gilbert JL, Black J, Galante JO. Composition and morphology of wear debris in failed uncemented total hip replacement. J Bone Joint Surg 76-B:60–67, 1994.

23. Shanbhag AS, Bailey HO, Hwang DS, Eror NG, Woo SL-Y, Rubash HE. Chemical and morphological characterization of wear debris associated with acetabular screw holes. Trans Soc Biomater 18:325, 1995.

24. Maloney WJ, Engh CA, Chandler H. Severe osteolysis of the pelvis in association with acetabular replacement without cement. J Bone Joint Surg 75-A:1627–1635, 1993.

25. Urban RM, Jacobs JJ, Gilbert JL, Galante JO. Migration of corrosion products from modular hip prostheses. Clin Orthop 76-A:1345–1359, 1994.

26. Margevicius KJ, Bauer TW, McMahon JT, Brown SA, Merritt K. Isolation and characterization of debris in membranes around total joint prostheses. J Bone Joint Surg 76-A:1664–1675, 1994.

27. Morscher EW, Hefti A, Aebi U. Severe osteolysis after third-body wear due to hydroxyapatite particles from acetabular cup coating. J Bone Joint Surg 80-B:267–272, 1998.

28. Hop JD, Callaghan JJ, Olejniczak JP, Pedersen DR, Brown TD, Johnston RC. The Frank Stinchfield Award. Contribution of cable debris generation to accelerated polyethylene wear. Clin Orthop 344:20–32, 1997.

29. Merchant KK, Rohr WL, Lintner WP, Bhambri SK. Orthopaedic implant surface debris. Trans Orthop Res Soc 20:164–164, 1995.

30. Willert HG, Semlitsch M. Tissue reactions to plastic and metallic wear products of joint endoprostheses. In: Gschwend N, Debrunner HU, eds. Total Hip Prosthesis. Baltimore, MD: Williams & Wilkins, 1976: 205–239.

31. Urban RM, Jacobs JJ, Sumner DR, Peters CL, Voss FR, Galante JO. The bone-implant interface of femoral stems with non-circumferential porous coating. J Bone Joint Surg 78-A:1068–1081, 1996.

32. Bobyn JD, Jacobs JJ, Tanzer M, Urban RM, Aribindi R, Sumner DR, Turner TM, Brooks CE. The susceptibility of smooth implant surfaces to periimplant fibrosis and migration of polyethylene wear debris. Clin Orthop 311:21–39, 1995.

33. Horikoshi M, Macaulay W, Booth RE, Crossett LS, Rubash HE. Comparison of interface membranes obtained from failed cemented cementless hip and knee prostheses. Clin Orthop 309:69–87, 1994.

34. Maloney WJ, Jasty MJ, Harris WH, Galante JO, Callaghan JJ. Endosteal erosion in association with stable uncemented femoral components. J Bone Joint Surg 72-A:1025–1034, 1990.

35. Tanzer M, Maloney WJ, Jasty MJ, Harris WH. The progression of femoral cortical osteolysis in association with total hip arthroplasty without cement. J Bone Joint Surg 74-A:404–410, 1992.

36. Haynes DR, Rogers SD, Hay S, App B, Pearcy MJ, Howie DW. The differences in toxicity and release of bone-resorbing mediators induced by titanium and cobalt-chromium-alloy wear particles. J Bone Joint Surg 75-A:825–834, 1993.

37. Shanbhag AS, Jacobs JJ, Black J, Galante JO, Glant TT. Human monocyte response to particulate biomaterials generated in vivo and in vitro. J Orthop Res 13:792–801, 1995.

38. Macaulay W, Shanbhag AS, Marinelli R, Stefanovic-Racic M, Rubash HE, Woo SL-Y. Nitric oxide release from murine macrophages when stimulated with particulate debris. Trans Soc Biomater 18:307, 1995.

39. Maloney WJ, Smith RL, Castro F, Schurman DJ. Fibroblast response to metallic debris in vitro. Enzyme induction, cell proliferation, and toxicity. J Bone Joint Surg 75-A:835–844, 1993.

40. Yao J, Glant TT, Lark MW, Mikecz K, Jacobs JJ, Hutchinson NI, Hoerrner LA, Kuettner KE, Galante JO. The potential role of fibroblasts in periprosthetic osteolysis: Fibroblast response to titanium particles. J Bone Miner Res 10:1417–1427, 1995.

41. Shanbhag AS, Jacobs JJ, Black J, Galante JO, Glant TT. Effects of particles on fibroblast proliferation and bone resorption in vitro. Clin Orthop 342:205–217, 1997.

42. Cohen J. Assay of foreign-body reaction. J Bone Joint Surg 41-A:152–166, 1959.

43. DiCarlo EF, Bullough PG. The biologic responses to orthopedic implants and their wear debris. Clin Mater 9:235–260, 1992.

44. Escalas F, Galante JO, Rostoker W, Coogan P. Biocompatibility of materials for total joint replacement. J Biomed Mater Res 10:175–195, 1976.

45. Goodman SB, Fornasier VL, Lee J, Kei J. The histological effects of the implantation of different sizes of polyethylene particles in the rabbit tibia. J Biomed Mater Res 24:517–524, 1990.

46. Horowitz SM, Doty SB, Lane JM, Burstein AH. Studies of the mechanism by which the mechanical failure of polymethylmethacrylate leads to bone resorption. J Bone Joint Surg 75-A:802–813, 1993.

47. Goodman SB, Fornasier VL, Kei J. The effects of bulk versus particulate polymethylmethacrylate on bone. Clin Orthop 232:255–262, 1988.

48. Goodman SB, Fornasier VL, Kei J. The effects of bulk versus particulate ultra-high-molecular-weight polyethylene on bone. J Arthrop 3(suppl):S41–S46, 1988.

49. Miller KM, Anderson JM. Human monocyte/macrophage activation and interleukin 1 generation by biomedical polymers. J Biomed Mater Res 22:713–731, 1988.

50. Gelb H, Schumacher HR, Cuckler J, Baker DG. In vivo inflammatory response to polymethylmethacrylate particulate debris. Effect of size, morphology, and surface area. J Orthop Res 12:83–92, 1994.
51. Glant TT, Jacobs JJ, Molnar G, Shanbhag AS, Valyon M, Galante JO. Bone resorption activity of particulate-stimulated macrophages. J Bone Miner Res 8:1071–1079, 1993.
52. Shanbhag AS, Jacobs JJ, Black J, Galante JO, Glant TT. Macrophage/particle interactions: effect of size, composition and surface area. J Biomed Mater Res 28:81–90, 1994.
53. Spector M, Shortkroff S, Hsu HP, Lane N, Sledge CB, Thornhill TS. Tissue changes around loose prostheses. A canine model to investigate the effects of an antiinflammatory agent. Clin Orthop 261:140–152, 1990.
54. Dowd JE, Schwendeman LJ, Macaulay W, Doyle JS, Shanbhag AS, Wilson S, Herndon JH, Rubash HE. Aseptic loosening in uncemented total hip arthroplasty in a canine model. Clin Orthop 319:106–121, 1995.
55. Hasselman CT, Kovach C, Keys B, Rubash HE, Shanbhag AS. Macrophage response to synergistic challenge with prosthetic wear debris. Trans Orthop Res Soc 22:739, 1997.
56. Miossec P, Cavender D, Ziff M. Production of interleukin 1 by human endothelial cells. J Immunol 136(7):2486–2491, 1986.
57. Vernon-Roberts B, Freeman MAR. Morphological and analytical studies of the tissues adjacent to joint prostheses. investigations into the causes of loosening prostheses. In: Schaldach M, Hohmann, D, eds. Advances in Artificial Hip and Knee Joint Technology. Berlin: Springer-Verlag, 1976:148–186.
58. Vernon-Roberts B, Freeman MAR. The tissue response to total joint replacement prostheses. In: Swanson SAV, Freeman MAR, eds. The Scientific Basis of Joint Replacement. New York: Wiley, 1977:86–129.
59. Charnley J. The reaction of bone to self-curing acrylic cement. J Bone Joint Surg 52-B:340–353, 1970.
60. Willert HG, Ludwig J, Semlitsch M. Reaction of bone to methacrylate after hip arthroplasty. J Bone Joint Surg 56-A:1368–1382, 1974.
61. Stauffer RN. Ten-year follow-up study of total hip replacement. J Bone Joint Surg 64-A:983–990, 1982.
62. Evans EM, Freeman MAR, Miller AJ, Vernon-Roberts B. Metal sensitivity as a cause of bone necrosis and loosening of the prosthesis in total joint replacement. J Bone Joint Surg 56B:626–642, 1974.
63. Brown GC, Lockshin MD, Salvati EA, Bullough PG. Sensitivity to metal as a possible cause of sterile loosening after cobalt-chromium total hip-replacement arthroplasty. J Bone Joint Surg 59-A:164–168, 1977.
64. Merritt K, Brown SA. Hypersensitivity to metallic biomaterials. In: Williams DF, ed. Systemic Aspects of Biocompatibility, vol II. Boca Raton, FL: CRC Press, 1981:33–48.
65. Rooker GD, Wilkinson JD. Metal sensitivity in patients undergoing hip replacement. J Bone Joint Surg 62-B:502–505, 1980.
66. Lalor PA, Revell PA, Gray AB, Wright S, Railton GT, Freeman MA. Sensi-

tivity to titanium. A cause of implant failure? J Bone Joint Surg 73-B:25–28, 1991.

67. Santavirta S, Konttinen YT, Bergroth V, Eskola A, Tallroth K, Lindholm TS. Aggressive granulomatous lesions associated with hip arthroplasty. J Bone Joint Surg 72-A:252–258, 1990.

68. Santavirta S, Konttinen YT, Hoikka V, Eskola A. Immunopathological response to loose cementless acetabular components. J Bone Joint Surg 73-B: 38–42, 1991.

69. Neumann L, Freund KG, Sorensen KH. Total hip arthroplasty with the Charnley prosthesis in patients fifty-five years old and less. J Bone Joint Surg 78-A:73–79, 1996.

70. Mulroy WF, Estok DM, Harris WH. Total hip arthroplasty with use of so-called second-generation cementing techniques. J Bone Joint Surg 77-A: 1845–1852, 1995.

71. Mulroy RD, Jr., Harris WH. The effect of improved cementing techniques on component loosening in total hip replacement. J Bone Joint Surg 72-B:757–760, 1990.

72. Maloney WJ, Galante JO, Anderson M, Goldberg V, Harris WH, Jacobs JJ, Kraay M, Lachiewicz P, Rubash HE, Schutzer S, Woolson ST. Fixation, polyethylene wear, and pelvic osteolysis in primary total hip replacement. Clin Orthop 369:157–164, 1999.

73. Engh CA, Hooten JP, Jr., Zettl-Schaffer KF, Ghaffarpour M, McGovern TF, Macalino GE, Zicat BA. Porous-coated total hip replacement. Clin Orthop 298:89–96, 1994.

74. Zicat B, Engh CA, Gokcen E. Patterns of osteolysis around total hip components inserted with and without cement. J Bone Joint Surg 77-A:432–439, 1995.

75. Fox GM, McBeath AA, Heiner JP. Hip replacement with a threaded acetabular cup. A follow-up study. J Bone Joint Surg 76-A:195–201, 1994.

76. Bruijn JD, Seelen JL, Feenstra RM, Hansen BE, Bernoski FP. Failure of the Mecring screw-ring acetabular component in total hip arthroplasty. A three to seven-year follow-up study. J Bone Joint Surg 77-A:760–766, 1995.

77. Clohisy JC, Harris WH. Primary hybrid total hip replacement, performed with insertion of the acetabular component without cement and a precoat femoral component with cement. An average ten-year follow-up study. J Bone Joint Surg 81-A:247–255, 1999.

78. Smith SE, Harris WH. Total hip arthroplasty performed with insertion of the femoral component with cement and the acetabular component without cement. Ten to thirteen-year results. J Bone Joint Surg 79-A:1827–1833, 1997.

79. Kim Y-H, Kim JS, Cho SH. Primary total hip arthroplasty with the AML total hip prosthesis. Clin Orthop 360:147–158, 1999.

80. Hellman EJ, Capello WN, Feinberg JR. Omnifit cementless total hip arthroplasty. A 10-year average followup. Clin Orthop 364:164–174, 1999.

81. Sakalkale DP, Eng K, Hozack WJ, Rothman RH. Minimum 10-year results of a tapered cementless hip replacement. Clin Orthop 362:138–144, 1999.

82. McLaughlin JR, Lee KR. Total hip arthroplasty in young patients. 8- to 13-year results using an uncemented stem. Clin Orthop 373:153–163, 2000.

83. Emerson RH, Jr., Sanders SB, Head WC, Higgins L. Effect of circumferential plasma-spray porous coating on the rate of femoral osteolysis after total hip arthroplasty. J Bone Joint Surg 81-A:1291–1298, 1999.

84. Christie MJ, DeBoer DK, Trick LW, Brothers JC, Jones RE, Vise GT, Gruen TA. Primary total hip arthroplasty with use of the modular S-ROM prosthesis. Four to seven-year clinical and radiographic results. J Bone Joint Surg 81-A: 1707–1716, 1999.

85. Dorr LD, Wan Z, Longjohn DB, Dubois B, Murken R. Total hip arthroplasty with use of the Metasul metal-on-metal articulation. Four to seven-year results. J Bone Joint Surg 82-A:789–798, 2000.

86. Yoon TR, Rowe SM, Jung ST, Seon KJ, Maloney WJ. Osteolysis in association with a total hip arthroplasty with ceramic bearing surfaces. J Bone Joint Surg 80-A:1459–1468, 1998.

87. Bizot P, Larrouy M, Witvoet J, Sedel L, Nizard R. Press-fit metal-backed alumina sockets: a minimum 5-year followup study. Clin Orthop 379:134–142, 2000.

88. Kim YH, Kim VE. Uncemented porous-coated anatomic total hip replacement. Results at six years in a consecutive series. J Bone Joint Surg 75-B:6–13, 1993.

89. Chiba J, Rubash HE, Kim KJ, Iwaki Y. The characterization of cytokines in the interface tisssue obtained from failed cementless total hip arthroplasty with and without femoral osteolysis. Clin Orthop 300:304–312, 1994.

90. Schmalzried TP, Kwong LM, Jasty MJ, Sedlacek RC, Haire TC, O'Connor DO, Bragdon CR, Kabo JM, Malcom AJ, Harris WH. The mechanism of loosening of cemented acetabular components in total hip arthroplasty. Clin Orthop 274:60–78, 1992.

91. Harris WH, Schiller AL, Scholler J-M, Freiberg RA, Scott R. Extensive localized bone resorption in the femur following total hip replacement. J Bone Joint Surg 58-A:612–618, 1976.

92. Anthony PP, Gie GA, Howie CR, Ling RSM. Localised endosteal bone lysis in relation to the femoral components of cemented total hip arthroplasties. J Bone Joint Surg 72-B:971–979, 1990.

93. Horikoshi M, Dowd J, Maloney WJ, Crossett L, Rubash HE. Activation of human fibroblasts and macrophages by particulate wear debris from failed total hip and total knee arthroplasty. Transactions of the Orthopaedic Research Society 19, 199–199. 1994. .

94. Kwong LM, Jasty M, Mulroy RD, Maloney WJ, Bragdon C, Harris WH. The histology of the radiolucent line. J Bone Joint Surg 74-B:67–73, 1992

95. Zimlich RH, Fehring TK. Underestimation of pelvic osteolysis. the value of the iliac oblique radiograph. J Arthrop 15:796–801, 2000.

96. Kim YH, Kim VE. Cementless porous-coated anatomic medullary locking total hip prostheses. J Arthrop 9:243–252, 1994.

97. Owen TD, Moran CG, Smith SR, Pinder IM. Results of uncemented porous-

coated anatomic total hip replacement. J Bone Joint Surg 76-B:258–262, 1994.

98. Mohler CG, Callaghan JJ, Collis DK, Johnston RC. Early loosening of the femoral component at the cement-prosthesis interface after total hip replacement [see comments]. J Bone Joint Surg 77-A:1315–1322, 1995.

99. Moyle DD, Klawitter JJ, Hulbert SF. Mechanical properties of the bone-porous biomaterial interface: Elastic behaviour. J Biomed Mater Res Symp 4: 363–382, 1973.

100. Schmalzried TP, Harris WH. The Harris-Galante porous-coated acetabular component with screw fixation. Radiographic analysis of eighty-three primary hip replacements at a minimum of five years. J Bone Joint Surg 74-A:1130–1139, 1992.

101. Schmalzried TP, Wessinger SJ, Hill GE, Harris WH. The Harris-Galante porous acetabular component press-fit without screw fixation. Five-year radiographic analysis of primary cases. J Arthrop 9:235–242, 1994.

102. Soto MO, Rodriguez JA, Ranawat CS. Clinical and radiographic evaluation of the Harris-Galante cup: Incidence of wear and osteolysis at 7 to 9 years follow-up. J Arthrop 15:139–145, 2000.

103. Clohisy JC, Harris WH. The Harris-Galante porous-coated acetabular component with screw fixation. An average ten-year follow-up study. J Bone Joint Surg 81-A:66–73, 1999.

104. Jasty MJ, Floyd WE, Schiller AL, Goldring SR, Harris WH. Localized osteolysis in stable, non-septic total hip replacement. J Bone Joint Surg 68A:912–919, 1986.

105. Goetz DD, Smith EJ, Harris WH. The prevalence of femoral osteolysis associated with components inserted with or without cement in total hip replacements. J Bone Joint Surg 76-A:1121–1129, 1994.

106. Heekin RD, Engh CA, Herzwurm PJ. Fractures through cystic lesions of the greater trochanter. A cause of late pain after cementless total hip arthroplasty. J Arthrop 11:757–760, 1996.

107. Heekin RD, Callaghan JJ, Hopkinson WJ, Savory CG, Xenos JS. The porous-coated anatomic total hip prosthesis, inserted without cement. J Bone Joint Surg 75-A:77–91, 1993.

108. Knight JL, Atwater RD, Guo J. Clinical results of the midstem porous-coated anatomic uncemented femoral stem in primary total hip arthroplasty: a five- to nine-year prospective study. J Arthrop 13:535–545, 1998.

109. Christie MJ, DeBoer DK, Trick LW, Brothers JC, Jones RE, Vise GT, Gruen TA. Primary total hip arthroplasty with use of the modular S-ROM prosthesis. Four to seven-year clinical and radiographic results. J Bone Joint Surg 81-A: 1707–1716, 1999.

110. Maloney WJ, Woolson ST. Increasing incidence of femoral osteolysis in association with uncemented Harris-Galante total hip arthroplasty. A follow-up report. J Arthrop 11:130–134, 1996.

111. Clohisy JC, Harris WH. The Harris-Galante uncemented femoral component in primary total hip replacement at 10 years. J Arthrop 14:915–917, 1999.

112. Jasty M, Maloney WJ, Bragdon CR, Haire T, Harris WH. Histomorphological studies of the long-term skeletal responses to well fixed cemented femoral components. J Bone Joint Surg 72-A:1220–1229, 1990.

113. Jasty M, Bragdon C, Jiranek W, Chandler H, Maloney W, Harris WH. Etiology of osteolysis around porous-coated cementless total hip arthroplasties. Clin Orthop 308:111–126, 1994.

114. Ohlin A, Johnell O, Lerner UH. The pathogenesis of loosening of total hip arthroplasties. The production of factors by periosthetic tissues that stimulate in vitro bone resorption. Clin Orthop 253:287–296, 1990.

115. Maloney WJ. Management of pelvic osteolysis. Transactions of the 26th Annual Hip Course. Boston: Harvard Medical School, 1996.

116. Paprosky W, Kronick JL, Barba ML. When to operate on femoral osteolysis. Transactions of the 26th Annual Hip Course. Boston: Harvard Medical School, 1996.

117. Rubash HE. Osteolysis; Clinical manifestation and management. Symposium at the 63th meeting of AAOS. Atlanta: 1996.

118. Schmalzried TP. Management of pelvic osteolysis. Transactions of the 26th Annual Hip Course. Boston: Harvard Medical School, 1996.

119. Rubash HE, Sinha RK, Shanbhag AS, Kim SY. Pathogenesis of bone loss after total hip arthroplasty. Orthop Clin North Am 29:173–186, 1998.

120. Dunbar MJ, Blackley HR, Bourne RB. Osteolysis of the femur: principles of management. Instr Course Lect 50:197–209, 2001.

121. Harris WH, Schiller AL, Scholler JM, Freiberg RA, Scott R. Extensive localized bone resorption in the femur following total hip replacement. J Bone Joint Surg 58-A:612–618, 1976.

122. Callaghan JJ, Salvati EA, Pellicci PM, Wilson PD, Jr., Ranawat CS. Results of revision for mechanical failure after cemented total hip replacement, 1979 to 1982. A two- to five-year follow-up. J Bone Joint Surg 67-A:1074–1085, 1985.

123. Rae T. The action of cobalt, nickel and chromium on phagocytosis and bacterial killing by human polymorphonuclear leucocytes; its relevance to infection after total joint arthroplasty. Biomaterials 4:175–180, 1983.

124. Sinha RK, Maloney WJ, Paprosky WG, Rubash HE. Surgical treatment of osteolysis. In: Callaghan JJ, Rosenberg AG, Rubash HE, eds. Adult Hip. Philadelphia-New York: Lippincott-Raven, 1998:1549–1570, 2001.

125. Hodgkinson JP, Shelley P, Wroblewski BM. The correlation between the roentgenographic appearance and operative findings at the bone-cement junction of the socket in Charnley low friction arthroplasties. Clin Orthop 228: 105–109, 1988.

126. Maloney WJ, Herzwurm P, Paprosky W, Rubash HE, Engh CA. Treatment of pelvic osteolysis associated with a stable acetabular component inserted without cement as part of a total hip replacement. J Bone Joint Surg 79-A:1628–1634, 1997.

127. Schmalzried TP, Fowble VA, Amstutz HC. The fate of pelvic osteolysis after reoperation. No recurrence with lesional treatment. Clin Orthop 350:128–137, 1998.

128. Paprosky. Size, shape, progrssion of acetabular progression and timing of acetabular surgery. Transactions of the 30th Annual Hip Course. Boston: Harvard Medical School, 2000.

129. Petrera P, Trakru S, Mehta S, Steed D, Towers JD, Rubash HE. Revision total hip arthroplasty with a retroperitoneal approach to the iliac vessels. J Arthrop 11:704–708, 1996.

130. McGann WA, Welch RB, Picetti GD, III. Acetabular preparation in cementless revision total hip arthroplasty. Clin Orthop 235:35–46, 1988.

131. Jacobs JJ, Kull LR, Frey GA, Gitelis S, Sheinkop MB, Kramer TS, Rosenberg AG. Early failure of acetabular components inserted without cement after previous pelvic irradiation. J Bone Joint Surg Am 77:1829–1835, 1995.

132. Goodman SB, Lee JS, Chin RC, Chiou SS. Modulation of the membrane surrounding particulate cement and polyethylene in the rabbit tibia. Biomaterials 12:194–196, 1991.

133. Schwarz EM, Lu AP, Goater JJ, Benz EB, Kollias G, Rosier RN, Puzas JE, O'Keefe RJ. Tumor necrosis factor-alpha/nuclear transcription factor-kappaB signaling in periprosthetic osteolysis. J Orthop Res 18:472–480, 2000.

134. Childs LM, Goater JJ, O'Keefe RJ, Schwarz EM. Efficacy of Etanercept for wear debris–induced osteolysis. J Bone Miner Res 16:338–347, 2001.

135. Ghivizzani SC, Oligino T J, Glorioso JC, Robbins PD, Evans CH. Gene therapy approaches for treating rheumatoid arthritis. Clin Orthop 379:288–299, 2000.

136. Wahl SM. Lymphocyte- and macrophage-derived growth factors. Methods Enzymol 163:715–731, 1988.

137. Shanbhag AS, Hasselman CT, Rubash HE. The John Charnley Award. Inhibition of wear debris mediated osteolysis in a canine total hip arthroplasty model. Clin Orthop 344;33–43, 1997.

138. Rubash et al. Osteolysis: surgical treatment. In: Cannon WD, ed. Instructional Course Lecture 47. Rosement, IL: American Academy of Orthopaedic Surgeons, 1997:321–330.

7
Revision Arthroplasty of the Acetabulum with Restoration of Bone Stock

Allan E. Gross
Mount Sinai Hospital, Toronto, Ontario, Canada

I. INTRODUCTION

Revision arthroplasty of the acetabulum is one of the most challenging problems in orthopaedic surgery today. The goals of acetabular revision are to restore anatomy and provide stable fixation for the new acetabular component. The *most important parameter* affecting the surgeon's ability to achieve this is *bone stock*. Bone stock deficiency must be identified and classified to plan appropriately for the surgery.

Bone stock deficiency can be classified as contained (cavitary) or uncontained (segmental). A contained defect is cavitary in that the acetabulum is ballooned out and weakened but the columns are intact. A contained defect may be localized to only part of the acetabulum or involve the entire acetabulum. An uncontained defect is segmental in that there is full-thickness loss of bone involving the acetabular rim and the adjacent anterior or posterior column.

Most bone defects can be defined by routine radiographs but on occasion Judet views are helpful to define the anterior and posterior columns (1). The final definition of the defect only can be made intraoperatively and may be more extensive than was anticipated (2). The surgeon must allow for this in planning for resource needs.

The author uses the following classification of acetabular defects, based on the degree of bone loss, for planning revision surgery.

A.   Classification of Acetabular Defects

Type I
No notable loss of bone stock. Amount of bone loss is less than that
which would require a revision component; there has been no migration of the primary component into the ilium, and both columns
are largely intact.

Type II
Contained loss of bone stock. There is cavitary or volumetric enlarge-
ment of the acetabulum. If the cup does extend beyond the ilioischial
line, it can be still considered a type II defect provided that the
columns are intact (i.e., protrusio).

Type III
*Uncontained (segmental) loss of bone stock involving less than 50%
of the acetabulum, primarily affecting either the (a) anterior or (b)
posterior column.* Bone loss is considered uncontained if it is not
amenable to treatment with morcellized bone graft. The sum of all
segments of bone loss in either the anterior or posterior column
allows greater than 50% cup coverage by host bone (as assessed
preoperatively with templates).

Type IV
*Uncontained (segmental) loss of bone stock greater than 50% of the
acetabulum affecting both anterior and posterior columns.* Type IV
is identical to type III except that the sum of the segmental bone
loss in the columns exceeds 50%. There is no pelvic discontinuity.
If there is greater than 50% loss of the acetabulum involving mostly
the medial wall but the columns are intact, then this type of defect
is considered a type II because of the availability of the columns
for reconstruction.

Type V
*Acetabular defect with uncontained loss of bone stock in association
with pelvic discontinuity.* Any pelvic discontinuity is considered a
type V defect regardless of the amount of bone loss.

Type I acetabular revisions, where there is no significant loss of bone
stock, can be managed by conventional cemented or cementless cups. Type
II contained defects can be treated with large uncemented cups if contact
can be made with 50% host bleeding bone or acetabular impaction grafting
with or without a protective ring (3–5) and a cemented cup. These techniques use morcellized allograft bone. Type III uncontained defects involving less than 50% of the acetabulum can be treated by a high hip center
(6–9) a structural allograft that supports less than 50% of the cup (10,11),
or an oblong cup (12,13).

Type IV uncontained defects involving more than 50% of the acetabulum can be treated under some circumstances by a high hip center (if contact can be made with bleeding host bone, the leg length discrepancy can be made up on the femoral side, and stability can be achieved), but they usually require a structural allograft (14).

Type V defects require a plate or reconstruction ring to stabilize the discontinuity. If there is an associated bone defect, morcellized or structural grafting may be necessary.

This chapter presents the author's techniques and results of restoring bone stock for contained and uncontained defects in acetabular revision surgery (see Table 1).

II. PRINCIPLES OF BONE GRAFTING

The spectrum of opinion regarding management of bone deficiency on the pelvic side of an arthroplasty varies from avoiding the use of bone graft, if at all possible (8), the use of morcellized bone only (15), to the use of complex structural grafts (16). There are situations where bone stock must be restored because the loss of bone is too extensive for alternatives such as a high hip center or so-called jumbo or asymmetrical cups. Posterior column defects or pelvic discontinuity with associated loss of bone stock

Table 1 Classification and Treatment Guide for Acetabular Revisions

Type I	No significant bone loss
	Conventional cemented or cementless cup
Type II	Contained bone loss
	Morcellized bone graft
	Contact with 50% host bone—cementless cup
	Contact with less than 50% host bone
	Protective ring and cemented cup
	Cemented cup (impaction grafting)
Type III	Uncontained (segmental) loss of less than 50% of acetabulum
	Structural graft (shelf) and cemented or uncemented cup
	High hip center
	Oblong cup
Type IV	Uncontained (segmental loss of greater than 50% of acetabulum)
	Structural graft and reconstruction ring with cemented cup
Type V	Pelvic discontinuity with or without bone loss
	Reconstruction ring and cemented cup with bone graft (morcellized or structural depending on defect)

are examples. In addition, patients who are facing further revision operations should have bone stock restored in order to facilitate another arthroplasty (16).

There is broad agreement that structural grafts on the pelvic side may have a guarded long-term prognosis and should be avoided if possible (7–10,14,16). Failure rates as high as 47% (14 of 30 hips) at 10 years have been reported (7). At the same time, there are situations where bulk allograft must be used; if used properly, it can provide successful clinical results without the need for revision for at least 5 years and provide bone stock for further procedures (16).

It is imperative that certain principles of bone grafting be understood and adhered to in order to optimize results.

Bone grafts may be classified into heterografts (bone from another species), allografts (bone from the same species), and autografts (bone taken from another part of the same individual). Often in the revision operations, because of the quantity and quality of bone required, allograft is more practical than autograft. There are, however, certain advantages and disadvantages associated with each type of graft.

Autograft has the advantage of not being immunogenic; even more importantly, it is best for inducing new bone formation by the host. Its main disadvantage is that the quantity available as well as its strength, shape, and form usually cannot duplicate the deficit encountered clinically.

Allografts, on the other hand, are available in large quantity, can have very good initial strength, and can duplicate very nearly any deficit. They are, however, costly, immunogenic (17–19), and not as effective as autografts for inducing new bone formation (17,18,20).

Allograft bone can be further classified accordingly to how it is used: (a) morcellized, or (b) structural (simulated or anatomical).

Morcellized bone (fragments of cancellous bone 3 to 5 mm in diameter) is indicated for contained defects, where it serves as a filler scaffold. It can undergo revascularization and remodeling, and it strengthens with time. If morcellized bone is used with a cementless cup, contact should be made with at least 50% of the host bone, and screws are usually necessary for cup fixation (5). If contact cannot be made with at least 50% of host bone, then a cemented cup with a roof reinforcement ring (16) or the technique of cementing into impacted bone (15) should be used.

Simulated structural graft is the term used when bone from another region is shaped to simulate the deficit. For example a distal femur can be sculpted to duplicate an acetabulum. The condyles can be reamed to accept an acetabular cup, while the metaphysis can provide bone for internal fixation to the ilium. Another option is the use of male or premenopausal female femoral heads, which can be sculpted to the desired shape.

Anatomical structural graft is the term used when the graft is the actual anatomical part being duplicated. For example, an acetabular allograft can be used in whole or in part to replace an acetabular defect. It is our experience that an anatomical graft is easier to shape to duplicate the defect and theoretically provides a more appropriate bone to withstand the subsequent biomechanical forces placed on it. We prefer an anatomical graft, but if that is not available, a simulated graft, such as a distal femur, is acceptable.

The advantages of a structural graft are restoration of anatomy and the potential to provide structural support for the implant. The disadvantage of a structural graft is that revascularization and remodeling can lead to resorption, collapse, or both; therefore it weakens with time.

Structural grafts are indicated for uncontained defects where it is necessary to restore anatomy and leg length and to provide bone support for the implant. An acceptable compromise to the anatomy and leg length is probably preferred to a structural graft if adequate bone stock is available, as through the use of a high hip center (8). If a high hip center is utilized, lateralization of the implant should be avoided, and there should be enough bone stock to allow a cementless or cemented component to be seated against healthy host bone (7,8). The leg-length discrepancy must be compensated by a long-neck prosthesis, and impingement of the femoral neck against the ischium must be avoided (8).

A structural allograft can fail by resorption or fragmentation (10,16). It is therefore important to protect these grafts by using implants that go from host bone to host bone, bridging and protecting the graft. It is also important to use strong bone for structural grafts. Allograft femoral heads obtained from postmenopausal females should be used in the morcellized form only. For structural grafting of the acetabulum, it has been our custom to use acetabular allografts, because they are strong and have the correct anatomical form and size for sculpting to fit segmental defects in this area. These grafts are fixed by cancellous screws and, if they support more than 50% of the cup, are protected by reconstruction rings. Alternatives to whole acetabular allografts include the use of excision arthroplasty (21) or perhaps the insertion of a custom implant.

When structural allografts are used, it is important to use morcellized autograft bone, which is usually available in the operative field, to bone graft host-allograft junctions, because allograft bone has poor bone induction properties (20).

Infection must be ruled out if it is suspected prior to allograft reconstruction and revision arthroplasty. A technetium, gallium, or indium scan and hip aspiration may be helpful (22–24). Even if these tests are negative, if, at the time of operation, the findings on gross examination, Gram stain, or frozen section are suspicious of infection, the reconstruction should be carried out in two stages *to avoid bone grafting into an infected site.*

III. METHODOLOGY

A. Approach and Graft Preparation

Reconstruction of the acetabulum with a contained defect can be carried out through any conventional approach, often without the need for trochanteric osteotomy. For structural defects, the author prefers to have access to the anterior and posterior columns and therefore uses a transtrochanteric approach. The trochanteric slide allows access to the posterior and anterior columns (25). This osteotomy is more stable than the transverse trochanteric osteotomy because the trochanter remains in continuity with the abductor and the vastus lateralis muscles and tendons making trochanteric migration unlikely. The trochanteric slide can be converted to a transverse osteotomy by releasing the vastus lateralis if more exposure is required. In the author's experience the prevalence of nonunion and trochanteric migration of 25% (32 of 130 hips) was unacceptably high with the classic transverse osteotomy (26).

A pin is inserted into the iliac crest and the distance between it and a fixed point on the resected trochanteric bed is measured as a reference for leg length. The sciatic nerve should be identified, particularly if leg lengthening of more than 3 cm is anticipated.

The acetabulum is prepared after the hip has been dislocated. After the acetabular component and cement have been removed, the interface membrane is excised gently. The defect then is defined by visualization, palpation, and the use of a trial cup. The defect is classified as contained or uncontained; then the decision is made as to what type of reconstruction and bone graft should be used. Much of this decision making can be done preoperatively based on the radiographs, but the final decision is based on the intraoperative findings.

The allograft bone, which is deep-frozen and irradiated (2.5 Mrad), is not opened until infection in the host joint has been ruled out by Gram's stain, frozen section, and visual inspection and the bone defect is defined. After the graft is unwrapped and cultured, it is thawed in a warm 50% solution of povidone-iodine (Betadine, Perdue Frederick Inc., Pickering Ontario, Canada) and saline. After the bone is thawed, it is prepared on a separate table. If morcellized bone is needed, morcellization may be done manually with rongeurs or by a bone mill. A bone mill that does not make the bone too mushy should be used. The morcellized bone pieces should be

5 to 10 mm in diameter. Alternatively, prepared morcellized bone can be obtained from some bone banks in freeze-dried or deep-frozen forms.

Structural grafts are prepared from acetabular allografts, male femoral heads, or distal femurs.

All bone is rinsed with a mixture of one-third 3% hydrogen peroxide, with two-thirds normal saline, and finally bacitracin (30,000 U in a 1000 mL of normal saline) before it is placed into the acetabular bed. This is the author's preferred mixture of cleansing solutions, but the author has no data to support this combination. Because the bone is dead and irradiated, these solutions should have no negative effect.

B. Surgical Technique

1. Type II Contained Defect (Cavitary)

A central or superomedial protrusio may be associated with a loose acetabular prosthesis (Figure 1A). The bone stock is restored by using impacted morcellized, cancellous allograft bone. Some of these defects are so large that two or three femoral heads may be necessary to obtain enough bone for morcellization. Female femoral heads should be used for morcellized

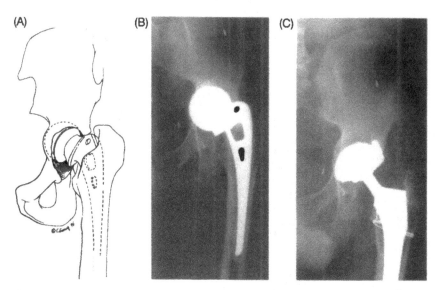

Figure 1   A. Drawing showing a contained (cavitary) defect. B. Radiograph of a 30-year-old man with a superomedial contained defect 10 years after a hemiarthroplasty for avascular necrosis of the femoral head. C. Patient seen 11½ years after revision surgery with morcellized allograft bone and an uncemented cup.

bone. There are several choices of acetabular implants that can be used, either uncemented or cemented.

For younger patients with higher demands, the author recommends impacted morcellized bone with an uncemented large-diameter cup. Contact with at least 50% host bone must be made. It is necessary to have some rim contact between the cup and the host (Figure 1B and C). Host-bone contact can be evaluated using a trial cup placed in the correct anatomical position and not in a high hip position. Some rim contact is important, particularly superiorly and posteriorly. It is optimal if the 50% host-bone contact is superior and posterior.

If contact cannot be made with 50% host bone, then the author recommends a roof reinforcement ring and a cemented cup. The ring must make rim contact with the host superiorly, posteriorly, and inferomedially and is fixed with at least three screws directed into the acetabular dome (Figure 2). If a contained defect is global, involving all quadrants of the acetabulum, then a reconstruction ring that goes from ilium to ischium must be used.

2. Type III Uncontained Defect (Segmental) Less Than 50% of the Acetabulum

In some acetabular revisions, it is difficult to obtain good coverage of the new cup because of superolateral bone loss attributable to loosening or failure to obtain good coverage during the primary procedure (Figure 3A). In

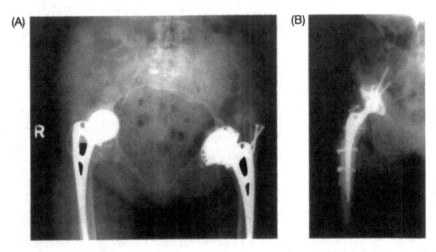

(A)   (B)

Figure 2 A. Radiograph of a 60-year-old woman with a contained defect several years after a hemiarthroplasty for a fracture. B. Radiograph obtained 5 years after revision surgery with a roof reinforcement ring and morcellized allograft bone.

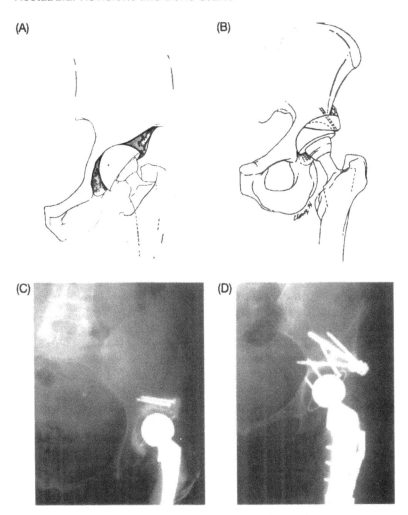

Figure 3 A. Drawing showing an uncontained defect involving less than 50% of acetabulum. B. Structural allograft (shelf or minor column) fixed by cancellous screws supports less than 50% of cup. Stippled area above shelf graft represents the "flying buttress" graft (morcellized autograft bone). C. Radiograph of a 32-year-old woman with bipolar arthroplasty for hip dysplasia and osteoarthritis. Poor coverage of the bipolar cup is seen. D. Radiograph obtained 12 years after revision surgery with minor column (shelf) allograft and an uncemented cup.

this situation, intact male femoral head segments or true acetabular allografts can be used to provide good coverage of the acetabular implant. These shelf or minor column grafts are fixed with 4.5-mm cancellous screws placed in an oblique to vertical direction (Figure 3B). The junction of the shelf allograft and the pelvic wall is autografted with cancellous bone (flying buttress graft). Cemented or uncemented acetabular implants can be used in combination with the shelf graft. There is contact with greater than 50% of host bone; therefore an uncemented cup can be used, but it is technically easier to use a cemented cup (Figure 3C and D).

3. Type IV Uncontained Defect (Segmental) Greater Than 50% of the Acetabulum

Major column defects are best restored with true acetabular allografts. These major column grafts are fixed to the host with cancellous screws and are protected by reconstruction rings that bridge the defect from host bone to host bone (Figure 4A and B). In this situation, the cup must be cemented because there is no contact with host bone. The reconstruction ring spans and protects the graft and also fixes a discontinuity if it exists. The ring goes from ilium to ischium. The ring is fixed by at least three cancellous screws inserted into the ilium, and two cancellous screws inserted into the ischium. If good screw fixation cannot be achieved into the ischium, then the inferior flange can be slotted into or buttressed against the ischium (Figure 4C and D).

In the author's experience, if stable fixation is achieved by screws in the ilium and ischium, the pelvic discontinuity is stabilized. If stable fixation cannot be achieved, particularly in the ischium, then additional fixation must be provided by a plate in addition to the ring. The author has had to do this in only one patient.

IV. AUTHOR'S RESULTS

Patients were evaluated prospectively using a modified Harris Hip Scoring System (26). Success was defined as a 20-point increase in the score, a stable cup (no migration of the cup or cement fractures), and no need for additional surgery on the acetabular side (10).

Allograft bone was assessed radiologically for union, as evidenced by trabecular bridging of the donor-host interface, for allograft fracture and fragmentation (for the structural grafts), and for graft resorption. Resorption was measured on anteroposterior pelvis radiographs and graded as minor (less than one-third of graft resorbed), moderate (one-third to one-half of

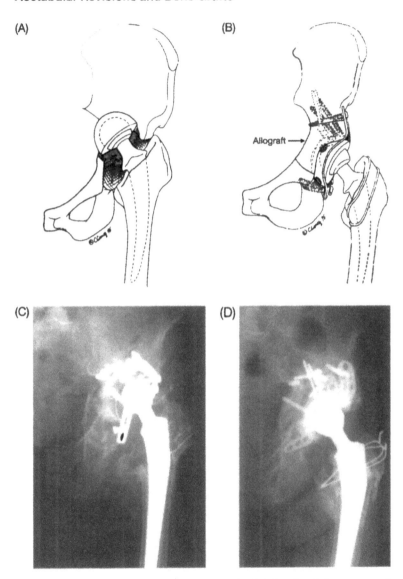

Figure 4 A. Drawing showing an uncontained defect involving greater than 50% of acetabulum with pelvic discontinuity. B. Reconstruction with structural allograft fixed by two cancellous screws and protected by reconstruction ring fixed to ilium and ischium. C. Radiograph of a 77-year-old man with a loose cemented cup and massive osteolysis of the right acetabulum involving greater than 50% of the acetabulum and pelvic discontinuity. D. Radiograph obtained 5 years after reconstruction with a major column allograft protected by a reconstruction ring that goes from host ilium to host ischium.

graft resorbed), and severe (more than one-half of graft resorbed). Migration was measured in superior and medial directions using the superolateral corner of the obturator foramen as a landmark. Loosening was defined as cup or ring migration of greater than 4 mm or a fracture of screws or the cement mantle. Radiographs were reviewed by two orthopaedic surgeons who were not blinded, and observer reliability was not assessed. As of October 1, 2000, a total of 676 hips have been revised using allograft bone during a period of 18 years at the author's institution. Of these, 575 have required acetabular revision.

A. Type II Contained Defects

Morcellized allograft bone has been used in 297 hips in 281 patients. Of these, 20 hips in 17 patients have required subsequent operations for a re-revision rate of 6.7%. In all, 7 were revised for recurrent dislocations and 13 were revised for cup loosening. In a study of 51 hips in 51 patients with at least 5 years follow-up (average, 6.8 years), the success rate was 90% (10). In 4 patients, 4 hips required an additional operation on the acetabular side.

    A total of 25 hips had uncemented cups (92% success rate); 16 hips had roof reinforcement rings (success rate 100%); and 10 hips had a bipolar acetabular component (success rate 70%). Severe resorption was seen in 2 of 25 hips with uncemented cups, which had to be revised, and in 3 of 10 bipolar cups, 2 of which had to be revised (10). In the four hips that were rerevised because of severe graft resorption, additional morcellized grafting was necessary.

    A more recent study was carried out on patients whose hips were reconstructed with morcellized allograft bone, a roof reinforcement ring, and a cemented cup because contact could not be made with 50% host bone. In this series of contained defects that were beyond the use of a cementless cup, one cup was found to have loosened at an average 5-year follow-up; this was revised. Four further hips were radiographically loose, demonstrating migration of the ring, but were asymptomatic (27).

B. Type III Uncontained Defects (Less than 50% of Acetabulum)

As of October 1 2000, a total of 74 hips in 69 patients had been revised with minor column allografts. Of these, 11 hips in 10 patients have required additional operations, for a rerevision rate of 15%. Seven hips were revised for cup loosening, 1 for infection, 1 for severe resorption, 1 for dislocation, and 1 for graft fracture. In 29 hips in 28 patients with a minimum of 5 years' follow-up (average, 7.1 years) the success rate as defined above was 86% (11). Of the total, 16 cups were uncemented porous-coated, 1 was a bipolar, 8 were cemented all-polyethylene, and 4 were cemented into roof reinforcement rings. In 4 patients, additional operations were required, 3 grafts had severe resorption, with 2 (1 cemented, 1 uncemented) requiring additional operations for cup loosening and only 1 of these 2 requiring additional grafting. One patient had an excision arthroplasty for loosening of a cemented cup, and one patient had exploration of the joint for pain but the graft was intact and the uncemented cup was solid. All but one graft united. There was no resorption in 9 patients, minor resorption in 17, and moderate resorption in 3.

In a more recent study, at an average follow-up of 10 years, of 47 patients in whom 51 hips were revised with minor column (shelf) allografts, 11 patients required additional surgery. Of these, 3 underwent excisional arthroplasty and 8 were successfully revised, with only 3 of the 8 requiring another structural graft. The cup aseptic survival was 80.4%, and the graft survival 94.1% (28).

C. Type IV Uncontained Defects (Greater than 50% of Acetabulum)

As of October 1, 2000, a total of 136 hips in 132 patients have been revised with major column allografts. Of these, 38 hips in 37 patients have required further surgery, for a rerevision rate of 28%; 11 hips in 10 patients have undergone excision arthroplasty and 27 have been revised successfully. 17 patients were revised for cup loosening, 9 for dislocation, and 1 explored for a sciatic nerve injury. Excision arthroplasty was done for nonunion in 1 patient, for cup loosening in 3 hips in 2 patients, for infection in 3 patients, for fracture in 1 patient, and for dislocation in 3 patients. In 33 hips in 32 patients with major column grafts and a minimum of 5 years' follow-up (average 7.1), 18 hips in 17 patients had a successful result, for a success rate of 55% (14). In the current study, success was defined as an increase in the hip score of at least 20 points, a stable cup with a united, structurally intact allograft and no additional operations related to the acetabulum. In 6 patients, 6 hips required additional operations for cup loosening, but the grafts were intact and united. One hip required exploration for a sciatic nerve injury. These hip replacements were considered partially successful because no additional grafting was necessary. The overall success rate, therefore, was 76%. Of 33 hips, 8 required additional operations because of graft failure, 7 having undergone severe resorption and 1 infection (14).

The acetabular implants used were 14 cemented polyethylene cups, 7 cementless cups, 4 bipolars, and 8 reconstruction rings with cemented cups. Of 8 reconstructions done with a ring and cemented cup, 7 were successful, with the only failure being the result of infection. Two of seven cementless cups and three of four bipolars had moderate or severe resorption requiring revision. Of 14 cups in 13 patients that were cemented directly into the allograft, 3 were associated with severe resorption and required additional surgery. Cup loosening occurred only when cementless or cemented cups were inserted directly into the allograft. Of the 15 hips in the 14 patients who required additional surgery, 7 required no additional grafting, 6 required additional grafting because of severe graft resorption, and 2 underwent excision arthroplasty.

V. DISCUSSION

The goals of revision arthroplasty of the hip are to restore the anatomy of the hip and to achieve a stable interface between implant and bone. This may be difficult to accomplish if there is loss of bone stock. Bone defects can be functionally classified as contained or uncontained. Contained defects are treated more easily than uncontained defects because by definition the acetabulum, although weakened and dilated, still has intact columns. Uncontained defects are segmental and there is loss of a part of the acetabular rim and the adjacent column.

Most orthopaedic surgeons throughout the world agree on the use of morcellized allograft bone to restore bone stock for contained defects (3,4,15,29–32). If contact can be made with 50% host bleeding bone, an uncemented cup can be used (3–5). This may require use of a jumbo cup. If contact cannot be made with 50% host bone, a cemented cup can be used with a roof reinforcement ring (10,31) or with a wire mesh (15,33). All of these techniques use impacted morcellized allograft bone and all have had excellent mid- to long-term results (3,4,15,29–32). For younger patients with high demands, the author's preference is to combine impacted allograft bone with an uncemented cup. If, however, contact cannot be made with 50% host bone, then a ring is used as a buttress to support the impacted bone and a cup is cemented into the ring. A roof reinforcement ring of the Müller (Sulzer, Baar, Switzerland) type is used if it can be stabilized against host bone superiorly and inferomedially. If the defect is a contained global defect affecting the entire acetabulum, then a reconstruction ring that extends from the ilium to the ischium should be used. If a roof reinforcement ring is seated entirely on morcellized allograft bone, it will toggle and fail; therefore it is necessary to use a device like the Burch-Schneider reconstruction ring (Sulzer), which extends from the ilium to the ischium.

The use of impacted morcellized bone for contained defects on the acetabular side has now gained universal acceptance, with the main variable being the choice of implant—cementless or cemented—and if cemented, with a ring or a mesh. The viability of the acetabular bone bed at revision surgery has been shown even after cemented primary arthroplasty (30). This provides a fertile base for remodelling of the morcellized allograft bone, which has been shown radiographically (33) and by biopsy (29).

Although the use of morcellized bone for contained defects is now well established, the treatment of uncontained defects remains controversial. Reports of structural graft failure have led to other methods for dealing with segmental acetabular defects (7). The use of large (5) or oblong cups (12,13) may be effective if adequate contact can be made with bleeding host bone. A high hip center is another alternative if adequate contact can be made with host bone (6–9). The leg-length discrepancy must be made up on the femoral side with long-neck or calcar-replacing femoral implants, which may lead to impingement against the ischium and instability. A high hip center may lead to a higher rate of component loosening (34,35) and does not restore bone stock for future surgery. However, despite these drawbacks, if a high hip center can be achieved without an unacceptable compromise to the anatomy, this may be the most practical solution for some patients. Impaction grafting with mesh to bridge segmental defects has also been used (33). The author's approach has been that restoration of bone stock should be one of he goals of revision surgery in the relatively younger patient facing additional revision surgery. If the bone defect is uncontained, then a structural graft may be necessary. There has been significant progress in tissue banking, so that a safer, stronger, higher-quality product is now available (36–43). Improvements in surgical techniques and implants to be used with allografts also have improved results (16). The author's experience has shown that even if additional surgery becomes necessary, the previously placed structural graft can often be salvaged, so that additional grafting may not be necessary. Thus, the goal of restoring bone stock for additional surgery is accomplished (14).

Structural acetabular grafts that support less than 50% of the acetabulum (minor column or shelf grafts) have a better prognosis than larger grafts. The success rate in the author's series is 86% at an average follow up of 7.1 years (11) and 80.4% at 10 years (28). These grafts are done using the same technique as shelf autografts in primary replacement for dysplasia and achieve similar results (44). They restore bone stock and anatomy and facilitate additional surgery. The success of these minor column or shelf grafts underlines the importance of striving for at least 50% contact between the cup and host bone, allowing the use of a minor rather than a major column graft.

Structural grafts that support greater than 50% of the acetabulum have a more guarded prognosis. These major column grafts in the author's entire series have a rerevision rate of 28%. A total of 32 grafts in 31 patients of 114 major column grafts required additional surgery, but 22 were revised successfully, with 16 requiring no additional bone grafting; 10 required excision arthroplasty. Moreover, this series includes all major column grafts using different techniques of fixation. However, when the technique described in this paper was used with protection of the graft by a reconstruction ring, the results were much better (7 of 8 being successful at an average followup of 7.5 years); the only failure was due to infection (14). The author now uses this technique for every major column graft. Major column grafts are indicated when the alternatives such as a high hip center or jumbo or oblong cups are not the optimal solution. Young patients with loss of 50% of the acetabulum and all patients with loss of 50% if the loss includes the dome and the posterior column with or without pelvic discontinuity are candidates for this procedure.

It is important to restore bone stock in revision arthroplasty of the hip especially in patients facing the possibility of additional revision surgery. A morcellized graft for contained defects has the best prognosis and is most widely accepted. Grafts that support less than 50% of the acetabulum also have a good prognosis. Grafts that support greater than 50% have a more guarded prognosis; therefore it is better to perform revisions when the defect still is contained or involves less than 50% of the acetabulum. If the defect becomes greater than 50% or is associated with a pelvic discontinuity, a major column graft may be necessary. Better-quality bone and improved surgical techniques have improved results in patients undergoing these complex reconstructions.

REFERENCES

1. Judet R, Judet J, Letournel E: Fractures of the acetabulum: classification and surgical approaches for open reduction. J Bone Joint Surg 46A:1615–1646, 1964.
2. Hozak WJ, Mesa JJ, Carey C, Rothman RH: Relationship between polyethylene wear, pelvic osteolysis and clinical symptomatology in patients with cementless acetabular components. J Arthrop 11:769–772, 1996.
3. Padgett DE, Kull L, Rosenberg A, Sumner DR, Galante JO: Revision of the acetabular component without cement after total hip arthroplasty. J Bone Joint Surg 75A:663–673, 1993.

4. Silverton CD, Rosenberg AG, Mitchell BS, et al: Revision of the acetabular component without cement after total hip arthroplasty. J Bone Joint Surg 78: 1366–1370, 1996.

5. Tanzer M, Drucker D, Jasty M, et al: Revision of acetabular components with an uncemented Harris-Galante porous-coated prosthesis. J Bone Joint Surg 74A:987–994, 1992.

6. Harris WH: Reconstruction at a high hip centre in acetabular revision surgery using a cementless acetabular component. Orthopaedics 21:991–992, 1998.

7. Kwong LM, Jasty M, Harris WH: High failure rate of bulk femoral head allografts in total hip acetabular reconstructions at 10 years. J Arthrop 8:341–346, 1993.

8. Russotti GM, Harris WH: Proximal placement of the acetabular component in total hip arthroplasty. A long-term follow-up study. J Bone Joint Surg 73A: 587–592, 1991.

9. Schutzer SF, Harris WH: High placement of porous coated acetabular components in complex total hip arthroplasty. J Arthrop 9:359–367, 1994.

10. Garbuz D, Morsi E, Mohamed N, Gross AE: Classification and reconstruction in revision acetabular arthroplasty with bone stock deficiency. Clin Orthop 324: 98–107, 1996.

11. Morsi E, Garbuz D, Gross AE: Revision total hip arthroplasty with shelf bulk allografts. J Arthrop 11:86–90, 1996.

12. De Boer DK, Christie MJ: Reconstruction of the deficient acetabulum with an oblong prosthesis. J Arthrop 13(6):674–680, 1998.

13. Koster G, Willert GH, Kohler HP, Dopkens K: An oblong revision cup for large acetabular defects. J Arthrop 13:559–569, 1998.

14. Garbuz D, Morsi E, Gross AE: Revision of the acetabular component of a total hip arthroplasty with a massive structural allograft. J Bone Joint Surg 78A: 693–697, 1996.

15. Slooff TJJH, Buma P, Schreurs BW, et al: Acetabular and femoral reconstruction with impacted graft and cement. Clin Orthop 323:108–115, 1996.

16. Gross AE, Duncan CP, Garbuz D, Elsayed Morsi ZM: Revision arthroplasty of the acetabulum in association with loss of bone stock. J Bone Joint Surg 80A:440–451, 1998.

17. Czitrom AA: Immunology of bone and cartilage allografts, in Czitrom AA, and Gross AE (eds): Allografts in Orthopaedic Practice. Baltimore, Williams & Wilkins, 1992, pp 15–25.

18. Czitrom A, Gross A, Langer F, et al: Bone banks and allografts in community practice. Instr Course Lect Am Acad Orthop Surg 37:13–24, 1988.

19. Langer F, Czitrom A, Pritzker KP, et al: The immunogenicity of fresh and frozen allogenic bone. J Bone Joint Surg 57A:216–220, 1975.

20. Goldberg VM, Stevenson S: Biology of bone and cartilage allografts, in Czitrom AA, and Gross AE (eds): Allografts in Orthopaedic Practice. Baltimore, Williams & Wilkins, 1992, pp 1–13.

21. Harris WH, White RE Jr: Resection arthroplasty for non-septic failure of total hip arthroplasty. Clin Orthop 171:62–67, 1982.

22. Barrack RL, Harris WH: The value of aspiration of the hip joint before revision total hip arthroplasty. J Bone Joint Surg 75A;1:66–76, 1993.

23. Gristina AG, Kolkin J: Current concepts review. Total joint replacement and sepsis. J Bone Joint Surg 65A:128–134, 1983.

24. Johnson JA, Christie MJ, Sandler MP, et al: Detection of occult infection following total joint arthroplasty using sequential technetium-99m HDP bone scintigraphy and indium-111 WBC imaging. J Nucl Med 29:1347–1353, 1988.

25. Glassman AH, Engh CA, Bobyn JD: A technique of extensile exposure for total hip arthroplasty. J Arthrop 2:11–21, 1987.

26. Gross AE, Hutchison CR, Alexeef M, et al: Proximal femoral allografts for reconstruction of bone stock in revision arthroplasty of the hip. Clin Orthop 319:151–158, 1995.

27. Wong P, Saleh KJ, King A, Gross AE: Acetabular revision with a roof reinforcement ring and impacted allograft bone. Hip Int 10(3):145–150, 2000.

28. Woodgate IG, Saleh KJ, Jaroszynski G, Agnidis Z, Woodgate MM, Gross AE: Minor column structural acetabular allografts in revision hip surgery. Clin Orthop Rel Res 371:75–85, 2000.

29. Heekin RD, Engh CA, Vinh T: Morsellized allograft in acetabular reconstruction. Clin Orthop 319:184–190, 1995.

30. Lamerigts NMP, Buma P, Sardar R, et al: Viability of the acetabular bone bed at revision surgery following cemented primary arthroplasty. J Arthrop 13:524–529, 1998.

31. Rosson J, Schatzker J: The use of reinforcement rings to reconstruct deficient acetabula. J Bone Joint Surg 74B:716–720, 1992.

32. Zehtner MK, Ganz R: Mid-term results (5.5 to 10 years) of acetabular allograft reconstruction with the acetabular reinforcement ring during total hip revision arthroplasty. J Arthrop 9:469–479, 1994.

33. Slooff TJ, Schimmel JW, Buma P: Cemented fixation with bone grafts. Orthop Clin North AM 24:667–677, 1993.

34. Kelley SS: High hip center in revision arthroplasty. J Arthrop 9,5:503–510, 1994.

35. Pagnano MW, Hanssen AD, Lewallen DG, Shaughnessey WJ: The effect of superior placement of the acetabular component on the rate of loosening after total hip arthroplasty. J Bone Joint Surg 78A:1004–1014, 1996.

36. Buck BE, Malinin TI, Brown MD: Bone transplantation and human immunodeficiency virus. An estimated risk of acquired immunodeficiency syndrome. Clin Orthop 24:129–136, 1989.

37. Campbell DG, Peng Li, Stephenson AJ, Oakeshott RD: Sterilization of HIV by gamma irradiation. Int Orthop 18:172–176, 1994.

38. Eastlund T: Infectious Hazards of Bone Allograft Transplantation: Reducing the Risk. In Czitrom A, Winkler H (eds): Orthopaedic Allograft Surgery. New York, Springer-Verlag, 1996, pp 11–28.

39. Fideler BM, Vangsness CT, Moore T, et al: Effects of gamma irradiation on the human immunodeficiency virus. A study in frozen human bone-patellar ligament-bone grafts obtained from infected cadavera. J Bone Joint Surg 76A: 1032–1035, 1994.

40. Jacobs NJ: Establishing a surgical bone bank. In Fawcett KJ, Barr HR (eds): Tissue Banking. Arlington VA, American Association of Blood Banks 1987, pp 67–96.

41. Pelker RR, Friedlaender GE, Markham TC: Biomechanical properties of bone allografts. Clin Orthop 174:54–57, 1983.

42. Mowe JC (ed): Standards for Tissue Banking. Arlington, VA, American Association of Tissue Banks 1984, revised 1985, 1987, 1988.

43. Tomford WW: Transmission of disease through transplantation of musculoskeletal allografts. J Bone Joint Surg 77A:1742–1754, 1995.

44. Morsi EZM, Garbuz D, Stockley I, Catre M, Gross AE: Total hip replacement in dysplastic hips using femoral head autografts. Clin Orthop 324:164–168, 1996.

8
Revision of the Femoral Component

Raj K. Sinha
University of Pittsburgh Medical Center, Pittsburgh, Pennsylvania

I. EVALUATION OF THE FAILED TOTAL HIP ARTHROPLASTY

Despite the widespread success of total hip arthroplasty, (THA), approximately 1% per year will fail, often requiring revision surgery (1). Given that approximately 125,000 THAs are performed annually in the United States, surgeons can expect that 1250 to 2000 revisons will need to be performed yearly (1). This chapter focuses upon evaluation and treatment of the failed femoral stem.

A. Causes of Failure

The reasons for failure of femoral stems are as diverse as are the number of stems currently available on the market. Certain design issues, mode of fixation, and surgical technique, among other factors, contribute to failure.

1. Aseptic Loosening

Stems designed for both cemented and cementless fixation are susceptible to loosening. Loosening can occur immediately after implantation or after a period of solid mechanical fixation. For cemented stems, immediate loosening is unusual unless some technical complication occurred at the time of implantation. This may include movement of the stem within the cement mantle before the cement has fully polymerized, cortical penetration or fracture during implantation, or distal migration of the cement restrictor during pressurization of the cement. Late loosening in cemented stems is usually an insidious process that leads to loss of interlock between the cement and cancellous bone or between the implant and the cement (Figure 1). Disruption of the cement-bone interface is typically the result of particulate debris that generates a penetrating fibrous tissue which invades the interface (2).

Alternatively, the interlock between the bone and the cement may succumb to the normal forces exerted upon the stem over time, leading to gradual loss of stability of the entire prosthesis-cement construct within the intramedullary canal (3). Osteopenic bone and cemented revisions into a smooth, sclerotic canal are susceptible to this mode of failure. In addition, certain design characteristics, such as precoating or macrotexturing, predispose stems to this mode of failure, as the strength of fixation at the prosthesis-cement interface is exceedingly rigid compared to that at the cement-bone interface (4).

Cementless stems, similarly, may become loose soon after implantation or after a period of initial strong mechanical fixation. Lack of initial stability

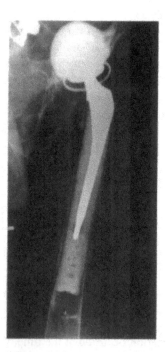

Figure 1   Example of an initially well-cemented stem that became loose two years after implantation. Note the circumferential radiolucency at the cement-bone interface.

often will result in failure of osseointegration (5). In this situation, loosening will be evident by change of stem position between the immediate postoperative radiograph and subsequent x-rays (Figure 2). In some situations, a stem will become fibrous-stable (6), in which circumstance the stem is not osseointegrated but not grossly unstable. These stems will cause intermittent thigh pain but will not demonstrably migrate on serial radiographs, thus often avoiding the need to remove them. Once a cementless stem becomes osseointegrated, it is uncommon for it to loosen, as survival rates exceed 95% for many different stem designs (7–9). Nevertheless, certain design features predispose to loosening, primarily due to particle-induced disruption of the interface. These features include less than circumferential porous coating, smooth portions at the proximal aspect that allow easy access to the diaphysis, anatomically shaped stems, and large-diameter heads (10,11). Rarely, a stem that achieves distal fixation but has no proximal contact may loosen due to bending stresses during repetitive loading.

2. Polyethylene Wear

The generation of polyethylene wear debris at the articular surface can lead to aseptic loosening of femoral stems but warrants separate mention. Certain

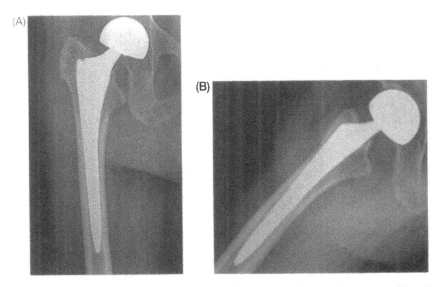

Figure 2 (A) Anteroposterior radiograph of a cementless stem that never achieved ingrowth because of lack of initial axial stability. Note that the proximo-medial aspect of the stem has subsided almost one centimeter below the level of the calcar, the level at which it was initially inserted. (B) Lateral radiograph of subsided stem.

design features, termed "particle generators," are known to cause large amounts of wear debris (12). These include 32-mm heads, scratched or burnished heads, titanium heads, poor congruency between the polyethylene liner and the acetabular component, and an inferior locking mechanism for the liner within the shell. Other design features will allow a well-fixed component to become loose after several years of service. For example, less than circumferential porous coating, which allows easy access of debris to the diaphysis, was commonly the culprit for the high failure rate of the HGP and APR-I stems (10,11). Though initially fixed, these stems would loosen in the face of large, ballooning osteolytic lesions that disrupted the osseointegrated surface. Similarly, circumferentially porous-coated stems may succumb to the aggressive osteolytic response incited by large amounts of wear debris (13). Avoidance of these features will generally lead to prolonged life for the femoral component (Figure 3).

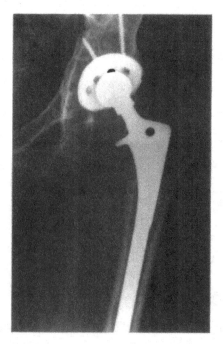

Figure 3 A cementless stem with patch-porous coating. Polyethylene debris was able to migrate along the smooth surfaces of the stem, leading to diaphyseal osteolysis and endosteal scalloping, with eventual loosening 11 years after insertion.

3. Infection

An infected arthroplasty will lead to pain and often loosening of the femoral stem. Effective treatment of the infection frequently requires removal of the component, resulting in bone loss that necessitates use of a revision component at the time of reimplantation. The diagnosis and treatment of infected THAs is thoroughly discussed in Chapter 10 of this text.

4. Dislocation

Removal of a well-fixed stem may be necessary due to component malposition, leading to recurrent dislocation. Most commonly, the stem was placed in excessive retroversion, leading to posterior dislocation during flexion, adduction, and internal rotation (Figure 4).

5. Periprosthetic Fracture

Fracture of the femur has been estimated to occur in 0.1% of THAs (14). Type I fractures (15), located adjacent to the stem, are often treated nonoperatively. If nonunion occurs, revision is necessary. In some situations, the type I fracture may lead to disruption of the osseointegrated interface, forcing component revision. Type II (extending beyond the tip of the stem) and type III (located entirely distal to the tip of the stem) fractures have been treated successfully with cable plates and allograft struts, with retention

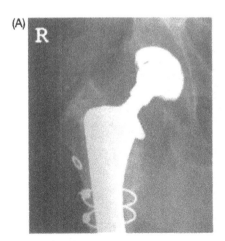 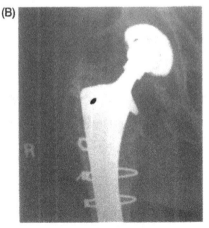

Figure 4   (A) Immediate postoperative film of a revision stem. (B) Radiograph of same stem 3 months postoperatively. The patient had suffered two dislocations, despite little change in radiographic apearance. At surgery, the stem was noted to have subsided and fallen into retroversion, resulting in instability.

of a well-fixed component (16,17). However, the author prefers removal of a well-fixed prosthesis followed by implantation of a long-stem prosthesis that bypasses the fracture, supplemented by an external strut graft and/or cable-plate fixation. This provides greater rotational stability of the fracture by virtue of both intra- and extramedullary fixation (Figure 5).

Periprosthetic fractures may also occur through osteolytic lesions in well-fixed stems or due to progressive endosteal cortical thinning caused by a chronically loose stem. These are almost always type II or III and are treated as described in the preceding paragraph.

6. Component Fracture

Breakage of a component is fortunately quite rare. It has been described as a mode of failure for cemented components since the 1970s (18), when

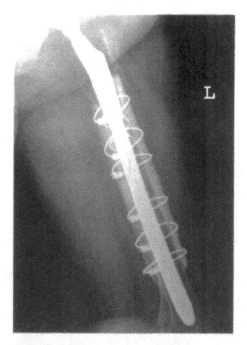

Figure 5 Example of a periprosthetic fracture nonunion treated by removal of the cemented stem, excision of the nonunion, apposition of the healthy proximal and distal femur, placement of two strut grafts, and implantation of a long-stem fully porous coated stem. This lateral radiograph, taken one year postoperatively, demonstrates osseointegration of the stem, healing of the nonunion, and incorporation of both strut grafts into host bone.

fatigue fractures of weaker stems were attributed to pistoning or inadequate proximal support (Figure 6). More recently, manufacturing techniques such as laser etching (19), the increased use of modular components, and stems of small diameter have been implicated.

7. Occult Pain

Painful THA without apparent radiographic or infectious reason for failure is difficult to treat. Exploration of an arthroplasty, with or without revision, has a poor rate of success (20). Thigh pain in a large-diameter stem has been related to modulus mismatch between the stiff metal alloy and the cortical bone, resulting in stress concentration in the bone adjacent to the tip of the stem (21). It is more commonly seen in straight cobalt-chrome stems and those greater than 17 mm in diameter. Treatment may include placement of an allograft strut to stiffen the bone (22) or revision of the component to a longer bowed stem that bypasses the area of stress concen-

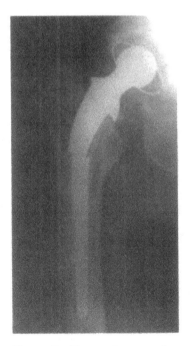

Figure 6   Fractured cemented stem 12 years after implantation. At revision surgery, the distal portion of the stem was well-fixed within the cement mantle, which was also well-fixed within the canal. The proximal portion of the stem and cement were grossly loose.

tration. Other possible sources of occult pain include iliopsoas tendon impingement, capsular impingement between the head and the cup, and galvanic corrosion between the arthroplasty and retained fixation devices from previous surgeries (e.g., screws in the trochanter or acetabulum) or between modular portions of the stem (Figure 7).

B. Radiographic Evaluation of Failed Stems

1. Cemented Stems

Specific criteria for loosening of a cemented stem have been described (23). These include stem fracture, cement mantle fracture, subsidence of greater than 5 mm, progressive radiolucency at the cement-bone interface, 2-mm radiolucency along greater than 50% of the cement-bone interface, and stem debonding from the cement. Recently, Berry et al. reported upon a series of debonded smooth stems that were not loose (24). Thus, debonding at the prosthesis-cement interface is acceptable in smooth, polished stems but is a harbinger of impending failure for textured or precoated stems (Figure 8).

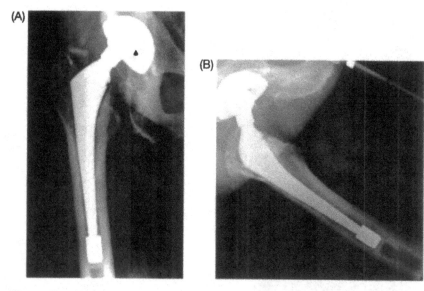

Figure 7 (A) Anteroposterior and (B) lateral radiograph of a modular stem that required revision due to persistent, disabling thigh pain. Despite the radiolucencies and distal pedestal, the stem was ingrown proximally, and the bullet tip was encapsulated by bone. In fact, this stem design is well-known to exhibit a pedestal even when ingrown. Revision to a fully porous coated stem that bypassed the level of pedestal resolved the patient's symptoms.

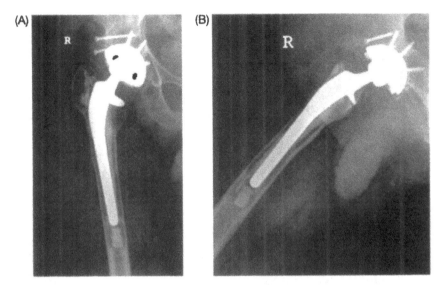

Figure 8 (A) Anteroposterior and (B) lateral radiograph of a precoated cemented stem 8 years after implantation. Note the circumferential radiolucencies, cement mantle fracture, loose cement restrictor, and subsided stem.

2. Cementless Stems

Criteria for loosening of cementless stems have been defined by Engh et al. (6). These include greater than 5-mm of subsidence, shedding of porous coating, radiolucency adjacent to the porous coating, cortical hypertrophy, and presence of a weight-bearing pedestal (Figure 9).

II. PREOPERATIVE PLANNING

A. Workup

Prior to revision surgery, the patient should have a thorough medical evaluation by an internist and the appropriate specialists. Infection can be reliably ruled out by checking an ESR and C-reactive protein. Normal values for both tests gives a negative predictive value of greater than 95% (25). Elevated values for one or the other give a positive predictive value for infection of greater than 90% (25). If there is any question whether a prosthesis may be infected, an aspiration should be performed to culture the joint fluid. Aspiration may need to be repeated if clinical suspicion is high and culture results are negative. Workup of a possibly infected THA is discussed in detail in Chapter 12 of this text.

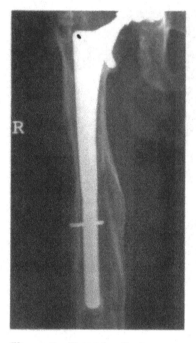

Figure 9   Example of a loose cementless stem. The stem has subsided and has a weight-bearing distal pedestal.

Femoral bone stock must be evaluated by full-length x-rays. Acetabular bone stock can be evaluated by Judet views and computed tomography (CT) scans when necessary. The appropriate components then can be ordered to address bone defects that are likely to be encountered during surgery. If limb lengthening greater than 2 cm is anticipated, the use of intraoperative somatosensory evoked potentials (SSEPs) is useful (26). Management of blood loss is controversial. The author favors preautologous donation coupled with intraoperative blood salvage and the use of autotransfusion drains postoperatively.

B.   Templating

Templating of preoperative x-rays is useful for several reasons. It provides the surgeon with the opportunity to dedicate time to planning and rehearsing the contemplated procedure. I have my residents and fellows make a tracing of the patient's x-rays that eliminates the implanted components (Figure 10). Sizing and positioning of the acetabular and femoral components can then

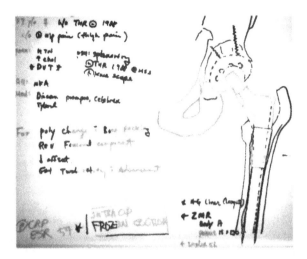

Figure 10 Template for a planned revision hip replacement. The template contains patient medical history, surgical plan, estimated sizes, and special considerations such as intraoperative frozen section.

be accomplished and often will highlight considerations such as placement of a high hip center cup, length of the stem required to bypass defects, depth of stem insertion to restore leg lengths, evaluation of offset compared to the opposite side, need for osteotomies for exposure or to restore alignment, the need for strut grafts, and the need for specialized equipment. A detailed discussion of templating for primary and revision hip replacement can be found in Chapter 13.

C. Surgical Exposure

1. Lateral Approach

I favor the Hardinge approach (27) to expose the hip joint. This and other anterior approaches have been associated with a lower dislocation rate (28). It can easily be converted to an extended trochanteric osteotomy but has the disadvantage of requiring a large amount of muscle stripping to do so. In addition, when the stem is severely retroverted, dislocation of the THA may be somewhat difficult. Nevertheless, with loose stems, this approach is adequate in the vast majority of cases.

2. Posterior Approach

Many authors favor the posterior approach (29). This approach is extensile and can easily be converted to an extended trochanteric osteotomy (30). It requires one less assistant but has the disadvantage of having a higher dislocation rate, presumably due to the tendency to retrovert both the acetabular and femoral component during implantation. I see no particular advantage of the posterior approach over the lateral except in terms of surgeon familiarity.

3. Extended Trochanteric Osteotomy

As described by Paprosky and associates (30), this technique is extremely useful for removing well-fixed cemented and cementless components. Mobilization of the lateral aspect of the greater trochanter and the proximal lateral femur allows easy access to the bone-cement or bone-prosthesis interface. Standard osteotomes can then be used to disrupt the interfaces. The distal canal is then easily accessible both for removal of cement and reaming for implantation of a straight component. Results with this technique have been extremely satisfying. The occasional complication includes nonunion or migration of the osteotomy fragment.

D. Removal of Implants

For loose components, extraction devices are very helpful in disrupting the fibrous tissue that tends to surround the prosthesis. Prior to the use of such devices, however, the lateral shoulder of the implant must be cleared of all capsule and overhanging trochanteric osteophyte. This avoids the devastating complication of fracture of the greater trochanter. Since the trochanter is often lytic, fixation with claw devices and standard wiring techniques is tenuous, with poor healing potential. Thus, fracture of the greater trochanter should be avoided at all costs.

Once the component is removed, standard hand chisels, curettes, drills, and burrs can be used to remove cement from within the canal. Alternatively, ultrasonic tools that melt the acrylic cement but do not penetrate bone are available for cement removal. On occasion, a femoral window may be necessary to remove a particularly recalcitrant cement restrictor or other debris. Fortunately, windows heal reliably (31). Finally, an extended trochanteric osteotomy simplifies removal of components and cement, as direct visualization of both is possible.

III. CHOOSING A STEM

A. Cemented Revision

Successful fixation of THA components was first reliably performed with acrylic polymethylmethacrylate (PMMA). Thus, when infection and mechanical loosening necessitated revision of femoral components, surgeons initially used cement for repeated fixation. Unfortunately, results were not encouraging, as discussed below.

1. Interface Mechanics

PMMA acts as a grout and is cohesive rather than adhesive. Cement must interdigitate with cancellous bone to achieve solid fixation. Simultaneously, cement bonds to metal femoral components by interdigitating with the microscopic irregularities in the surface of metal. Alternatively, when a polished, tapered stem is used, the cement forms an exact mold of the component, allowing it to remain stable even though the bond between the cement and the metal is relatively weak.

When femoral stems loosen, the motion of the stem and cement within the canal leads to the formation of a smooth and sclerotic endosteal surface. This surface does not allow for adequate interdigitation of cement within bone; thus, the bond to bone is significantly reduced. In fact, the shear strength of the cement-bone interface in a revision femoral canal is only 21% of that in a primary situation (32). In a repeat revision, the shear strength drops to only 6%.

2. Clinical Results

Given the unfavorable mechanical situation when using cement in a revision situation, it is not surprising that results have been worse than with primary THA. Pellici et al. (33) revised 110 stems with cement. At 3.4-year follow-up, 15 of 110 (14%) stems had loosened. By 1985, this same group of patients had been followed for 8.1 years, with a 29% mechanical failure rate (34). Similarly, Callaghan et al. reported a 15.8% failure rate of cemented revision stems after only 3.6 years of follow-up (35). The authors suggested that young, active patients had a higher chance for failure. Marti et al. (36) revised 60 stems with cement in elderly, low-demand patients. Although survivorship was 85% at 8.9 years, 19 of 60 (32%) stems were loose. Finally, Engelbrecht et al. (37) reported that 43 of 193 (22%) stems were loose after 7.4 years of follow-up. Thus, stem revision using first-generation cementing techniques historically has been associated with poor durability.

Improved cementing techniques have increased survivorship of primary stems. Second-generation techniques include the use of an intramedullary plug and cement gun to deliver the cement in a doughy state. Third-generation technique includes the use of pulsatile lavage to clean the bone bed of debris and porosity reduction of the cement by vacuum-mixing or centrifugation. These improved techniques have been utilized for revision of the femoral stem with cement and reported upon by several authors. Using second-generation cement technique, Pierson and Harris reported a 14% failure rate in 29 patients after 8.5 years (38). Similarly, Raut et al. (39) found that the use of an intramedullary cement block decreased the rate of loosening at 6.3 years from 17% (3 of 18) to 2% (2 of 88). However, Mulroy and Harris (40) reported that 26% of stems inserted using second-generation cement technique at the time of revision were loose at average 15-year follow-up. Poor proximal femoral bone stock at the time of revision was felt to contribute to the loosening rate. Hultmark et al. (41) used second- and third-generation techniques to revise 109 femoral components. They reported that 7 of 21 standard-length cemented revision stems were loose at mean 7.6-year follow-up, while only 1 of 88 long stem prostheses were loose. Similarly, third-generation cement techniques were applied to revision arthroplasties using a Charnley prosthesis (42). Of 74 stems, 39% were loose at 3.6-year follow-up. The quality of the cement-bone interface was the only radiographic factor that predicted stem durability.

Thus, it appears that cemented revision is best reserved for elderly, low-demand patients with good femoral bone stock and short expected life-spans (Figure 11). The cement technique used seems less critical, although longer stems with neutral alignment and good-quality cement mantles are likely to provide the best results.

B. Monoblock Cementless Revision

1. Clinical Results

Many different types of cementless stems have been designed and used for the revision of failed stems. As one might expect, several of these designs were unsuccessful for various reasons, from design flaws to poor choice of materials.

This section discusses successful designs only, focusing on common stem characteristics that make for success.

a. Proximal Fixation. In situations where there is minimal loss of proximal femoral bone, a primary stem can be used for revision. However, the issues of stem choice arise when there is significant loss or deformity of femoral bone. One revision stem with good intermediate- to long-term follow-up is the Mallory-Head Calcar (43). This stem is a monoblock titanium alloy stem with a proximal plasma spray porous coating and distal corundumization. It has a calcar buildup proximally. Head et al. reported a 96% survivorship rate at 10-year follow-up, with minimal thigh pain (43). All bone-type deformities were treated.

b. Hydroxyapatite Stems. Several recent stem designs with proximal HA or HA-TCP coating have been introduced (44). Long-term data are

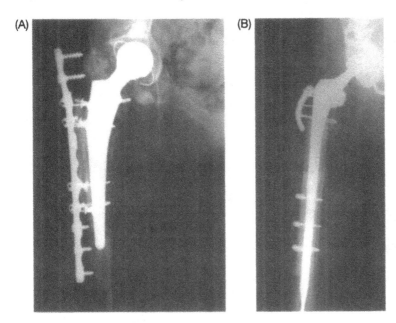

Figure 11 (A) Radiograph showing nonunion of a periprosthetic fracture treated with a lateral plate. In addition, the cemented stem is loose. (B) Immediate postoperative film of revision THA. Because the patient was elderly and had very low functional demands, the hip was reconstructed with a long-stem cemented stem and strut graft.

scarce. The general impression is that HA coating allows quicker osseointegration and may increase bone stock, particularly in contained defects.

c. Distal Fixation

AML. The Anatomic Medullary Locking (AML, Depuy, Inc., Warsaw, IN) stem and its revision stem, the Solution, have been available for revision arthroplasty since 1983 (Figure 12). This stem is made of cobalt-chromium-molybdenum alloy and is circumferentially porous-coated with cobalt-chrome beads along its entire length. The stem is intended to gain fixation in the diaphyseal portion of the femur. Engh et al. (45) reported on 127 patients with failed cemented stems who were revised with AML stems. At average 6.6-year follow-up, 84% were bone-ingrown and 12% were stably fibrous-ingrown. The fixation failure rate was only 4%. The authors noted that optimal fill of the diaphysis was important for osseous ingrowth

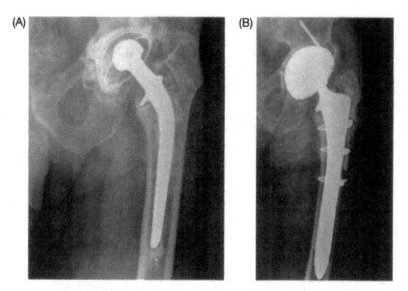

Figure 12 (A) Failed cemented THA. (B) Postoperative radiograph of cementless revision THA. A fully porous coated Solution cup and stem (Depuy, Inc, Warsaw, IN) were utilized. In addition, an extended trochanteric osteotomy was utilized to facilitate removal of the failed implant.

to occur. Similarly, revision of 21 failed cementless stems to a larger cementless stem met with good results. Of 21 stems, none were radiographically loose and Harris hip scores improved from 42 to 84 at average 6.3-year follow-up (46). In addition, Paprosky et al. (47) reported their results with the AML for revision at minimum 10-year follow-up: 82% were osseointegrated and 14% had stable fibrous fixation. The mechanical failure rate was 4%. Stress shielding was greatest in stems over 16.5 mm in diameter. Disadvantages include the possibility of gaining distal fixation only, thigh pain, and intraoperative fracture. When distal fixation only can be achieved, the proximal femur is susceptible to stress shielding, occasionally leading to fracture of the trochanter (48). When stress shielding is severe, revision of a well-fixed AML often leaves few choices for reconstruction except for a tumor-type of prosthesis. Thigh pain is related to the diameter of the stem, and an incidence of up to 25% has been reported (49). Intraoperative fracture may occur when large-diameter stems are inserted within femurs having thin cortices. Also, fractures may occur when long, straight stems are inserted into bowed femurs.

C. Modular Cementless Revision

1. Advantages of Modularity

Despite the widespread use of monoblock revision stems, several problems have been identified, as described above. Chief among these are proximal stress shielding and thigh pain. In order to gain proximal bone contact, modular components were developed. These stems allow broaching and sizing of the proximal femur that is independent from diaphyseal reaming and sizing. Trial body and stem components can then be assembled to gain bone contact proximally, distally, or both. Advantages include the ability to reconstruct a wide variety of types of femoral bone loss and deformity, the ability to change stem version without compromising fixation, proximal stress transfer to decrease the risk of stress shielding, and the ability to use curved stems to decrease the risk of thigh pain.

2. Disadvantages of Modularity

There are several disadvantages to modular components. Cost can be significantly increased due to increased complexity and tolerances in design. Because of the extra interface between the proximal body and stem, fretting corrosion may be increased (50). In addition, the stems are weaker at the junction, and if the proximal body does not achieve ingrowth, bending forces are concentrated at the junction, creating the risk of stem fracture (51).

3. Clinical Results

   a. S-ROM. The S-ROM revision stem (J&J, Warsaw, IN) has a series of proximal sleeves that can be fitted to the proximal femoral metaphysis to gain a large area of surface contact. The sleeves have a graduated surface with a circumferential porous coating. There is a circular hole through the sleeves that allow a non-porous-coated, bowed or straight, fluted stem to be inserted into the diaphysis. The two components are mated via a Morse taper junction. The stem provides initial rotational and axial stability, so that the proximal sleeve can achieve ingrowth.

   Smith et al. (52) reported on 66 consecutive revisions with 2- to 5-year follow-up. Eighty-nine percent of patients were satisfied with their results, and the average Harris hip score improved from 44 to 83. Fifty-two of 66 stems (79%) had bony ingrowth, while 7 were fibrous-stable and 5 were loose. Although the 5-year survival rate, as defined by revision, was 96%, the mechanical failure rate was 8%. Although this modular stem provides the ability to address a wide variety of bone-loss situations, the mechanical loosening rate is higher than that of the AML. Further evaluation will determine the relative value of the S-ROM stem in revision arthroplasty.

b. Modular Mallory-Head. Another modular version of revision stems is the modular Mallory-Head (Biomet, Inc., Warsaw, IN). This stem has a circumferentially plasma-sprayed titanium proximal body that is coupled to a plasma-sprayed titanium stem via a Morse taper and screw. The proximal body has a calcar loading configuration, one offset, three body heights, and six circumferences. The stems may be straight or bowed and come in a variety of lengths.

To my knowledge, there are no published papers on results with this stem. However, I have implanted 33 modular Mallory-Head stems with a minimal 2-year follow-up. Three intraoperative fractures occurred, all treated successfully with cerclage fixation. Six patients had a single dislocation; all were treated successfully with 6 weeks of bracing. All stems have achieved radiographic evidence of osseointegration with no detectable subsidence. Long-term follow-up is necessary to determine whether any adverse effects will occur as a result of the modularity.

c. ZMR. A recently introduced modular revision stem is the ZMR (Zimmer Holdings, Inc, Warsaw, IN). This system has four proximal body configurations (tapered, cone, calcar, spout) with two offsets, three body heights (34, 45, and 55 mm), and six diameters. There are multiple stem options: grit-blasted tapered, straight smooth, straight fully porous coated, bowed smooth, and bowed fully porous-coated.

Again, no long-term data are available. I have implanted 48 ZMR stems with minimal 3-month follow-up. Forty-seven stems have achieved ingrowth, two have dislocated (both treated with bracing), and four intraoperative fractures have occurred. Longer follow-up will provide more information (Figure 13).

IV. SPECIAL CONSIDERATIONS

A. Periprosthetic Fracture

1. Stem Revision Required

When the periprosthetic fracture is associated with a loose stem or occurs at the tip of the stem, I favor revision with a long-stem fully porous-coated prosthesis that passes the fracture site and is supplemented with an external cortical strut allograft or cable plate (Figure 14). Often, the fracture can be stabilized with the strut or plate, and then the canal can be prepared for stem insertion as if the femur were intact. Incavo et al. reported on 14 cases of periprosthetic fracture associated with a loose, cemented stem (53). Each case was treated with revision to a long-stem prosthesis with supplemental

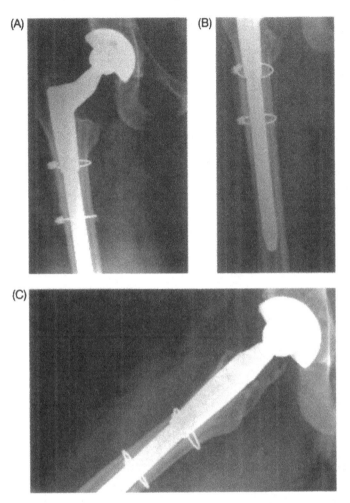

Figure 13 (A–B) AP radiograph of modular ZMR revision stem (Zimmer Holdings, Inc, Warsaw, IN). (C) Lateral radiograph. Note the excellent proximal and distal fill that can be achieved independently with a modular stem.

cortical graft fixation. Three prostheses became loose, likely due to the fact that the prostheses used in these cases had no distal porous coating. Thus, based upon my experience, these prostheses probably never provided adequate rotational stability to the fracture.

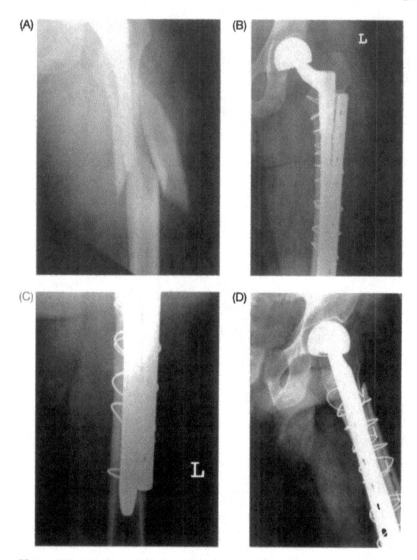

Figure 14 (A) Comminuted periprosthetic fracture adjacent to a cementless stem. (B–D) Postoperative radiographs of reconstruction using a long-stem prosthesis that bypassed all fracture fragments. Fixation of the fracture was achieved with a cable-plate and cortical strut graft.

2. No Revision Required

When a fracture occurs well distal to a well-fixed stem, open reduction and internal fixation (ORIF) with plates and cortical strut grafts can be successfully accomplished (16,17). Biomechanical studies suggest that unicortical and bicortical screws through the plate, with or without cerclage cables, are superior to cerclage cables only (54). In addition, two locations of fixation (e.g., strut and plate, two struts, two plates) are superior to just one. In addition, I believe that rigid fixation over a long length of the femur is critical to fracture healing when the stem is not revised.

B. Massive Proximal Bone Loss

Loosening of primary components often results in a large amount of proximal metaphyseal bone loss. When the cortex is intact circumferentially, impaction grafting may be used. However, when the cortex is damaged, and distal fixation is not possible due to an excessively large diaphyseal diameter, proximal allografts are necessary for reconstruction. Alternatively, massive endoprostheses may be used.

1. Allograft

Haddad et al. (55) reported their results with the use of proximal femoral allografts in 40 cases at minimum 5-year follow-up. Nonunion of the graft-host junction occurred in 8% of patients and was treated successfully with autograft in two-thirds of the cases. Four cases had dislocations, all after trochanteric nonunion. Trochanteric nonunion occurred in 46% of patients. Harris hip scores improved from 39 to 79. Important lessons learned included retention of the proximal host bone with wrapping of the host bone around the graft-host junction, trochanteric slide rather than formal osteotomy, and the press-fitting of stems into distal host bone whenever possible.

Gross et al. (56) reported their results with 168 structural femoral allografts. At 5-year follow-up, there was an 85% success rate (increase of greater than 20 points of the clinical score). There have been 17 revisions (10%): 3 for infection, 8 for dislocation, 5 for nonunion, and 1 for pain. These authors have recommendations similar to those of Haddad et al.

2. Proximal Femoral Replacement

Advantages of proximal femoral replacement endoprostheses include better soft tissue reattachment, multiple options for restoring leg length and soft tissue tension, and ease of insertion. Disadvantages include limitations in distal fixation, and high rates of dislocation and infection. Clinical results suggest 81% survivorship at 10 years (57), with approximately 20% dislocation rates. In addition, because of soft tissue loss or abductor deficiency, constrained acetabular components are frequently required (Figure 15). As such, the use of proximal femoral replacement prostheses should be limited to elderly, low-demand patients.

3. Impaction Grafting

Another option to deal with loss of proximal femoral bone stock is impaction grafting (Figure 16). This technique attempts to restore proximal bone by tightly impacting morcelized cancellous bone within the proximal femur. A tapered and polished component is then cemented within the impacted graft bed. The design of the stem is such that it allows further compaction of the allograft bone. In order for impaction grafting to be considered, the proximal femoral bone must be intact circumferentially. In addition, impaction grafting is contraindicated when a periprosthetic fracture is associated with proximal bone loss.

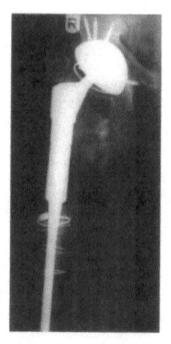

Figure 15 Proximal femoral replacement stem used for excessive proximal bone loss.

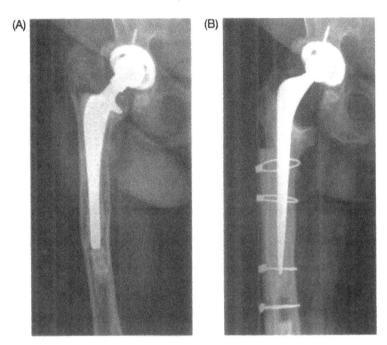

Figure 16 (A) Failed cemented stem with resulting patulous canal. (B) The hip was reconstructed using impaction grafting and a long, polished tapered stem.

Gie et al. reported upon 60 hips treated with impaction grafting and evaluated at average 2.5-year follow-up (58). There was a 4% failure rate requiring further surgery and subsidence of 1 to 4 cm occurred. Similarly, Elting et al. (59) reported a 10% failure rate at 2 to 5 years, with 2 to 8 mm of subsidence in half the patients. Histological data from Mikhail et al. (60) suggest that there is limited restoration of viability of the morcelized allograft.

Importantly, Leopold and coworkers attempted to perform impaction grafting with precoated, textured stems in order to decrease subsidence (61). The failure rate was 12% at 5-year follow-up. Indications and limitations for impaction grafting continue to evolve. The technique is quite labor-intensive and results appear to be correlated with the quality of the graft mantle that is created.

V. SUMMARY

Revision of the femoral component is most successfully accomplished by use of circumferentially and fully porous coated stems that achieve fixation in the diaphysis. Cemented revision is infrequently indicated. Newer modular designs may improve upon the experience with distal fixation stems by preserving proximal bone stock and decreasing thigh pain. Less common techniques such as impaction grafting, proximal femoral replacement prostheses, and allograft-prosthesis composites are useful alternatives in unusual cases of massive proximal femoral bone loss.

REFERENCES

1. Hip and pelvis reconstruction. In: Kasser JP, ed. Orthopaedic Knowledge Update 5. Chicago: American Academy of Orthopaedic Surgeons, 1996.
2. Schmalzried TP, Jasty M, Harris WH: Periprosthetic bone loss in total hip arthoplasty: polyethylene wear debris and the concept of the effective joint space. J Bone Joint Surg 74A:849–863, 1992.
3. Dowd JE, Cha CW, Trakru S, Kim SY, Yang IH, Rubash HE: Failure of total hip arthroplasty with a precoated prosthesis. Clin Orthop Rel Res 355:123–136, 1998.
4. Charnley J: The Use of Acrylics in Orthopaedics Surgery. London: Churchill Livingstone, 1970:19–20.
5. Galante JO, Jacobs JJ: Clinical performance of ingrowth surfaces. Clin Orthop Rel Res 276:41–49, 1992.
6. Engh CA, Bobyn JD, Glasman AH: Porous coated hip replacement. The factors governing bone ingrowth, stress shielding and clinical results. J Bone Joint Surg 69B:45–55, 1987.
7. Engh CA and Culpepper WJ: Femoral fixation in primary total hip arthroplasty. Orthopedics 20:771–773, 1997.
8. Burt CF, Garvin KL, Otterberg ET, Jardon OM: A femoral component inserted without cement in total hip arthroplasty. A study of the Trilock component with an average 10-year duration of follow-up. J Bone Joint Surg 80-A:952–960, 1998.
9. Purtill JJ, Rothman RH, Hozack WJ, Sharkey PF: Total hip arthroplasty using two different tapered cementless stems. Clin Orthop Rel Res 393:121–127, 2001.
10. Smith E, Harris WH: Increasing prevalence of femoral lysis in cementless total hip arthroplasty. J Arthrop 10:407–412, 1995.
11. Dorr LD, Lewonowski K, Lucero M, Harris M, Wan Z. Failure mechanisms of the anatomic porous replacement—I. Cementless total hip replacement. Clin Orthop Rel Res 334:157–167, 1997.
12. Rubash HE, Sinha RK, Maloney WJ, Paprosky WG: Osteolysis: surgical treatment. In: Cannon, WD, ed. Instructional Course Lectures. Vol 47. Chicago: American Academy of Orthopaedic Surgeons, 1997.
13. Kim YH, Kim VE: Uncemented porous coated anatomic total hip replacement: results at six years in a consecutive series. J Bone Joint Surg 75-B:6–13, 1993.

14. Mont MA, Maar DC: Fractures of the ipsilateral femur after hip arthroplasty. J Arthrop 9:511–519, 1994.

15. Johannson JE, McBroom R, Barrington TW, Hunter GA: Fracture of the ipsilateral femur in patients with total hip replacement. J Bone Joint Surg 63-A: 1435–1442, 1981.

16. Schwartz JT, Mayer JG, Engh CA: Femoral fracture during non-cemented total hip arthroplasty. J Bone Joint Surg 71-A:1135–1142, 1989.

17. Stern RE, Harwin SF, Kulick RG: Management of ipsilateral femoral shaft fractures following hip arthroplasty. Orthop Rev 20:779–785, 1991.

18. Gruen TA, McNeice GM, Amstutz HC: Modes of failure of cemented stem-type femoral components: a radiographic analysis of loosening. Clin Orthop Rel Res 141:17–27, 1979.

19. Woolson ST, Milbauer JP, Bobyn JD, Yue S, Maloney WJ: Fatigue fracture of a forged cobalt-chromium-molybdenum femoral component inserted with cement. A report of ten cases. J Bone Joint Surg 79-A:1842–1848, 1997.

20. Mont MA, Serna FK, Krackow KA, Hungerford DS: Exploration of radiographically normal total knee replacements for unexplained pain. Clin Orthop Rel Res 331:216–220, 1996.

21. Kawamura K, Dunbar MJ, Murray P, Bourne RB, Rorabeck CH: The porous coated anatomic total hip replacement. A 10 to 14 year follow-up study of a cementless total hip arthroplasty. J Bone Joint Surg 83-A:1333–1338, 2001.

22. Domb B, Hostin E, Mont MA, Hungerford DS: Cortical strut grafting for enigmatic thigh pain following total hip arthroplasty. Orthopedics 23:21–24, 2000.

23. Harris WH Schiller AL, Scholler JM, et al.: Extensive localized bone resorption in the femur following total hip replacement. J Bone Joint Surg 58-A:612–618, 1976.

24. Berry DJ, Harmsen WS, Ilstrup DM: The natural history of debonding of the femoral component from the cement and its effect on long-term survival of Charnley total hip replacements. J Bone Joint Surg 80-A:715–721, 1998.

25. Spangehl MJ, Masri BA, O'Connell JX, Duncan CP: Prospective analysis of preoperative and intraoperative investigations for the diagnosis of infection at the sites of 202 revision total hip arthroplasties. J Bone Joint Surg 81-A:672–683, 1999.

26. DeHart MM, Riley LH: Nerve injuries in total hip arthroplasty. J Am Acad Orthop Surg 7:101–111, 1999.

27. Hardinge K: The direct lateral approach to the hip. J Bone Joint Surg 64-B: 17–19, 1982.

28. Demos HA, Rorabeck CH, Bourne RB, MacDonald SJ, McAlden RW: Instability in primary total hip arthroplasty with the direct lateral approach. Clin Orthop Rel Res 393:168–180, 2001.

29. Hoppenfeld SA, DeBoer P: Surgical Approaches in Orthopaedics. Philadelphia: Lippincott, 1984:335–348.

30. Miner TM, Momberger NG, Chong D, Paprosky WL: The extended trochanteric osteotomy in revision hip arthroplasty. A critical review of 166 cases at mean 3 year, 9 month follow-up. J Arthrop 16:188–194, 2001.

31. Klein AH, Rubash HE: Femoral windows in revision total hip arthroplasty. Clin Orthop Rel Res, 291:164–170,1993.

32. Dohmae Y, Bechtold JE, Sherman RE, Puno RM, Gustilo R: Reduction in cement-bone interface shear strength between primary and revision arthroplasty. Clin Orthop Rel Res 236:214–220, 1988.

33. Pellici, PM, Wilson PD, Sledge CB, Salvati EA, Ranawat CS, Poss R: Revision total hip arthroplasty. Clin Orthop Rel Res 170:34–41, 1982.

34. Pellici, PM, Wilson PD, Sledge CB, Salvati EA, Ranawat CS, Poss R, Callaghan JJ: Long-term results of revision total hip replacement. J Bone Joint Surg 67-A:513–516, 1985.

35. Callaghan JJ, Salvati EA, Pellici, PM, Wilson PD, Ranawat CS: Results of revision for mechanical failure after cemented total hip replacement, 1979–1982. J Bone Joint Surg 67-A:1074–1085, 1985.

36. Marti RK, Schuller HM, Besselaar PP, Haasnoot ELV: Results of revision hip arthroplasty with cement. J Bone Joint Surg 77-A:346–354, 1990.

37. Engelbrecht DJ, Weber FA, Sweet MBE, Jakim I: Long term results of revision total hip arrthoplasty. J Bone Joint Surg 72-B:41–45, 1990.

38. Pierson JL, Harris WH: Cemented revision for femoral osteolysis in cemented arthroplasties. J Bone Joint Surg 76-B:40–44, 1994.

39. Raut VV, Sidney PD, Wroblewski BM: Cemented Charnley revision arthroplasty for severe femoral osteolysis. J Bone Joint Surg 77-B:362–365, 1995.

40. Mulroy WF, Harris WH: Revision total hip arthroplasty with use of so-called second generation cementing techniques for aseptic loosening of the femoral component. J Bone Joint Surg 78-A:325–330, 1996.

41. Hultmark P, Karrholm J, Stromberg C, Herberts P, Mose CH, Malchau H: Cemented first-time revisions of the femoral component: prospective 7 to 13 years' follow-up using second-generation and third-generation technique. J Arthrop 15:551–561, 2000.

42. Eisler T, Svensson O, Iyer V, Wejkner B, Schmalholz A, Larsson H, Elmstedt E: Revision total hip arthroplasty using third-generation cementing technique. J Arthrop 15:974–981, 2000.

43. Head WC, Malinin TI, Emerson RH Jr, Mallory TH: Restoration of bone stock in revision surgery of the femur. Int Orthop. 24:9–14, 2000.

44. Dorr LD, Wan Z, Song M, Ranawat A: Bilateral total hip arthroplasty comparing hydroxyapatite coating to porous coated fixation. J Arthrop 13:729–736, 1998.

45. Engh CA, Glassman AH, Griffin WL, Mayer JG: Results of cementless revision for failed cemented total hip arthroplasty. Clin Orthop Rel Res 235:91–110, 1988.

46. Engh CA, Culpepper WJ, Kassapidis E: Revision of loose cementless prostheses to larger porous-coated components. Clin Orthop Rel Res 347:168–178, 1998.

47. Paprosky WG, Greidanus NV, Antoniou: Minimum 10-year results of extensively porous-coated stems in revision arthroplasty. Clin Orthop Rel Res 369: 230–242, 1999.

48. Heekin RD, Angh CA, Herzwurm PJ: Fractures through custic lesions of the greater trochanter: J Arthrop 11:757–760, 1996.

49. Moreland JR, Bernstein ML: Femoral revision hip arthroplasty with uncemented, porous-coated stems. Clin Orthop Rel Res 319:141–150, 1995.

50. Urban RU, Jacobs JJ, Gilbert JL, Galante JO: Migration of corrosion products from modular hip prostheses. J Bone Joint Surg 76-A:1345–1359, 1994.

51. Shilling JW, Sharkey PF, Hozack WJ, Rothman RH: Femoral revision hip arthroplasty: modular versus nonmodular femoral component for severe femoral deficiency. Op Tech Orthop 10:133–137, 2000.

52. Smith JA, Dunn HK, Manaster BJ : Cementless femoral revision arthroplasty. 2- to 5-year results with a modular titanium alloy stem. J Arthrop 12:194–201, 1997.

53. Incavo SJ, Beard DM, Pupparo MD, Ries M, Wiedel J: One-stage revision of periprosthetic fractures around loose cemented total hip arthroplasty. Am J Orthop 27:35–41, 1998.

54. Dennis MG, Simon JA, Kummer FH, Koval KJ, DiCesare PE: Fixation of periprosthetic femoral shaft fractures occurring at the tip of the stem: a biomechanical study of 5 fixation techniques. J Arthrop 15:523–528, 2000.

55. Haddad FS, Garbuz DS, Masri BA, Duncan CP: Structural proximal femoral allografts for failed total hip replacements. J Bone Joint Surg 82-B:830–836, 2000.

56. Gross AE, Hutchison CR, Alexeef M, Mahomed N, Leitch K, Morsi E: Proximal femoral allografts for reconstruction of bone stock in revision arthroplasty of the hip. Clin Orthop Rel Res 319:151–158, 1995.

57. Malkani AL, Simm FH, Chao EY: Custom made segmental femoral replacement prostheses in revision total hip arthroplasty. Orthop Clin North Am 24:727–733, 1993.

58. Gie GA, Linder L, Ling RS, Simon JP, Sloof TJ, Timperly AJ: Impacted cancellous allografts and cement for revision total hip arthroplasty. J Bone Joint Surg 75-B:14–21, 1993.

59. Elting JJ, Zicat BA, Mikhail WEM: Impaction grafting: preliminary report of a new method for exchange femoral arthroplasty. Orthopedics 18:107–112, 1995.

60. Mikhail WEM, Weidenheim LRA, Wretenberg P, Mikhail MN, Bauer TW: Femoral bone regeneration subsequent to impaction grafting during hip revision. J Arthrop 14:849–853, 1999.

61. Leopold SS, Berger RA, Rosenberg AG, Jacobs JJ, Quigley LR, Galante JO: Impaction grafting with cement for femoral component revision using a collared precoated femoral component at four year minimum follow-up. J Bone Joint Surg 81-A:1080–1092, 1999.

9

Surface Arthroplasty of the Hip Revisited: Current Indications and Surgical Technique

Paul E. Beaulé and Harlan C. Amstutz
Joint Replacement Institute at Orthopaedic Hospital, Los Angeles, California

I. INTRODUCTION

The concept of surface arthroplasty (SA) of the hip has always been appealing because of its conservative nature and adherence to the basic principle of replacing only diseased bone. These principles date back to Smith-Petersen's initial mold arthroplasty of the hip that, however, was not fixed to the bone (1). Haboush was the first to implant a surface type arthroplasty of the hip using a metal-on-metal bearing as well as acrylic cement to fix the prosthesis to the bone (2). Later on, Charnley experimented with the same concept using two concentric shells made out of polytetrafluoroethylene (3), but he abandoned it because of the concern of ischemic necrosis of the femoral head remnant as well as the higher frictional torque of the larger head sizes (4). Despite this, in the early 1970s, investigators from different countries developed several designs that initially showed encouraging results (5–9) and appeared a promising alternative to total hip replacement (THR) for the young patient. Unfortunately, this was not the case, and failure rates of 15–33% were reported by multiple centers at a mean follow-up of 3 years (10–12). Also, when socket loosening occurred, some centers reported major acetabular defects at conversion surgery (13–15).

Therefore one may ask: Why do we need to revisit such a poor experience, given the current results of THR? On the other hand, why are we still considering young patients for procedures such as pelvic osteotomies

(16,17) and hip arthrodesis (18) to delay or prevent a THR if the results of THR are so good? Unfortunately, the long-term results (10 to 15 years) of THR in this patient population have been disappointing, with revision rates between 33 and 45% (19–22). In all of these studies, patients with unilateral hip disease secondary to avascular necrosis and osteoarthritis, and who had a high activity level (23), did worse than those patients with inflammatory conditions.

While improved survivorship is being achieved with cementless fixation (24) and alternate bearings [highly crosslinked polyethylenes (25), metal-on-metal (26)], which may reduce the extent of periprosthetic bone loss and wear debris induced osteolysis (27), neither has sufficient long-term clinical data to assure increased durability of THR in young patients. Proximal femoral bone stock is always compromised after THR due to adaptive bone remodeling (stress shielding) and the actual removal of bone at the time of implantation (28). Therefore, with time, this periprosthetic osteoporosis may cause an increasing incidence of periprosthetic fractures (29) and may affect long-term fixation of the prosthesis. Thus, in treating a young patient, lack of long-term fixation and the prospect of multiple revisions remain significant concerns for both patient and surgeon (30).

While hip arthrodesis will always have a role in the treatment of end-stage hip arthritis in the young patient (18), an alternative bone-preserving procedure such as surface arthroplasty of the hip would be a tremendous gain for the patient. While there is no long-term data on the current generation of SA (hybrid fixation with metal-on-metal bearing), its capacity to restore hip mobility and permit a return to a normal active lifestyle comparable to total hip replacement (14,31) would certainly meet initial patient expectations (32). Additionally, its bone preserving nature will always be advantageous for any further hip surgery.

II. HISTORY AND DEVELOPMENT OF SURFACE ARTHROPLASTY OF THE HIP

In several countries, initial enthusiasm for surface arthroplasty of the hip was strong and the procedure was perceived as possibly the next major evolution in hip surgery after low-friction hip arthroplasty. However, unlike the introduction of Charnley's low-friction hip arthroplasty, surface arthroplasty of the hip was geared to the young and active patient; had multiple designs, bearings, and fixation methods; and had no standard surgical approach. More importantly, surface arthroplasty of the hip, because of its smaller fixation area on the femoral head, was technically more demanding and less forgiving than THR surgery. These factors inevitably led to the

higher early failure rate as seen in other new implants when initially introduced to the community. Many factors were suspected for these high failure
rates: ischemic necrosis (11,33), neck fractures (10), and higher frictional
torque (11). Not all centers reported such high initial failure rates (34–37).

With the THARIES implant (total hip articular replacement with internal eccentric shells), Amstutz and associates reported survivorships of 77
and 53% at 5 and 7 years, respectively (38). Howie et al. reported similar
results with the Wagner resurfacing, with 70 and 40% survivorship at 5 and
8 years, respectively. These results are important, because 6 and 7 years
after implantation, the failure rate dramatically increased. On the other hand,
Mesko and associates, using the total articular replacement arthroplasty
(TARA), reported survivorships of 87 and 84% at 7 and 9 years (37). This
discrepancy between the TARA and THARIES or Wagner prostheses may
be related to the presence of a femoral stem on the TARA (Figure 1), which
provides additional fixation. In these three series, the acetabular socket loosenings posed the greatest difficulties because of the major bone loss associated with them. In examining the underlying hip etiologies and failure rate
(39), patients with osteonecrosis (ON), hip dysplasia (DDH), and rheumatoid
arthritis (RA) did comparatively worse than those with osteoarthritis. The
primary mode of failure for ON was femoral loosening; for DDH, acetabular
loosening and presence of femoral head cysts; and for RA, both acetabular

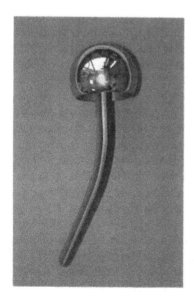

Figure 1   Femoral component of a total articular replacement arthroplasty (TARA).

and femoral loosening, also with a significant number of femoral neck fractures. These data illustrate the critical role of the bone quality and quantity in the outcome of cemented SA of the hip using a metal-on-polyethylene bearing. This clinical information should also be carefully considered in selecting patients for SA of the hip using new designs, which will require a sufficient length of follow-up (5 years and longer) before being considered as a viable alternative to THR in the young patient.

It was not until the role of polyethylene wear debris became evident in prosthetic loosening for both THR and SA (12,40–42) that the focus on the failure of SA shifted from implant design to the bearing surface. Because SA of the hip consistently used larger head sizes than conventional THR, the amount of volumetric wear debris produced was 4 to 10 times higher than with a 28-mm head (43). Additionally, because of the smaller fixation area of SA compared to THR, the area to be undermined before prosthetic loosening occurred was smaller, and thus loosening occurred sooner. In that respect, patients with larger femoral components in the THARIES series had significantly better survivorships at 11 years of follow-up compared with the smaller sizes: 59 versus 39% (44). Frictional torque was not a factor, confirming the retrieval studies of failed SA of the hip demonstrating polyethylene wear debris (40,41) as the primary cause of both femoral and acetabular component loosenings. Subsequent studies also failed to identify major osteonecrotic lesions within the remaining femoral heads (45,46).

Only a handful of surgeons continued to implant SA of the hip, altering implant design and fixation methods in order to improve long-term survivorship. As in THA, SA evolved to cementless fixation on both the acetabular and femoral sides (47–49). However, the use of modular acetabular components had to be combined with thinner polyethylene liners, which at that time were gamma-sterilized in air. As we know now, the wear characteristics of such polyethylenes are poor (50), and with the larger femoral head sizes of hip resurfacing, the amount of polyethylene wear was increased. This, unfortunately, led to even worse results (48), with a loosening rate of 45% and 91% at 5 and 10 years, respectively (Figure 2). Interestingly, the vast majority of failures occurred on the femoral side, with the cementless socket maintaining its fixation, which was contrary to the cemented design. We have recently reported the fate of 82 consecutive well-fixed cementless sockets after revision surgery at a mean follow-up of 7.5 years, with an average time in situ of 11.6 years, and found only one socket loosening. It appears that the advent of cementless fixation on the acetabular side has resolved the problems associated with the cemented design—i.e., loosening and significant loss of bone stock—but that wear debris induced osteolysis remained as the key issue (Figure 3). While SA with a polyethylene bearing was abandoned, the use of only the femoral component with-

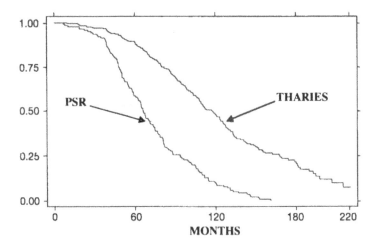

Figure 2 Kaplan-Maier survivorship curve showing the clinical performance of the THARIES and PSR.

out the acetabular component (51–53) was still retained in cases of osteo-necrosis of the hip.

III. BRIDGING THE TWO GENERATIONS: HEMIRESURFACING ARTHROPLASTY FOR OSTEONECROSIS OF THE HIP

A. Overview on the Treatment of Osteonecrosis of the Hip

The results of THR for osteonecrosis continue to be inferior to THR for other etiologies (54–56). Ortiguera and associates (20) reported a mechanical failure of 79% at a mean follow-up of 17.8 years. This is why alternative, more conservative procedures such as hemiresurfacing have been advocated in these patients (57), who are usually in their midthirties (58).

The success of joint-preserving procedures relies on the minimal involvement of the acetabular cartilage once collapse of the head has occurred in Ficat stage III and IV. These joint and bone-preserving procedures encompass different biological treatment strategies designed to preserve the femoral head, such as proximal femoral osteotomies (59–62) (intertrochanteric or transtrochanteric) as well as decompression and grafting procedures such as the trapdoor procedure (63,64). Although a proximal femoral osteotomy preserves the patient's own joint, the poor predictable pain relief

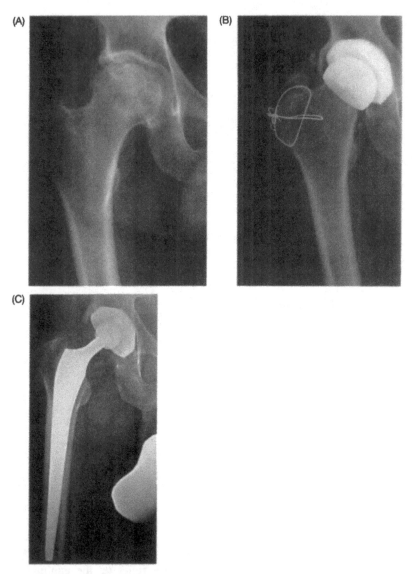

Figure 3 A. 51-year-old male with ON. B. 4 years post porous surface replacement. Development of osteolysis on the femoral side led to revision. C. 10 years post revision of the femoral component to ATH long stem uncemented. The well-fixed PSR socket was left in place during revision and the liner replaced with a 28-mm ID step-down liner. His UCLA hip score for pain, walking, and function are: 10, 8, 7, and 7, respectively.

achieved as well as survivorship of only 70% at 5 years (59,65), its limited indications (Kerboull angle of <200 degrees and age below 45 years) (66) and adverse effects on the long-term survivorship of THR (67,68) make it a less favorable option. The trapdoor procedure, which requires an arthrotomy so that the necrotic segment of the head can be curetted out through a cartilage window and iliac crest bone graft placed instead, lacks long-term follow-up and again has limited indications (64).

The senior author (52,69) as well as others (70,71) have favored a conservative prosthetic solution, namely hemiresurfacing hip arthroplasty, when bone quality is adequate and acetabular articular cartilage is relatively normal, as in cases of Ficat stage III or early stage IV osteonecrosis and failed free-vascularized fibular graft. One must distinguish hemiresurfacing from full-surface arthroplasty. In the former, almost no wear debris is produced, since the hemiresurfacing component directly articulates with the acetabular cartilage. Unlike cup arthroplasty, hemiresurfacing relies on a precision fit of the component to the remaining acetabular cartilage, which is not reamed, and the component is fixed with cement to the reamed femoral head.

Using a variety of designs, several centers reported survivorship of 79– 92% at 5–6 years follow-up (70–74). These five centers reported on a total of 215 hips treated with hemiresurfacing arthroplasty for hip osteonecrosis. In all but 5 hips (4 of which were in patients with sickle cell disease), the failures were due to increasing pain secondary to wearing of the acetabular cartilage. In none of these studies did the size of the necrotic lesion (Kerboull angle) affect femoral component fixation. Also, probably because of the small number of hips studied in each of the centers, only sickle cell disease showed a higher incidence of failures, while the other underlying etiologies of osteonecrosis showed no adverse effect on outcome. In order to improve the predictability of hemiresurfacing outcomes, Beaulé et al (74) reviewed a series of 37 hips with a mean follow-up of 6.5 years (range 2 to 18 years), where the acetabular cartilage involvement was graded (Table 1) at the time of the operative procedure. It was found that a longer duration of preoperative symptoms (17 versus 12 months, respectively) was associated with a worse acetabular grading and an earlier time to conversion to total hip replacement. Proper component sizing and acetabular cartilage quality, which are directly related to duration of symptoms, are probably the most important factors affecting outcome.

The limited data regarding conversion of hemiresurfacing to THR from the three reports mentioned above showed no adverse effect of hemiresurfacing on THR survivorship and indicated a relative ease in performing the conversion procedure. Ash et al. (75) reported on 58 hips converted to cemented total hip replacements after cup arthroplasty. Survivorship after con-

Table 1 Grading of Acetabular Cartilage in Osteonecrosis of the Hip

Grade I:	Minimal changes with localized softening with some or no break in the surface
	A blunt instrument pressed on the surface may sink into the cartilage
	The cartilage may be appearing slightly discolored and soft
Grade II:	Area of fissuring and an irregular surface
Grade III:	*A: no osteophytes; B: with non calcified osteophytes*
	Definite fibrillation with fissuring extending down to subchondral bone.
Grade IV:	Exposure and/or erosion of subchondral bone

Source: From Ref. 74.

version was 92% at 10 years and 74% at 20 years. Acetabular and femoral bone grafts were not required; no fractures occurred intraoperatively, and there were no cases of femoral loosening. Thus, with proper patient selection and good surgical technique, hemiresurfacing hip arthroplasty is a valid bone-preserving procedure with minimal penalties for a young patient who will eventually require a total hip replacement. One of the most difficult challenges will remain the accurate assessment of the acetabular cartilage and its potential durability against the hemiresurfacing component.

B. Hemiresurfacing Arthroplasty of the Hip: Clinical Indications and Surgical Technique

1. Clinical Evaluation

The age of the patient at presentation should be considered carefully; the younger the patient, the more strongly hemiresurfacing should be considered, since it is very likely that he or she will require another operative procedure in their lifetime. With the use of anteroposterior (AP) and frog-leg lateral x-ray views, the Ficat (76) classification can serve for the initial staging of disease. In addition, we recommend measuring the Kerboull angle (77), which represents the size of the necrotic segment and is the sum of the angles subtended from the center of the head to the edges of the necrotic segment as measured on the radiographs. While the Kerboull angle is subject to some observer variability, no other methods have proven superior, including magnetic resonance imaging (78). However, Mitchell et al. (79) have suggested that the presence of joint effusion and diffuse signal abnormality of the head and neck distal to the focal lesion indicate a high likelihood of preexisting collapse, even if they are not apparent radiographically. These findings in a patient having hip pain even in the absence of radiographic collapse should be considered as strong evidence of collapse of the femoral head.

There are many factors that can affect the long-term survivorship of the acetabular cartilage in patients with osteonecrosis: activity level, patient weight, age, and condition of the cartilage at surgery. Both Steinberg (80) and Beaulé (74) have demonstrated acetabular involvement with osteonecrosis of the femoral head. We suggest that the quality of the acetabular cartilage be evaluated at the time of the operative procedure; if significant damage is identified (exposure and/or erosion of subchondral bone) in an older patient, other options such as THR must be considered.

2. Current Indications

Ideal candidates are patients less than 50 years old with Ficat stage III and early stage IV or failed free-vascularized fibular graft, in whom the acetabular grade is III or less. For patients with an acetabular grade of IV who are below 50 years of age, results are less predictable. In older patients with grade IV cartilage, THR with alternate bearing [metal-on-metal (26) highly crosslinked polyethylene (81)] is the treatment of choice at this time, with metal-on-metal SA a promising alternative. Once collapse has occurred, we recommend that the patients refrain from weight bearing from the point of identification onward to minimize further damage to the articular cartilage. Because the quality of the cartilage is directly related to the duration of symptoms and ultimately dictates the outcome of this procedure, early intervention is recommended. We have extended our indications of hemiresurfacing to patients with Ficat stage II disease with Kerboull angles >200 degrees. This is based on the inability of procedures such as core decompression and free-vascularized fibular graft to address the full extent of the lesion and prevent collapse (82,83). In our practice, the underlying pathogenesis of osteonecrosis has not been a contraindication in considering patients for hemiresurfacing. However, in Nelson's (84) series of 21 patients, 4 out of 7 failures occurred in patients with sickle cell disease or trait.

3. Surgical Technique

The detailed surgical technique has been described elsewhere (86). Preoperatively, the approximate size and orientation of the prosthesis should be determined. Using a caliper and/or the scaled x-ray templates provided with the instrumentation, the dimension of the femoral neck, the center of the femoral head, and the approximate size of the hemiresurfacing component should be estimated (head size plus one-half of the cartilage space based on the normal contralateral hip), with final selection of prosthesis size made at the time of surgery (Figure 4).

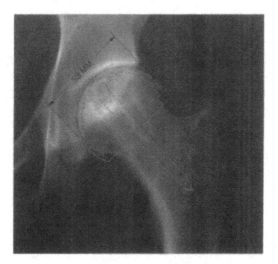

Figure 4 Selecting the target component size: scaled templates are superimposed on preoperative x-rays to estimate the final component size and orientation.

We prefer the posterior approach with a hockey-stick–shaped skin incision (Figure 5). With this approach, visualization of the entire circumference of the femoral head and neck and the acetabulum can be accomplished. To mobilize the proximal femur and the femoral head, the gluteus maximus tendon needs to be released distally, the quadratus femoris and the ligamen-

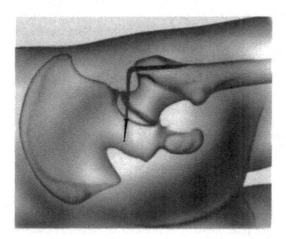

Figure 5 The hockey-stick–shaped skin incision used for the posterior approach to the hip facilitates femoral neck visualization.

tum teres should be sectioned. The array of instruments needed is displayed in Figure 6. We do attempt to preserve the labrum. The femoral head is delivered into wound by flexion, internal rotation, and adduction. Sizing-ring gauges are then used to estimate femoral head size, trying to obtain a tight fit at the widest part of the head (Figure 7).

Preparation of the femoral head can then begin. First, the pin-centering guide should be placed firmly about the superior and inferior femoral neck with the wide mobile grip placed inferiorly. A 3.2-mm Steinmann pin should then be inserted to a depth of approximately 30 to 50 mm, usually slightly anterior and superior on the head. A drill guide is a helpful adjunct to ensure a correct starting point. Pin alignment in the femoral neck axis should be assessed visually in two planes. We recommend using a goniometer to ensure

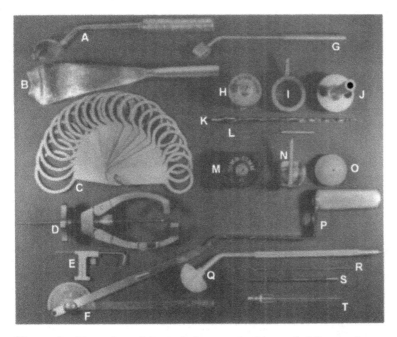

Figure 6 Illustration of the main instrumentation needed for metal-on-metal sur-face arthroplasty. A. Ligamentum Teres sectioner. B. Femoral neck elevator. C. Siz-ing ring gauges. D. Pin-centering guide. E. Cylindrical reamer gauge. F. Goniometer. G. Pin relocator guide. H. Cylindrical reamer. I. Saw cutoff guide. J. Tower align-ment guide. K. Tapered stem reamer. L. Chamfer guide. M. Chamfer cutter. N. Component template. O. Femoral head protector. P. Right-angle retractor. Q. Trans-lucent acetabular gauge. R. 1.5-mm drill bit. S. Tapered suction for central hole. T. Starter guide.

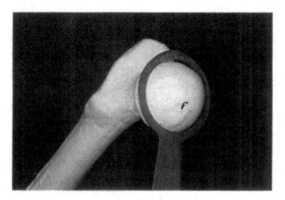

Figure 7   Sizing ring gauge placed onto the widest portion of the femoral head.

proper placement of the femoral component at approximately 135 to 140 degrees (Figure 8). One should avoid excessive valgus where notching of the femoral neck is more likely or excessive varus where excessive tension stresses on the superior aspect of the femoral neck cortex could possibly lead to premature fracture of the femoral neck or loosening of the component. One should note that pin placement does not correspond to the center of the head, since the head overlaps the neck cortex most prominently posteriorly, as does the greater trochanter and its crest. As stated by Harty (86),

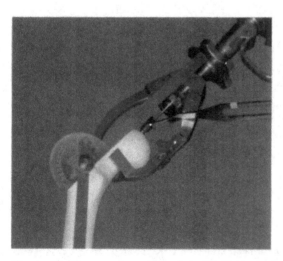

Figure 8   Pin-centering guide placed onto the femoral neck with goniometer to verify correct alignment. Use drill guide to prevent errant skiving of the pin.

this combination increases the curved outline of the neck, which must be considered during operative intervention. The pin-centering guide must often be forced anteriorly to correct against the tendency to retrovert the pin. The hip is then placed in neutral rotation, and with the hip flexed, proper version of the pin is assessed by verifying that it is parallel to the anterior femoral neck.

Correct positioning of the pin should then be checked using the appropriate estimated final size of cylindrical reamer gauge by rotating it around the pin to confirm that there is equal clearance around the femoral neck (Figure 9). This verifies that the pin is positioned down the central axis of the neck. If the tip of the cylindrical reamer gauge impinges against the femoral neck, either the central guide pin should be relocated or a larger component size should be selected. If the correction is about the width of the pin, the relocation guide should be used, leaving the first pin in situ (Figure 10). A new pin can then be inserted in the proper orientation without fear of inserting it down the original hole. The relocation guide has two holes, with one having the width of two pins, permitting simultaneous angle (maximum of 5 degrees) and position change. By using the cylindrical reamer gauge, proper pin placement can be achieved, and selection of a reamer that is smaller than the femoral neck can be prevented. Moreover, displacement of the cylindrical reamer from the neck axis, which could result in notching of the femoral neck during reaming, can also be prevented.

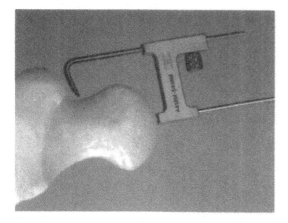

Figure 9 Checking pin placement and reamer size. The cylindrical reamer gauge, rotated about the Steinmann pin, assesses the accuracy of pin centering and ensures that the cylindrical reamer will have sufficient clearance to avoid notching the femoral neck.

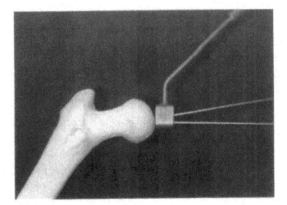

Figure 10   Using the relocator guide one can adjust alignment as well as position.

It is necessary to check both visually and by palpation that there are no positioning errors and that the reamer will not violate the neck. As the cylindrical reamer advances, the surgeon should use his free hand to palpate the location of the vibrations and avoid notching the neck (Figure 11). There is a subcapital recess (86)—usually located on the inferior head-neck junction but occasionally located superiorly—that allows extra space to avoid notching the neck during reaming. Successive reaming should be made with appropriate, smaller-sized reamers until the final reamed head diameter is reached. Each reamer has an intrinsic dome stop anthropometrically de-

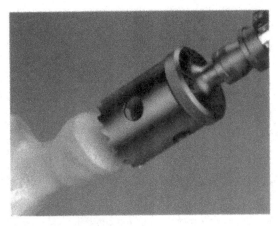

Figure 11   Cylindrical reaming. Bone is removed equidistant around the central axis of the femoral neck, guided by the Steinman pin.

signed to prevent notching. These stops are effective when the largest cylindrical reamer used is no more than two sizes greater than the target reamer size. However, as the reamer is advanced, regular visual inspection and finger palpation is advised to avoid neck invasion. For the femoral dome resection, a cutoff guide, which corresponds to the size of the last cylindrical reamer used, should be secured onto the femoral head (Figure 12) with two pins. The femoral head dome is then resected with a saber or oscillating saw.

The hole for the short neck stem of the component is made with the tapered reamer by mounting the tower alignment drill guide onto the saw cutoff guide and firmly seating it by clearing all debris. Improper seating will result in putting the hole off center and inability to properly place the component onto the reamed femoral head (Figure 13). The chamfer cutter (Figure 14), which corresponds to the size of the final component, should then be used to give the femoral head its final shape, significantly increasing the available fixation area on the femoral head. It should be advanced until it "bottoms out." All remaining friable, yellow, nonviable necrotic bone should be removed with a curette or high-speed burr. We do not remove the dense reactive sclerotic bone but instead cancellize it with a 1.5-mm drill bit (Figure 15). The size of the femoral head should then be confirmed by rotating the component template that matches the inner dimension of the femoral component (Figure 16). The bone at the distal tip of the template should be marked to indicate complete seating of the femoral component

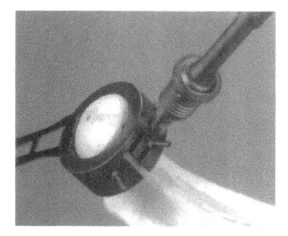

Figure 12 Resecting the femoral head dome. The saw cutoff guide stabilized with two short pins, and a saber or oscillating saw are used to prepare the base of the chamfer.

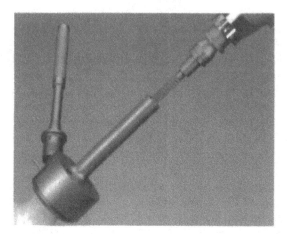

Figure 13 Preparing the stem hole. The tower alignment guide is mounted onto the cutoff guide. Use the starter drill to ensure accurate central axis placement for the tapered stem reamer.

during impaction. Residual areas of poorly vascularized, sclerotic bone and remaining cysts should be curetted out and the bone cleaned with saline, using pulsatile lavage.

With the femoral head protector on, a pocket for the head is created anteriorly and superiorly to the acetabulum using a periosteal elevator and

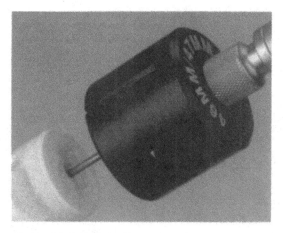

Figure 14 Chamfered reaming. After the chamfer guide is inserted into the stem hole, it guides the progress of the chamfered reamer, which gives the femoral head its final shape.

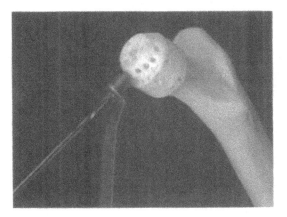

Figure 15 Femoral head with drill holes to add fixation area.

sharp dissection to release the reflected head of rectus femoris. With a right-angle retractor placed on the anterior wall of the acetabulum, the cartilage can be fully visualized. The translucent acetabular gauge (Figure 17) should then be inserted into the acetabulum and pressed against the acetabular cartilage to visualize the contact areas. A careful evaluation of the cartilage's quality should be done at this time, especially in the superior weight-bearing dome area. In order to optimize contact with the best remaining cartilage,

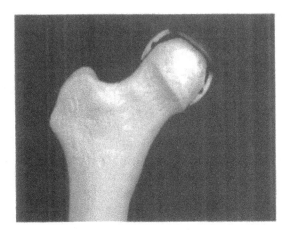

Figure 16 Checking the femoral head preparation. The femoral head template, when placed on the resurfaced area, is used to assess the accuracy of the bone preparation.

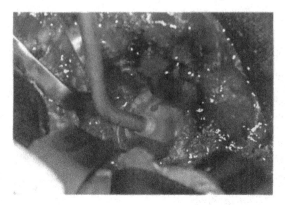

Figure 17 Precision fitting the component. A series of translucent acetabular gauges is pressed against the acetabular cartilage to determine which size maximizes contact with the best remaining acetabular cartilage.

several trials with larger or smaller acetabular gauges should be performed. For central defects, a slightly larger component provides rim contact; for peripheral defects, a smaller component provides central or polar contact. Generally, we recommend using the next largest size when the dimensions fall between millimeter increments in order to provide peripheral or rim contact.

After cleansing of the reamed femoral head using pulsatile lavage, the acrylic bone cement should be mixed and poured in a low-viscosity state into the component up to the circumferential recess (Figure 18). Once the reamed femoral head has been properly dried off with the tapered suction tip, which is placed into the central hole, the femoral component containing the doughy cement should be pressed onto the prepared femoral surface and rigidly held until polymerization is complete. For sizes greater than 50 mm and femoral heads with large lesions, 1½ packages of cement should be mixed. It is our preference, where there is good bone quality, to avoid cementing the stem of the implant by reinserting the chamfer guide temporarily into the dome hole for the stem during initial application and finger pressurization of bone cement into the cancellous bone, especially the cylindrically reamed bone. The hip should then be reduced and checked for range of motion and stability. Standard closure for a total hip replacement is done as well as antibiotic therapy and thromboprophylaxis. Ambulation should begin on the first postoperative day, allowing weight bearing as tolerated, then using crutches for 4–6 weeks. A cane may be used for an additional 2–3 weeks. Sports are permitted at 4 months postoperatively.

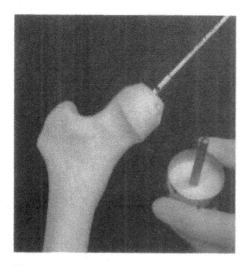

Figure 18 The tapered femoral suction is used to dry the bone before insertion of the femoral component, which is filled up to the circumferential recess with cement and pressurized onto the reamed femoral head.

4. Case Illustration

A 23-year-old male with right osteonecrosis of the hip who underwent hemi-resurfacing arthroplasty (Figure 19). The hip was staged as a Ficat stage III with 12 months' duration of symptoms. The Kerboull angle was 260 degrees and acetabular cartilage was graded as III. The patient's UCLA hip score improved from 5, 5, 6, 6 to 6, 8, 8, 4 for pain, walking, function, and activity, respectively. At this point 2 years have passed since his surgery and he is doing well.

IV. METAL-ON-METAL SURFACE ARTHROPLASTY OF THE HIP

A. Rationale for Metal on Metal

During the 1990s, polyethylene wear debris was identified as the main cause of aseptic loosening of THRs including SA of the hip (87), and reduction in its production has become the focus of much current research. In 1990, Jacobsson and associates (89) reported survivorship of metal-on-metal and metal-on-polyethylene THR at a mean follow-up of 11–12 years as 82.2 and 89.5%, respectively. These data, combined with the personal observations of surgeons in Europe (89), led to the reintroduction of metal-on-metal bear-

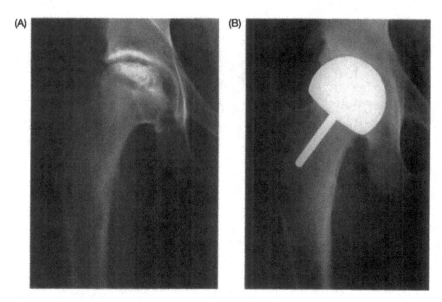

Figure 19 A. 23-year-old male with idiopathic ON ficat stage III, Kerboul angle 260°, acetabular cartilage grading IIIA, symptomatic for 12 months. B. 18 months post Conserve™ Hemiresurfacing.

ings in total hip arthroplasty. This enthusiasm was also supported by retrieval analysis of on long-term metal-on-metal THRs, which showed extremely low wear rates with absence of corrosion (90,91). Metal-on-metal bearings were used in SA of the hip in late 1960s by Professor Muller, using a press-fit design (93), and by Gérard (6), using double cups that were not fixed to the bone. Muller abandoned it in favor of low-friction hip arthroplasty (93) and Gérard's results were associated with high rates of loosening (94).

Two European centers were the first to reintroduce metal-on-metal SA of the hip (95,96). The Wagner cementless design came in four sizes, with a rough-blasted Ti surface for fixation. The initial series was in 35 patients with a mean age of 36 years and follow-up of 20 months. Clinical results were comparable to THR, with five conversions to THR for four femoral loosenings and one neck fracture. The femoral loosenings were attributed to the threaded design of the femoral component. At the same time, McMinn and his group (95) developed several pilot designs starting with an uncemented, uncoated, press fit on both sides, followed by a fully hydroxyapatite (HA)-coated design. The third design was fully cemented, and with the final version being hybrid: HA-coated on the acetabular side and cemented on the femoral side. With minimal data on the final version, this initial pilot series (first three designs) (95), with a mean follow-up of 50.2 months, had 9 patients reoperated on for socket loosenings—6 in the press-fit and 3 in the cemented. More recently, McMinn (98) reported 6- to 7-year results in 1324 cases using the HA-coated acetabular component and cemented femoral side with a survivorship of 97.1%. Revision surgery was secondary to four neck fractures, three socket loosenings, three infections, and two femoral neck collapses. However there were two different designs (smooth versus porous cup), making it too difficult to decipher which acetabular component is superior, since we did not know if both components had comparable follow-up. However, it does appear that the metal-on-metal bearing has led to a significant improvement in the medium-term follow-up. These findings are also corroborated by recent retrieval analysis from THR on the currently used metal-on-metal bearings, with a 60-fold reduction in the amount of volumetric wear (26). Additionally, clinical studies on the current generation have demonstrated results that are similar to those of total hip replacements with a metal-on-polyethylene articulation (98).

We have recently reviewed our initial experience with the Wagner and McMinn metal-on-metal SA in 46 hips. At a mean follow-up of 6.8 years (5.0–8.1) our survivorship was 87% with conversion to THR as the endpoint. Six hips (all McMinns) had to be reoperated on for acetabular loosening, of which three were converted to THR. Five of these six sockets were cemented; all dissociated at the implant cement interface at less than 25 months. The other socket loosening occurred in a hydroxyapatite-coated implant secondary to debonding of the coating. There was one femoral neck fracture. The mean time to reoperation was 30.3 months. There was no major loss of acetabular bone stock, and three of these cases were maintained as SA using the double-socket technique (99) (Figure 20). As we enter the era of low wear, alternative bearing surfaces such as metal-on-metal, implant fixation and design will be the critical determinants of implant survivorship for both THR and SA (100). This is certainly evident with the McMinn design of the acetabular component. Based on this initial experience (101) and our long-term results with hemiresurfacing for hip osteonecrosis (74), a hybrid design was adopted, the Conserve Plus (Wright Medical Technology, Inc., Arlington, TN). The device is now in a FDA Investigational Device Exemption multicenter trial.

2. Current Implant Design and Preliminary Results

The Conserve Plus acetabular shell is hemispherical (170 degrees) with a sintered porous coating for cementless fixation (Figure 21). The femoral component is of the same design as the one used for hemiresurfacing, employing a short stem to ensure accurate alignment with a uniform cement

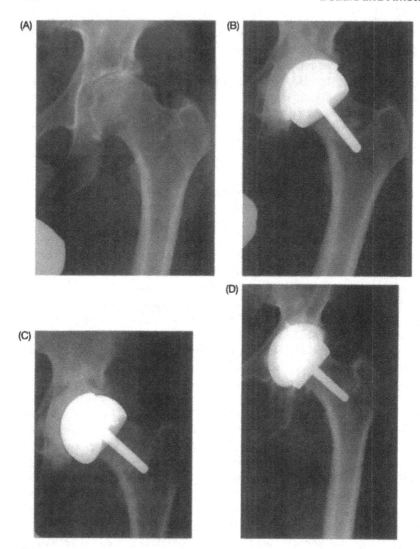

Figure 20   A. 40-year-old male with OA. B. 1 month post all cemented McMinn metal-on-metal surface arthroplasty. C. 25 months post surgery, loosening of the acetabular component at the cement-implant interface. D. 63 months post revision of the acetabular component to a double socket construct. His UCLA hip score for pain, walking, and function are: 7, 10, and 7, respectively.

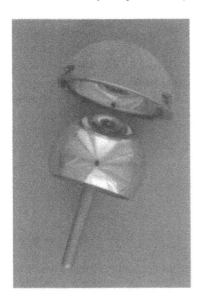

Figure 21   Conserve® Plus hybrid metal-on-metal resurfacing prosthesis.

mantle around the resurfaced femoral head. However, the tolerances for sphericity and surface finish are significantly tighter in order to permit adequate diametral clearances for the metal-on-metal bearing. There are 10 sizes with the components coming in 2-mm increments, with a 10-mm difference in size between the acetabular (range, 46–64) and femoral components (range, 36–54). All components are made of a cast F75 cobalt chrome molybdenum alloy.

Our preliminary experience with our first 100 (of 520) in 89 patients with hybrid metal-on-metal Conserve Plus has a 3- to 5.5-year (4.1-year mean) follow-up. The mean age was 49 years. There were 68% males and 32% females. The primary diagnosis was osteoarthritis in 65, osteonecrosis in 19, developmental dysplasia of the hip in 7, spondylitis in 3, rheumatoid arthritis in 2, and 1 each of slipped capital femoral epiphysis, Legg-Calvé-Perthes disease, melorheostosis, and epiphyseal dysplasia. Ten percent had prior surgery such as coring, osteotomy or hemiresurfacing arthroplasty. UCLA hip scores improved from 3.7 to 9.4 for pain, 6.1 to 9.5 for walking, 5.6 to 9.2 for function, and 4.6 to 7.6 for activity. Range of motion normalized. Complications have included one subluxation, one wire removal, one heterotopic ossification, and one subluxation due to impingement. Four cases have been converted to THR: three for femoral loosenings, and one due to persistent subluxation.

We have observed six patients with small areas of presumed osteolysis. Two have acetabular and femoral lesions and four have either femoral or acetabular lesions. Only one has progressed. Metal-on-metal devices produce less wear, which should lead to a reduced incidence and magnitude of osteolysis; this was the primary failure mode of surface arthroplasty with polyethylene. However, longer-term follow-up is essential, as the failure rate of metal-on-polyethylene surface arthroplasty increased significantly with time (34,36).

C. Surgical Technique and Clinical Applications

1. Radiographic Evaluation

The AP and the true lateral (Johnson or shoot-through) (Figure 22) radiographs are used to define the anatomy of the femoral neck and for appropriate sizing. The AP radiograph is used for templating of the acetabulum. The placement of the acetabular shell is at level of the teardrop with an abduction angle of 45 degrees. The femoral neck component is fitted to the femoral neck for a close fit and placed in slight valgus alignment (135 to 140 degrees) in order to minimize tension stresses on the lateral aspect of the femoral neck (102). In the cases of long-standing end-stage arthritis,

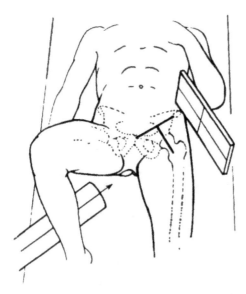

Figure 22 Johnson lateral x-ray is used to assess the femoral neck bone quality and version both pre- and postoperatively.

where the hip is subluxed laterally the unloaded portion of femoral neck can become quite osteopenic. In these cases, measurement of bone mineral density of the proximal femur may be advisable. However, there are no established guidelines on the extent of osteopenia, which may significantly compromise femoral fixation.

2. Indications for Surface Arthroplasty of the Hip

Ideal candidates are patients less than 55 years old with end-stage osteoarthritis or in whom hemiresurfacing hip arthroplasty is not indicated—i.e., acetabular cartilage damage. The only reservation we have is in patients with compromised renal function, since metal ions generated from the metal-on-metal bearing are excreted through the urine and the lack of clearance of these ions may lead to excessive levels in the blood (103). At this time we have limited experience with older patients and those who have severe osteopenia of the femoral neck. However, these patients would be expected to be at increased risk for femoral neck fractures because of the stress distributions under the femoral component (104).

3. Surgical Technique

The technique for the femoral head preparation differs from that previously described for hemiresurfacing. With the full-surface arthroplasty, the femoral reaming reduces the head size to that of the largest dimension of the femoral neck in order to preserve acetabular bone stock (85). The diameter of the femoral component for full-surface arthroplasty will be 4 to 6 mm smaller than that of the normal femoral head with articular cartilage or its replication with a hemiresurfacing arthroplasty.

Preoperatively, the approximate size and orientation of the prosthesis is determined. Using the scaled x-ray templates provided, the dimension of the femoral component should closely fit the femoral neck when placed in anatomic or slight valgus orientation (135–140 degrees) on the AP radiograph (Figure 23A). The diameter of the femoral neck in its widest plane is observed in the medial/lateral perspective, but anteversion and bone quality of the femoral neck should also be viewed with a "Johnson lateral" x-ray (Figure 23B).

One will often notice a large anterior osteophyte on the true lateral x-ray, which, if not removed, will make placement of the component in the proper version (i.e., short stem parallel to the anterior cortex) quite unreliable and may lead to perforation of the anterior neck by the stem. The surgical approach is as described for the hemiresurfacing.

The entire capsule must be removed in order to mobilize the proximal femur for preparation of the acetabular cavity. The retroacetabular portion

(A)

(B)

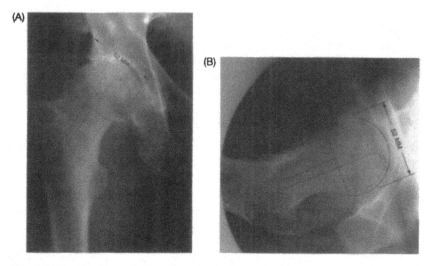

Figure 23 Total resurfacing. Templates are used with respect to head and neck size both on A) AP and B) Johnson lateral radiographs.

of the gluteus minimus must be elevated or partially sectioned in order to gain full access to the capsule. Once the posterior capsule has been removed, release of the superior capsule facilitates the dislocation of the femoral head. The femoral head is delivered into the wound by flexion, internal rotation, and adduction. The remainder of the anterior and inferior capsule is then removed, and the reflected head of the rectus femoris is released using a Cobb elevator; a pocket to accept the femoral head is created superiorly and anteriorly. One may then choose to prepare the femoral head or the acetabulum first. It has been our preference lately to prepare the acetabulum first, since it most often dictates the final component size. This facilitates conservation of acetabular bone; therefore, one must be careful not to excessively undersize (i.e., greater than one size) from the original femoral templating. Another useful option is to debulk the femoral head with the cylindrical reamer, removing all osteophytes and synovium so that the actual size of the neck can be ascertained. Then the acetabulum can be prepared.

   a. Acetabular Preparation. The leg should be brought to a neutral position. With lateral traction and external rotation of the femur, the femoral head is placed anteriorly and superiorly. With a right angle retractor placed on the anterior wall of the acetabulum to displace the femur anteriorly and a wide retractor in the infracotyloid notch, the acetabular cavity can be fully visualized. Carefully assess the wall thickness initially and subsequently as you proceed with the reaming in order to preserve as much bone stock as possible. Acetabular preparation does not differ significantly from that of press-fit acetabular components for a THR. We usually start reaming with a size 8–10 mm smaller than the templated component and begin removing the central acetabular osteophytes down to the floor of the cotyloid fossa, exposing some cancellous bone. We recommend undersizing by 1 mm when the quality of the bone is good or 1½–2 mm if it is osteopenic. Acetabular cysts should be curetted and the sclerotic floor drilled and grafted. By pressing the translucent acetabular gauge, as for hemiresurfacing, against the reamed acetabular cavity, one observes a thin film of fluid, by which one can assess the sphericity and depth of the reaming. The depth of each translucent gauge corresponds to the depth of the acetabular component, whose outside diameter is 2 mm larger than the gauge (i.e. acetabular gauge of 56 mm OD has the same depth as the 58-mm acetabular shell). A final check is made with the ring gauges inserted in two planes to assess roundness and size (Figure 24). The acetabular shell, rigidly mounted on the coupling device (Figure 25) is ready for insertion. We recommend inserting the acetabular component in 25–30 degrees of anteversion and in 45 degrees of abduction. Again if you are uncertain that you can match your acetabular component size with the femoral component (10 mm smaller than the acetabulum), proceed with preparation of the femoral head.

   b. Femoral Head Preparation. With the femoral head well mobilized, the femoral neck elevator is then placed carefully so that the femoral

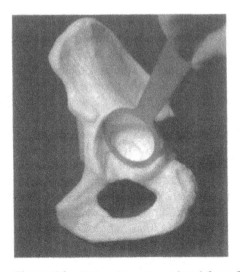

Figure 24   Sizing ring gauge placed for a final check of roundness and size.

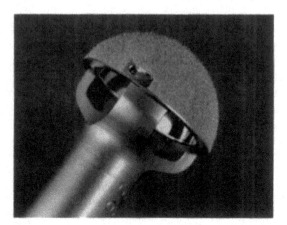

Figure 25   Acetabular shell mounted on the coupling device before insertion.

head/neck can be inspected. The femoral neck elevator not only facilitates the inspection of the proximal femur but also protects the sciatic nerve posteriorly. One must then debulk the osteophytes at the head/neck junction, especially anteriorly and superiorly, using small curved osteotomes or a cebatome burr. When accomplishing this, the assistant is asked to adduct and internally rotate the leg with flexion to gain access to excise the remaining anterior capsule as well as to view the superior and anterior femoral neck. Then, by hip extension, internal rotation, and adduction, the surgeon can visualize the inferior neck and capsule. By completing this visualization of the femoral neck and with the removal of the osteophytes, one can identify the true dimensions of the neck, which will facilitate accurate pin placement down the central axis of the neck and preparation of the femoral head.

The sequence for femoral head preparation is similar to hemiresurfacing. However, with the metal-on-metal SA, the femoral component is reamed very closely to the remaining neck; thus notching can occur more easily than with the hemiresurfacing. If the template is too snug to the neck and does not rotate freely, the chamfer guide is repositioned, and the area of inadequate clearance is reamed using the last cylindrical reamer. Residual areas of sclerotic bone are drilled using a 1.5-mm drill bit into more vascular bone to a depth of approximately 3 mm (Figure 26). Remaining cysts should be curetted out, and the bone should be cleaned with pulsatile lavage. If the acetabular component has not been inserted, the resurfaced femoral head should then be placed superiorly and anteriorly after the femoral head protector has been applied.

The femoral component is cemented in the same fashion as for hemiresurfacing. The hip should then be reduced and checked for range of motion

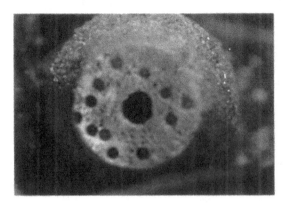

Figure 26 Femoral head after preparation. Note the drilled holes for increased fixation.

and possible impingement. When the impingement occurs in flexion and internal rotation, there may be a residual anterior femoral neck osteophyte or prominence of the superior acetabular rim. These should be resected. The other potential source of impingement is between the posterior aspect of the greater trochanter and the posterior acetabular rim or ischium when the hip is placed in extension and external rotation. In those circumstances removing the posterior projection of the greater trochanter (5–8 mm of bone) is usually sufficient. Rarely, in cases of dysplasia, where the offset is reduced due to increased valgus, we have had to remove bone from the ischium.

The wound should then be closed with one or more suture drains. Prophylactic antibiotics and chemical antithromboembolic medications are given (our preference is an adjusted low-dose of warfarin beginning on the night of surgery). All patients receive a 5-day course of indomethacin for prevention of heterotopic ossification (HO), beginning with 50 mg the night before surgery and 25 mg tid for 5 days. For patients undergoing simultaneous bilateral surgery or who have had a predisposition of forming HO on previously operated contralateral hip, we follow Letournel's protocol (105) of single-dose radiation and indomethacin. Ambulation should begin on the first postoperative day, allowing weight bearing as tolerated, and using crutches for 4–6 weeks. A cane may be used for an additional 2–3 weeks. Sports are generally permitted at 4 months postoperatively.

4. Case Illustration

A 50-year-old female presented with end-stage osteoarthritis of the hip and was treated with SA (Figure 27). Her UCLA hip score improved from 4, 9,

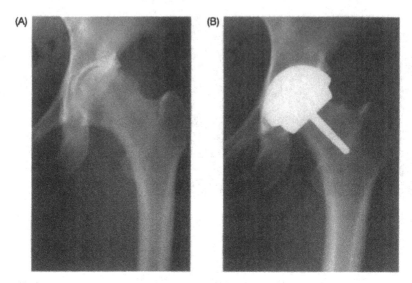

Figure 27   A. Highly active 50-year-old female with OA. B. 40 months post Conserve® Plus metal-on-metal surface arthroplasty.

8, 9 to 10, 10, 10, 10 for pain, walking, function, and activity, respectively. At this point, 3.3 years have passed since her SA of the hip, and she is participating regularly in various sporting activities, including tennis, every day.

V. CONCLUSION

The concept of SA to date has always been appealing because of its bone-preserving nature and ease of revision on the femoral side. As we look ahead to the future applications of SA of the hip, the long-term results will be especially critical for the metal-on-metal design. We can safely say that hemiresurfacing arthroplasty of the hip is a reproducible and excellent alternative to THR for a young, active population. The clinical results of hemiresurfacing are good and comparable to the outcomes of THR; however, the quality of the pain relief is not as predictable as in THR. The method should be considered as a component of a lifelong treatment plan in the young patient with osteonecrosis despite the potentially better initial performance of conventional THR. Because the predictability of results deteriorates with time and acetabular cartilage damage, non-weight-bearing and early surgery are recommended. The younger the patient, the more acetabular cartilage damage is considered acceptable to buy time in order to defer THR with SA, with a metal-on-metal as a promising alternative.

The last symposium published on SA of the hip concluded that it should not be considered a standard arthroplasty and should be performed only by surgeons with considerable experience in hip reconstruction. It should be considered to be in the stage of evaluation (106). For SA of the hip to be considered a viable alternative to THR, certain goals must be met: it must show a survivorship of close to 90% at 5 to 10 years, demonstrate that it is a reproducible technique, and prove its ease of conversion to THR. The longevity of this implant will rely mainly on the femoral side, where the bone stock may be compromised by long-standing disease. When in doubt, we recommend a THR or cementing of the short stem based on patient's age and expectations.

REFERENCES

1. Smith-Petersen MN. Evolution of mold arthroplasty. Clin Orthop Rel Res 1978; 134:5–21.
2. Haboush EJ. A new operation for arthroplasty of the hip based on biomechanics, photoelasticity, fast-setting dental acrylic, and other considerations. Bull Hosp Joint Dis 1953; 14:242–277.
3. Charnley J. Surgery of the hip-joint. Present and future developments. Br Med J 1960; 821–826.
4. Charnley J. Low Friction Arthroplasty of the Hip: Theory and Practice. New York: Springer-Verlag, 1979.
5. Amstutz HC, Graff-Radford A, Gruen TA, Clarke IC. THARIES surface replacements: A review of the first 100 cases. Clin Orthop 1978; 87–101.
6. Gerard Y. Hip Arthroplasty by Matching Cups. Clin Orthop Rel Res 1978; July/August:25–35.
7. Wagner H. Surface replacement arthroplasty of the hip. Clin Orthop Rel Res 1978; 134:102–130.
8. Capello WN, Ireland PH, Trammell TR, Eicher P. Conservative total hip arthroplasty. A procedure to conserve bone stock. Clin Orthop Rel Res 1978; 134:59–74.
9. Freeman MAR, Cameron HU, Brown GC. Cemented double cup arthroplasty of the Hip: A 5 year experience with ICLH prosthesis. Clin Orthop Rel Res 1978; 134:45–52.
10. Jolley MN, Salvati EA, Brown GC. Early results and complications of surface replacement of the hip. J Bone Joint Surg 1982; 64A:366–377.
11. Head WC. Wagner surface replacement arthroplasty of the hip. J Bone Joint Surg 1981; 63A:420–427.
12. Bell RS, Schatzker J, Fornasier VL, Goodman SB. A study of implant failure in the Wagner resurfacing arthroplasty. J Bone Joint Surg 1985; 67A:1165–1175.

13. Head WC. The Wagner surface replacement arthroplasty. Orthop Clin North Am 1982; 13:789–797.

14. Ritter MA, Gioe TJ. Conventional versus resurfacing hip arthroplasty. J Bone Joint Surg 1986; 68A:216–225.

15. Treuting RJ, Waldman D, Hooten J, Schmalzried TP, Barrack RL. Prohibitive failure rate of the total articular replacement arthroplasty at five to ten years. Am J Orthop 1997; 26:114–118.

16. Siebenrock KA, Scholl E, Lottenbach M, Ganz R. Bernese periacetabular osteotomy. Clin Orthop 1999; 363:9–20.

17. Leunig M, Siebenrock KA, Ganz R. Rationale of periacetabular osteotomy and background work. J Bone Joint Surg 2001; 83A:438–448.

18. Beaulé PE, Mast JW, Matta JM. Hip Arthrodesis: Current indications and techniques. J Am Acad Orthop Surg 2002. In press.

19. Dorr LD, Luckett M, Conaty JP. Total hip arthroplasties in patients younger than 45 years. A nine- to ten-year follow-up study. Clin Orthop Rel Res 1990; 260:215–219.

20. Ortiguera CJ, Pulliam IT, Cabanela ME. Total hip arthroplasty for osteonecrosis: Matched-pair analysis of 188 hips with long-term follow-up. J Arthrop 1999; 14:21–28.

21. Sochart DH, Porter ML. Total hip arthroplasty with cement in patients less than twenty years old. Long-term results [letter; comment]. J Bone Joint Surg 1998; 80A:1397–1398.

22. Torchia ME, Klassen RA, Bianco AJ. Total hip arthroplasty with cement in patients less than twenty years old. J Bone Joint Surg 1996; 78A:995–1003.

23. Feller JA, Kay PR, Hodgkinson JP, Wroblewski BM. Activity and socket wear in the Charnley low-friction arthroplasty. J Arthrop 1994; 9:341–345.

24. McLaughlin JR, Lee KR. Total hip arthroplasty in young patients. Clin Orthop Rel Res 2000; 373:153–163.

25. McKellop H, Shen F-W, Lu B, Campbell P, Salovey R. Development of an extremely wear-resistant ultra high molecular weight polyethylene for total hip replacements. J Orthop Res 1999; 17:157–167.

26. Sieber H-P, Rieker CB, Kottig P. Analysis of 118 second-generation metal-on-metal retrieved hip implants. J Bone Joint Surg 1999; 81B:46–50.

27. Schmalzried TP, Callaghan JJ. Wear in total hip and knee replacements. J Bone Joint Surg Am 1999; 81:115–136.

28. Rubash HE, Sinha RK, Shanbhag AS, Kim S-Y. Pathogenesis of bone loss after total hip arthroplasty. Orthop Clin North Am 1998; 29:173–186.

29. Radl R, Aigner C, Hungerford MW, Pascher A, Windhager R. Proximal femoral bone loss and increased rate of fracture with a proximally hydroxyapaptite-coated femoral component. J Bone Joint Surg 2000; 82B:1151–1155.

30. Robinson AH, Palmer CR, Villar RN. Is revision as good as primary hip replacement? J Bone Joint Surg Br 1999; 81:42–45.

31. Amstutz HC, Thomas BJ, Jinnah R, Kim W, Grogan T, Yale C. Treatment of primary osteoarthritis of the hip. A comparison of total joint and surface replacement arthroplasty. J Bone Joint Surg 1984; 66A:228–241.

32. Wright JG, Young NL. The patient-specific index: asking patients what they want. J Bone Joint Surg Am 1997; 79:974–983.

33. Bogoch ER, Fornasier VL, Capello WN. The femoral head remnant in resurfacing arthroplasty. Clin Orthop Rel Res 1982; 167:92–105.

34. Amstutz HC, Dorey F, O'Carroll PF. THARIES resurfacing arthroplasty. Evolution and long-term results. Clin Orthop Rel Res 1986; 213:92–114.

35. Capello WN, Misamore GW, Trancik TM. The Indiana conservative (surface replacement) hip arthroplasty. J Bone Joint Surg 1984; 66A:518–528.

36. Howie DW, Campbell D, McGee M, Cornish BL. Wagner resurfacing hip arthroplasty. The results of one hundred consecutive arthroplasties after eight to ten years. J Bone Joint Surg 1990; 72A:708–714.

37. Mesko JW, Goodman FG, Stanescu S. Total articular replacement arthroplasty. A three- to ten-year case-controlled study. Clin Orthop Rel Res 1994; 300: 168–177.

38. Amstutz HC, Dorey F, O'Carroll PF. THARIES resurfacing arthroplasty. Evolution and long-term results. Clin Orthop Rel Res 1986; 213:92–114.

39. Amstutz HC, Kabo JM, Dorey FJ. Surface replacement arthroplasty: Evolution of today's ingrowth-fixed design. In: Reynolds, D, and Freeman, MAR, eds. Osteoarthritis in the Young Adult Hip. Edinburgh: Churchill Livingstone, 1989, pp 251–275.

40. Howie D, Cornish BL, Vernon-Roberts B. Resurfacing hip arthroplasty. Classification of loosening and the role of prosthetic wear particles. Clin Orthop Rel Res 1990; 255:144–159.

41. Amstutz H, Campbell PA, Kossovsky N, Clarke IC. Mechanism and clinical significance of wear debris-induced osteolysis. Clin Orthop Rel Res 1992; 276:7–18.

42. Schmalzried TP, Jasty M, Harris WH. Periprosthetic bone loss in total hip arthroplasty: The role of polyethylene wear debris and the concept of the effective joint space. J Bone Joint Surg 1992; 74A:849–863.

43. Kabo J, Gebhard JS, Loren G, Amstutz HC. In vivo wear of polyethylene acetabular components. J Bone Joint Surg 1993; 75B:254–258.

44. Mai M, Schmalzried TP, Amstutz HC. The contribution of frictional torque to loosening at the cement-bone interface in Tharies hip replacements. J Bone Joint Surg 1996; 78A:505–511.

45. Campbell PA, Mirra J, Amstutz HC. Viability of femoral head treated with resurfacing arthroplasty. J Arthrop 2000; 15:120–122.

46. Howie DW, Cornish BL, Vernon-Roberts B. The viability of the femoral head after resurfacing hip arthroplasty in humans. Clin Orthop Rel Res 1993; 291: 171–184.

47. Amstutz HC, Kabo M, Hermens K, O'Carroll PF, Dorey F, Kilgus D. Porous surface replacement of the hip with chamfer cylinder design. Clin Orthop Rel Res 1987; 222:140–160.

48. Nasser S, Campbell PA, Kilgus D, Kossovsky N, Amstutz HC. Cementless total joint arthroplasty prostheses with titanium-alloy articular surfaces. A human retrieval analysis. Clin Orthop 1990; 261:171–185.

49. Buechel F. Hip resurfacing revisited. Orthopedics 1996; 19:753–756.

50. McKellop H, Shen F-W, Lu B, Campbell PA, Salovey R. Effect on sterilization method and other modifications on the wear resistance of acetabular cups made of ultra-high molecular weight polyethylene. J Bone Joint Surg 2000; 82A:1708–1725.

51. Townley CO. Hemi and total articular replacement arthroplasty of the hip with the fixed femoral cup. Orthop Clin North Am 1982; 13:869–894.

52. Tooke SM, Amstutz HC, Delaunay C. Hemiresurfacing for femoral head osteonecrosis. J Arthrop 1987; 2:125–133.

53. Scott RD, Urse JS, Schmidt R. Use of TARA hemiarthroplasty in advanced osteonecrosis. J Arthrop 1987; 2:225–232.

54. Salvati EA, Cornell CN. Long-term follow-up of total hip replacement in patients with avascular necrosis. Instr Course Lect 1988; 37:67–73.

55. Piston RW, Engh CA, De Carvalho PI, Suthers K. Osteonecrosis of the femoral head treated with total hip arthroplasty without cement. J Bone Joint Surg Am 1994; 76:202–214.

56. Kantor SG, Huo MH, Huk OL, Salvati EA. Cemented total hip arthroplasty in patients with osteonecrosis. A 6-year minimum follow-up study of second-generation cement techniques. J Arthrop 1996; 11:267–271.

57. Mont MA, Jones LC, Sotereanos DC, Amstutz HC, Hungerford DS. Understanding and treating osteonecrosis of the femoral head. Instr Course Lect 2000; 49:169–188.

58. Mankin HJ. Nontraumatic necrosis of bone (osteonecrosis). N Engl J Med 1992; 326:1473–1479.

59. Mont MA, Fairbank AC, Krackow KA, Hungerford DS. Corrective osteotomy for osteonecrosis of the femoral head [see comments]. J Bone Joint Surg 1996; 78A:1032–1038.

60. Langlais F, Fourastier J. Rotation osteotomies for osteonecrosis of the femoral head. Clin Orthop Rel Res 1997; 343:110–123.

61. Dean MT, Cabanela ME. Transtrochanteric anterior rotational osteotomy for avascular necrosis of the femoral head. Long-term results. J Bone Joint Surg 1993; 75B:597–601.

62. Sugioka Y. Transtrochanteric rotational osteotomy in the treatment of idiopathic and steroid-induced femoral head necrosis, Perthes' disease, slipped capital femoral epiphysis, and osteoarthritis of the hip. Indications and results. Clin Orthop Rel Res 1984; 277:12–23.

63. Merle D'Aubigné R, Postel M, Mazabraud A, Massias P, Gueguen J. Idiopathic necroisis of the femoral head in adults. J Bone Joint Surg 1965; 47B: 612–633.

64. Mont MA, Einhorn TA, Sponseller PD, Hungerford DS. The trapdoor procedure using autogenous cortical and cancellous bone grafts for osteonecrosis of the femoral head. J Bone Joint Surg 1998; 80B:56–62.

65. Dinulescu I, Stanculescu D, Nicolescu M, Dinu G. Long-term follow-up after intertrochanteric osteotomies for avascular necrosis of the femoral head. Bull Hosp Joint Dis 1998; 57:84–87.

66. Mont MA, Hungerford DS. Non-traumatic avascular necrosis of the femoral head. J Bone Joint Surg 1995; 77A:459–474.

67. Ferguson GM, Cabanela ME, Ilstrup DM. Total after failed intertrochanteric osteotomy. J Bone Joint Surg 1994; 76B:252–257.
68. Boos N, Krushell R, Ganz R, Muller ME. Total hip arthroplasty after previous proximal femoral osteotomy. J Bone Joint Surg 1997; 79B:247–253.
69. Amstutz HC, Grigoris P, Safran MR, Grecula MJ, Campbell PA, Schmalzried TP. Precision-fit surface hemiarthroplasty for femoral head osteonecrosis. Long term results. J Bone Joint Surg 1994; 76B:423–427.
70. Nelson CL, Walz BH, Gruenwald JM. Resurfacing of only the femoral head for osteonecrosis. Long-term follow-up study. J Arthrop 1997; 12:736–740.
71. Hungerford MW, Mont MA, Scott R, Fiore C, Hungerford DS, Krackow KA. Surface replacement hemiarthroplasty for the treatment of osteonecrosis of the femoral head. J Bone Joint Surg 1998; 80A:1656–1664.
72. Langlais F, Barthas J, Postel M. Les cupules ajustees pour necrose idiopathique. Bilan radiologique. Rev Chir Orthop 1979; 65:151–155.
73. Sedel L, Travers V, Witvoet J. Spherocylindric (Luck) cup arthroplasty for osteonecrosis of the hip. Clin Orthop Rel Res 1987; 219:127–135.
74. Beaulé PE, Schmalzried TP, Campbell PA, Dorey F, Amstutz HC. Duration of symptoms and outcome of hemiresurfacing for hip osteonecrosis. Clin Orthop Rel Res 2001; 385:104–117.
75. Ash SA, Callaghan JJ, Johnston RC. Revision total hip arthroplasty with cement after cup arthroplasty. J Bone Joint Surg 1996; 78A:87–93.
76. Ficat RP. Idiopathic bone necrosis of the femoral head. Early diagnosis and treatment. J Bone Joint Surg 1985; 67B:3–9.
77. Kerboull M, Thomine J, Postel M, d'Aubigne RM. The conservative surgical treatment of idiopathic aseptic necrosis of the femoral head. J Bone Joint Surg 1974; 56B:291–296.
78. Kim Y-M, Ahn JH, Kang HS, Kim HJ. Estimation of the extent of osteonecrosis of the femoral head using MRI. J Bone Joint Surg 1998; 80B:954–958.
79. Mitchell DG, Rao VM, Dalinka MK, Spritzer CE, Gefter WB, Axel L, Steinberg ME, Kressel HY. MRI of joint fluid in the normal and ischemic hip. AJR 1986; 146:1215–1218.
80. Steinberg ME, Corces A, Fallon M. Acetabular involvement in osteonecrosis of the femoral head. J Bone Joint Surg 1999; 81A:60–65.
81. McKellop H, Shen F-W, Lu B, Campbell P, Salovey R. Development of an extremely wear-resistant ultra high molecular weight polyethylene for total hip replacements. J Orthop Res 1999; 17:157–167.
82. Steinberg ME, Bands RE, Parry S, Hoffman E, Chan T, Hartman KM. Does lesion affect the outcome in avascular necrosis. Clin Orthop Rel Res 1999; 367:262–271.
83. Bozic KJ, Zurakowski D, Thornhill T. S. Survivorship analysis of hips treated with core decompression for nontraumatic osteonecrosis of the femoral head. J Bone Joint Surg 1999; 81A:200–209.
84. Nelson CL, Walz BH, Gruenwald JM. Resurfacing of only the femoral head for osteonecrosis. Long-term follow-up study. J Arthrop 1997; 12:736–740.
85. Beaulé PE, Amstutz HC. Hemiresurfacing arthroplasty for osteonecrosis of the hip. Op Tech Orthop 2000; 10:123–132.

86. Harty M. Surface Replacement Arthroplasty of the Hip. Anatomic considerations. Orthop Clin North Am 1982; 13:667–679.

87. Schmalzried T, Callaghan JJ. Wear in total hip and knee replacements. J Bone Joint Surg 1999; 81A:115–136.

88. Jacobsson SA, Djerf K, Wahlstrom O. A comparative study between McKee-Farrar and Charnley arthroplasty with long-term follow-up periods. J Arthrop 1990; 5:9–14.

89. Weber B. Experience with the Metasul total hip bearing system. Clin Orthop 1996; 329S:S69–S77.

90. Schmalzried T, Peters PC, Maurer BT, Bragdon CR, Harris WH. Long duration metal-on-metal total hip replacements with low wear of the articulating surfaces. J Arthrop 1996; 11:322–331.

91. McKellop H, Park SH, Chiesa R, Doorn P, Lu B, Normand P, Grigoris P, Amstutz H. In vivo wear of three types of metal on metal hip prostheses during two decades of use. Clin Orthop 1996; 329S:S128–S140.

92. Muller ME, Boltzy X. Artificial hip joints made from PROTOSOL. Bull Assoc Study Int Fixation 1968; 1–5.

93. Muller ME. The benefits of metal-on-metal total hip replacement. Clin Orthop Rel Res 1995; 311:54–59.

94. Gérard Y, Chelius P, Legrand A. Hip arthroplasty using non-cemented paired cups. 14-year experience. Rev Chir Orthop 1985; 71(suppl 2):82–85.

95. McMinn D, Treacy R, Lin K, Pynsent P. Metal on metal surface replacement of the hip: Experience of the McMinn prosthesis. Clin Orthop 1996; 329S: S89–S98.

96. Wagner M, Wagner H. Preliminary results of uncemented metal on metal stemmed and resurfacing hip replacement arthroplasty. Clin Orthop 1996; 329S:S78–S88.

97. McMinn D, Pynsent P. Metal/Metal Hip Resurfacing with Hybrid fixation: Results of 1000 cases. San Francisco: American Academy of Orthopedic Surgeons, 2001.

98. Dorr LD, Wan Z, LongJohn DB, Dubois B, Murken R. Total hip arthroplasty with use of the Metasul metal-on-metal articulation. J Bone Joint Surg 2000; 82A:789–798.

99. Beaulé PE, Ebramzadeh E, Prasad R, Amstutz HC. Biomechanical Evaluation and Preliminary Clinical Results of Re-cementing Liner into a Well-Fixed Acetabular Socket in Revision Hip Surgery. London, Ontario, Canada, Canadian Orthopedic Research Society, 2001.

100. Mjoberg B. Theories of wear and loosening in hip prostheses. Wear-induced loosening vs loosening-induced wear-a review. Acta Orthop Scand 1994; 65: 361–371.

101. Beaulé PE, Dorey FJ, Amstutz HC. Wagner and McMinn Metal-on-Metal Surface Arthroplasty of the Hip. Minimum 5 year follow-up. London, Ontario, Canada, Canadian Orthopedic Association, 2001.

102. Freeman MAR. Some anatomical and mechanical considerations relevant to the surface replacement of the femoral head. Clin Orthop Rel Res 1978; 134: 19–24.

103. Jacobs J, Skipor AK, Doorn PF, Campbell PA, Schmalzried TP, Black J, Amstutz H. Cobalt and chromium concentrations in patients with metal on metal total hip replacements. Clin Orthop Rel Res 1996; 329S:S256–S263.

104. Watanabe Y, Shiba N, Matsuo S, Higuchi F, Tagawa Y, Inoue A. Biomechanical study of the resurfacing hip arthroplasty. Finite element analysis of the femoral component. J Arthrop 2000; 15:505–511.

105. Moed B, Letournel E. Low dose irradiation with indomethacin for the prevention of heterotopic ossification. J Bone Joint Surg 1993; 76B:895–900.

106. Steinberg ME. Summary and conclusions: Symposium on surface replacement arthroplasty of the hip. Orthop Clin North Am 1982; 13:895–902.

10
Treatment of the Infected Total Hip Arthroplasty

David J. Dunlop, Bassam A. Masri, Donald S. Garbuz, Nelson V. Greidanus, and Clive P. Duncan
University of British Columbia, Vancouver, British Columbia, Canada

I. INTRODUCTION

A.   The Scope of the Problem: Incidence, Cost, Sequelae

Total hip arthroplasty has evolved to become an extremely successful procedure for the majority of patients. Those who experience no complications can expect dramatic improvement in their quality of life after surgery (1). Deep infection, unfortunately, remains one of the most serious complications for the patient and also has dramatic implications due to the significant burden that it imposes on the cost of health care delivery (2).

The first total hip arthroplasty was performed more than a century ago by Gluck in Germany, in 1890, using cemented ivory femoral and acetabular components. However, the modern era dates back roughly 40 years to the pioneering work of Sir John Charnley. Initially between 1959 and 1961, Charnley had a high infection rate of 8.9% (3), which he worked arduously to decrease to 1% by 1970 by employing a variety of strategies, emphasizing particularly the importance of reducing air contamination in the operating room (4). Multiple measures—including prophylactic antibiotics, ultraclean air in operating rooms, and careful patient—selection have contributed to maintaining acceptably low infection rates (5). Specialist units where a large volume of joint replacements are performed generally record infection rates under 1% (6).

There are several well-accepted risk factors for infection after total hip arthroplasty, and it may be that large population studies will give a more accurate figure for the overall rate of infection rather than smaller individual series. Data from all Medicare patients who underwent total hip replacement in the United States between 1986 and 1989 showed that 2.2% became infected (5370 of 236,140) (2). Kreder looking at the Washington State Department of Health data set, reported a 0.8% infection rate in 1 year (67 of 8774), although some infections would still be undeclared at only 1 year of follow-up from surgery (7). Recent data from a Regional Arthroplasty Register in the United Kingdom showed an infection rate of 1.4% at 5 years (8).

There is some concern that the low level of infection achieved during the British Medical Research Council trial (9), as low as 0.3%, has not always been sustained (10) despite widespread knowledge of the problems of infection, technological advances, and refinement of surgical technique. If the true overall rate of infection lies closer to 2% than under 1%, this has profound implications, in that Sculco calculated in 1993 the annual cost to treat 3500–4000 infected hip arthroplasties in the United States is between $150 and $200 million, with each case averaging $50,000–$60,000 (2).

Appropriate diagnosis of an infected total hip arthroplasty is crucial but can be difficult. No single test is currently available that can accurately distinguish septic from aseptic loosening. The preoperative diagnosis depends on interpretation of a combination of an appropriate history, careful physical examination, radiological examination, laboratory investigations including erythrocyte sedimentation rate (ESR) and C-reactive protein (CRP), hip joint aspiration where appropriate (11), and occasionally nuclear imaging. At revision, the diagnostic yield can be increased with appropriate tissue samples and newer techniques of molecular biology. It has recently been suggested that improved microbiological techniques—including immunofluorescence microscopy and polymerase chain reaction (PCR) amplification—show that the current incidence of prosthetic joint infection is a gross underestimate (12). The full clinical significance of these findings are not yet known. Misdiagnosis of infection as aseptic loosening can easily lead to inappropriate surgery, with a high failure rate. Further surgery will then be required, which is disheartening for the patient and often more difficult for the surgeon owing to loss of bone stock; it also means a further unnecessary expense for the health care payer.

II. PATHOGENESIS OF INFECTION

A. Routes of Infection

There are four routes by which infecting organisms can reach the periprosthetic space: contamination at the time of surgery, direct or contiguous spread, hematogenous spread, and reactivation of infection in a previously infected hip.

Contamination at the time of surgery is well recognized. Charnley emphasized the importance of reducing the air contamination in the operating room (4). In the early stages of his work, he showed that by introducing 10 air exchanges per hour, his infection rate was halved from 7% to 3.5%, and the bacterial colonies measured in 6 petri dishes fell from 18–2.5/ft^3. Increasing the number of air changes to 300/hr reduced his infection rate to 1.5%. He did, however, accept that further increasing the air cleanliness would, by itself, be unlikely to reduce the infection rate below 1.5%. Reviewing the data from the Medical Research Council's prospective trial of ultraclean operating room air, Lidwell showed the association between infection rates and bacterial counts in the operating room, with a progressive decline in the incidence of joint infection being associated with reduction of air contamination (13). Salvati looked at the effect of horizontal laminar flow on both hip and knee replacements and found a statistically significant decrease in infection rates for hip replacements from 1.4–0.9% but an increase in infection rates for knee replacements from 1.4–3.9% (14). The reason for the increased infection rate in knee replacements was thought to be related to the interposition of members of the surgical team between the source of the clean air and the open wound.

The second route through which infection reaches the hip joint is by direct or contiguous spread. Although accepted to be a more common problem with joints close to the surface, like the knee and the elbow, it can also occur in the hip. The organisms migrate to the hip joint from a more superficial infection. Schmalzried reported on 47 deep infections from a series of 3051 total hip arthroplasties. Two of these patients had infection from direct or contiguous spread; one, who had urethral strictures, developed a deep perineal abscess that drained into the hip (15). Surin reviewed 34 deep infections from a consecutive series of 803 hip replacements (16). They found that the 115 hips with a superficial postoperative wound discharge had a 3.2 times increased risk of deep infection presenting later (11 of 115) with a minimum follow-up of 3 years. The unanswered question from their study was whether an initially sterile hematoma became cross-infected on the ward, and subsequently caused a deep infection by contiguous spread, or whether the deep infection was established from the time of surgery but not fully declared initially. More recently, Gaine reported no increase in deep wound infection in the subgroup of 56 patients with a superficial infection as compared with those who had no wound problems from their group of 301 total hip arthroplasties at a mean follow-up of 26 months (17). They had a rate of 1.3% (4 of 301) early deep infections, which they state has subsequently decreased with the installation of a laminar airflow system.

The third mechanism is via the hematogenous route, enabling a remote infection to seed and cause a deep periprosthetic infection. The commonest sources for these blood-born infections have been reported to be skin infections (31 of 67, or 46%) followed by dental infection or manipulation (10 of 67, or 15%), and urinary tract infections (9 of 67, or 13%) (18).

The fourth mode of infection is reactivation of infection in a previously infected hip. This was the mechanism in 13 of 47 infected cases from Schmalzried's series of 3051 arthroplasties (15). The total number of previously infected hips that were operated on was not given, so the prevalence of recurrent sepsis could not be calculated.

B. Classification of Periprosthetic Hip Infections

A variety of classification systems have been developed for periprosthetic infections. Coventry (19), from the Mayo Clinic, initially described phase 1a infections as acute suppurative infections usually occurring in the first 3 weeks after surgery. Phase 1b represented an early hematoma with questionable infection. Phase 2 infections were the low-grade, creeping, insidious infections, which usually occurred between 2 months and 1 year after operation. He also described infections occurring more than 2 years from surgery as being most likely to be of hematogenous origin. Two years later, the same Mayo Clinic group (20) divided infections into three stages, which were slightly altered from Coventry's original phases as described:

Stage I (acute fulminating infection) occurs within 3 months of the procedure. The presentation includes systemic symptoms such as fever, chills, sepsis, and increasing pain, particularly at rest and at night. Local signs include wound drainage, erythema, swelling, and abscess formation.

Stage II (delayed sepsis) develops as a creeping, indolent infection within the first 26 months after surgery. These infections are also thought to originate from the time of surgery, but due to either a smaller inoculum or to the lower virulence of the infecting organism, the presentation is delayed by months to years after the procedure. This is the most common presentation of infection after total hip arthroplasty and the most difficult to diagnose.

Stage III (late hematogenous infections). These infections were the least common in Fitzgerald's series (20). They are metastatic infections caused by hematogenous spread from a focus of infection elsewhere. The presentation is usually that of an acute infection, with features similar to those of a stage I infection in a patient with a previously asymptomatic hip. The diagnosis is usually obvious on history and physical examination. Seeding of infection can occur regardless of the status of fixation of the components.

Tsukayama (21) described four different clinical settings for infection. Overall, these are similar to Coventry and Fitzgerald's work but include a fourth group for patients with positive intraoperative cultures at the time of revision surgery.

1. Positive intraoperative cultures if at least 2 of 5 samples taken at the time of revision surgery were positive.
2. Acute infections presented within 1 month of surgery.
3. Chronic infections developed 1 month or more after surgery and with an insidious course.
4. Acute hematogenous infections occurring with an acute onset of symptoms following a documented or suspected antecedent infection.

C. Risk Factors for Infection

There are several well-established risk factors for infection and a variety of prophylactic steps that can be taken to reduce the risk of infection. These can be broken down into patient factors, the operating room environment, surgical factors, and factors related to perioperative care.

1. Patient Factors

Patients with rheumatoid arthritis, diabetes, previous renal or liver transplants, dialysis patients, and those with sickle cell anemia have been shown to be at increased risk of infection. Fitzgerald (20) showed rheumatoid arthritis to roughly triple the risk of infection, as compared with degenerative joint disease, from 0.8–3.1% for previously unoperated hips and 2.2–6.5% for previously operated hips. Poss (22) showed that patients with rheumatoid arthritis had a 1.8 times increased risk of infection following total hip arthroplasty as compared with patients with osteoarthritis. In Maderazo's series of 24 patients with infected total hip or knee arthroplasties, all 7 of the rheumatoid patients who became infected were taking steroids (18).

The Norwegian hip register (23) showed that patients taking antidiabetic medication, either insulin or oral hypoglycemics, had almost double (odds ratio 1.9) the risk of infection compared with nondiabetics. Patients who have had a previous renal or liver transplant have an extremely high (19%) reported rate of infection (24). Furthermore, 13% of patients on long-term dialysis became infected in a series of 15 hips implanted in patients with end-stage renal failure (25). Sickle-cell anemia has been reported to have a high infection rate of 23% (3 of 13) for primary hip replacements (26), 18% (3 of 17) for primary and revision operations (27), and 20% (7 of 35) for primary and revision procedures (28).

Poor nutrition has been implicated as a cause of delayed wound healing (29). The authors reviewed 103 total hip replacements and found that the preoperative and postoperative serum transferrin and postoperative serum albumin levels were significantly lower in the group of 34 patients with delayed wound healing as compared with those who healed uneventfully. They did not, however, report on the incidence of subsequent deep infection.

2. Operating-Room Environment

The environment in which the surgery takes place has a vital impact on contamination of the surgical wound. The impact of laminar airflow has already been discussed. The bacteria in the air of the operating room come from people, with each individual shedding between 1000 and 10,000 viable bacteria per minute. It is characteristics of the individual, rather than hair length or type of head cover, that appears to affect the number of viable organisms shed (30). Ritter also showed a reduction of overall environmental contamination by 69% with the use of a helmet aspirator in a conventional operating room but no difference between a helmet or a hood in conditions of laminar airflow (30). The Medical Research Council trial showed that the lowest infection rate of 0.3% was achieved when a body exhaust suit was used in conditions of ultraclean air (31). Sterile helmet aspirator suits are also advantageous in reducing the potential for contamination, which can exist during a revision procedure when cement fragments hit an unsterile face mask and fall back into the wound.

An alternative method of reducing airborne contamination is the use of ultraviolet light in the operating room. Berg et al. (32) showed this to significantly reduce the number of bacteria during hip surgery when compared with a sham blue light. In a subsequent study, Berg et al. (33) showed ultraviolet light to be more effective at reducing bacterial counts than an ultraclean air enclosure with 30 air changes per hour. Ultraviolet light has also been shown to reduce the incidence of deep infection following hip replacement surgery. Lowell (34) reported a reduced rate of infection of 0.5% for 2389 hips after the introduction of ultraviolet light in 1973, compared with 3% of 621 hips performed without ultraviolet light before 1973.

The use of an unscrubbed ungowned leg holder during skin preparation in hip and knee replacement surgery was associated with 4.4 times higher bacterial air counts than during the operation itself. This was reduced to 2.4-fold with the use of a scrubbed and gowned leg holder. However, on occasions, the standards for ultraclean air, of 10 colony forming units per cubic meter (CFU/m^3) within 30 cm of the wound, and not more than 20 CFU/m^3 at the level of the operating table in the rest of the clean air area, were exceeded (35). The explanation for these increased counts is almost certainly

the increased number of people moving around during preparation and draping; the authors suggest, as originally taught by Charnley, that instruments
should not be exposed at this stage.

There are many other potential sources of intraoperative bacterial contamination. A study of 100 primary hip and knee arthroplasties showed rates
of contamination of 11.4% for the sucker tips, 14.5% for light handles, 9.4%
for skin blades, 3.2% for inside blades, and 28.7% of gloves used during
skin preparation (36). Skin preparation of the patient in the anesthetic room
and the use of a scrubbed "leg holder" significantly reduced the contamination of the gloves used during final preparation of the patient ($p < 0.05$).
Overall, 63% of operations showed contamination in the field of operation,
although there was only one deep infection at a minimum 2-year follow-up.
The deep infection was with *Staphylococcus aureus*, but the only contami-
nant during the original procedure had been *Staphylococcus albus* from the
front of the surgeon's gown. Based on this information, it is recommended
that, whenever possible, skin preparation be performed by gloved and
gowned personnel, and that gloves be changed frequently during the procedure. Strict aseptic technique should be observed during all joint replacement procedures.

3. Surgical Factors and Technique

Previous hip surgery has been shown to increase the infection rate from
0.9–2.3% (20). Specifically, revision total hip arthroplasty was previously
associated with much higher rates of infection. In the early 1980s, a review
by James et al. (37) showed an infection rate of 12% for revision of uninfected cases. Better results have since been achieved both for infected revisions, with a 4% reinfection rate (38), and revisions for aseptic loosening,
with a 2.5% reinfection rate (39). Revision cases where structural femoral
allografts have been used have a slightly higher reported infection rate of
5% (40). Although not frequently performed conversion of an arthrodesis to
a total hip arthroplasty still has a very high reported infection rate of 10–
13% (41,42).

Charnley (4) showed that, even under conditions of very low air contamination, with 300 air changes per hour, it was still possible to have one
colony in six petri dishes exposed for 1 hr. Extrapolating from this suggests
that an increased surgical time will be associated with an increased risk of
infection. Although prolonged operating time is widely considered to be a
risk factor for deep infection following total hip arthroplasty, Fitzgerald et
al. (20) demonstrated only a trend toward a higher infection rate, which did
not reach statistical significance.

Surin et al. (16) reviewed 34 deep infections from a consecutive series
of 803 hip replacements. They found that the 115 hips with a superficial

discharge had a 3.2 times increased risk of later deep infection (11 of 115). It is therefore important to have careful wound closure to avoid areas of wound necrosis, large hematomas, and reoperations. Tissue trauma is an important predisposing factor in the development of infection due to bacterial binding to fibronectin. Tissue damage exposes collagen, basement membrane proteins, and clots to the bloodstream. All of these are associated with fibronectin. Circulating *S. aureus* binds specifically and avidly to the N-terminal portion of fibronectin; therefore, with increased tissue trauma, more fibronectin becomes available to provide a favorable environment for staphylococcal proliferation. Tissue trauma is unavoidable during surgery; but with meticulous handling of the soft tissue, this can be minimized. Subinhibitory concentrations of penicillin and cephalothin have even been shown to enhance this binding in vitro, which could further potentiate infection in clinical practice (43).

There are some prospective data on the benefit of antibiotic-impregnated bone cement. Josefsson (44) prospectively randomized patients undergoing total hip replacement to either systemic antibiotics or gentamicin-containing bone cement. At 8–12 year follow-up, the deep infection rate was 13 of 835 patients with systemic antibiotics (1.6%) compared with 9 of 853 patients with gentamicin cement (1.1%). This difference was not statistically significant, although it had previously been significantly in favor of the antibiotic-loaded cement at both 2- and 5-year follow-up.

Data from the Scandinavian Hip Registries supports the use of antibiotic-loaded cement. The Norwegian Hip Register (45) shows that the combination of both systemic antibiotics and antibiotic cement led to the fewest revisions for both septic and aseptic reasons. The Swedish Hip Register (46) shows that of all cement types, Palacos with gentamicin has the lowest risk ratio for revision. A retrospective review of 1542 Charnley total hip arthroplasties without systemic antibiotics showed no benefit for gentamicin cement over plain cement for primary arthroplasties (47). The same study did show a significant benefit for gentamicin cement in patients who had undergone previous hip surgery other than arthroplasty, with 5 of 125 (4%) in the plain cement group becoming infected compared with 1 of 55 (1.82%) with antibiotic cement. Clearly, with the increasing use of cementless implants, this becomes irrelevant.

4. Perioperative Care

Perioperative systemic antibiotic use continues to be the most important factor in the prevention of infection. The use of perioperative antibiotic prophylaxis is supported by randomized trials. The timing of antibiotic administration was investigated by Bowers (48). In an animal model, cephaloridine could sterilize a bacterial innoculum if given preoperatively but not if started 6 hr or more after contamination. Hill (49) showed a significant reduction in infections from 3.3% (placebo) to 0.9% (5 days cefazolin) in a double-blind, randomized, placebo-controlled trial on 2137 patients undergoing hip replacement. They also found infections to be less common in the four centers with hypersterile operating rooms; the benefits of antibiotics were restricted to patients having hip replacements in conventional operating rooms. Unfortunately, the large Medical Research Council trial did not control for antibiotic use, but it was associated with a lower incidence of sepsis than in patients who received no antibiotic prophylaxis (0.4 versus 2.3%). Subsequently, Nelson (50) demonstrated the efficacy of a shorter 1-day course of antibiotics in a randomized comparison to 7 days of antibiotics in 358 patients.

The use of a drain postoperatively remains controversial. There are few data to support the perceived benefits of reducing postoperative hematoma, prolonged drainage, delayed healing, and ultimately infection (51). Willett et al. (52) prospectively studied a series of 120 hip replacements divided into three groups depending on the time of removal of their suction drains. They found that 90.9% of the total loss occurred in the first 24 hr. Removal of the drain in the earliest group at 24 hr was not associated with a higher incidence of wound haematoma than the other two groups, at either 48 or 72 hr after surgery. In seven cases there was a positive deep wound culture identical to skin organisms cultured from that patient. All seven of these cases had their drain removed at 48 or 72 hr. Thus the risk of ingress of skin organisms was found to be statistically significant if the drain remained in situ for more than 24 hr.

Beer et al. (51) prospectively randomized patients undergoing bilateral hip or knee replacements to receive a drain on one side but not the other. Their group comprised 76 knees but only 24 hips. They found no differences between the two groups with regard to swelling or persistent discharge and recommended that the routine use of suction drains after uncomplicated total joint arthroplasty was unnecessary. Kim et al. (53) prospectively studied 48 patients (96 hips) undergoing bilateral hip replacement, randomizing one side to be drained and the other to be undrained. They found a significant increase in drainage, soaked dressings, and erythema in the undrained group but no correlation with other wound complications, pain, hip score, range of motion, or infection at 1-year follow-up.

It would appear, therefore, that routine use of a drain is not required, but it may reduce the requirement for dressing changes. If used, the drain should be removed at 24 hr to minimize the risk of deep contamination by skin organisms. If not used, the nursing staff should pay meticulous attention to wound management and dressing changes because of the increased prevalence of soaked dressings when a drain is not used.

Postoperative urinary retention requiring catheterization has been shown by Wroblewski (54) to be a risk factor for infection. He reported a 6.2% risk of deep infection in a series of 195 men who suffered from postoperative urinary retention requiring catheterization and in some cases subsequent prostatectomy. This was compared with an overall rate of 0.5% from his unit. Although not all these infections definitely originated from the urinary tract at least 3 of the 12 almost certainly did so. Of the patients who required only catheterization in Wroblewski's series, 59% received antibiotic coverage and 67 of 70 patients who went on to have a prostatectomy were given prophylactic antibiotics.

A short-term indwelling urinary catheter placed in the operating room and removed within 24–48 hr postoperatively has been shown to have a lower incidence of urinary retention than intermittent catheterization as required without increasing the rate of urinary infection (55,56). Unfortunately, neither of these papers looked at effect of the alternative catheterization protocols on the incidence of deep hip infection.

It is therefore recommended that any patient with urological symptoms should have these treated before hip arthroplasty surgery to help avoid this increased risk of periprosthetic infection. It is also accepted but not proven that antibiotic prophylaxis should be given for urinary tract manipulation in the immediate postoperative period to help reduce the risk of a transient bacteremia, which could seed the joint and cause a periprosthetic infection.

III. BASIC SCIENCE OF INFECTION

A. Susceptibility of the Periprosthetic Space to Infection and Mechanisms of Bacterial Adherence

The periprosthetic space is susceptible to infection for several reasons. Foreign bodies produce an inflammatory and necrotic tissue response. This is greater around articulating than static implants and especially so when associated with high levels of wear debris (57). The foreign-body presence of metal and bone cement can reduce host defenses. Polymethylmethacrylate reduces the chemotaxis, phagocytosis and killing ability of polymorphonuclear leukocytes (58,59). The effect of various metal implants on macrophage activity has also been investigated (60). Elevated levels of lactate dehydrogenase and glucose-6-phosphate dehydrogenase were used as a marker for cell damage and diminished activity in an in vitro study in macrophagic tissue near particles from metal implants. Low enzyme levels were found near titanium, molybdenum, and chromium implants, but raised enzyme levels indicating reduced macrophage activity were found near cobalt, nickel, and cobalt-chromium alloy implants. In a rabbit model, implants made of cobalt-chromium were found to be more conducive to infection than titanium implants and porous surfaces more conducive than polished (61).

The situation can also change with time. Failing cemented and cementless implants can be associated with an osteolytic response with significant bone destruction and debris generation from aggressive granulomatous lesions (62,63). This can then predispose to infection in the presence of microorganisms.

Infecting organisms can be divided into those that exist in planktonic forms as individual free-floating cells and sessile forms that exist within a biofilm of glycocalyx. This biofilm, or slime layer, is formed from polysaccharides synthesized by the bacteria as well as a range of host molecules (64). Organisms that produce biofilms can adhere to and survive on synthetic surfaces and are provided with protection from antibiotics, complement activation, and ingestion by neutrophils.

Gristina (65) looked at the significance of biofilms in clinical sepsis. Tissue from 25 biomaterial infections was studied, and in 76% of cases the causative bacteria grew in a glycocalyx-enclosed biofilm. They also showed that accurate microbiological sampling was difficult with conventional techniques, often yielding only one species from what was shown by electron microscopy to be a polymicrobial population. This suggests that relying on the results of a simple aspiration and routine culture to decide on the proper antibiotics may be inappropriate, as not all of the bacterial species present in the biofilm will be identified (65). Biofilms require time to form after the inoculation of an infecting organism; if the prosthesis becomes stable and covered with living tissue, the surface is less vulnerable to the adherence of bacteria. Gristina has introduced the phrase 'the race for the surface' and antibiotics may be effective while the organism is still in the planktonic phase before the biofilm has developed.

Many types of *S. aureus* and *Staphylococcus epidermidis* produce slime, whereas most gram-negative organisms except the *Pseudomonas* species are poor slime producers. Pseudomonal infections are also difficult to eradicate due to their slow rates of replication and natural resistance to many antibiotics (64). It is sometimes contended that other gram-negative organisms are more difficult to eradicate. However, as discussed later in more detail, there is evidence that this is not so. Tsukayama et al. (21) successfully treated all 13 hips infected with a gram-negative bacillus, in the majority of cases after one course of therapy. They attributed this high rate of success to, among other things, the use of newer antimicrobial agents and tobramycin-impregnated polymethylmethacrylate beads, which can achieve high local concentrations of antibiotic. The properties of antibiotic-loaded bone cement are now well understood and there is some clinical evidence that such cement may reduce the infection rate following primary total hip arthroplasty at up to 10 years (44).

B. Antibiotic-Loaded Bone Cement

Animal experiments (66) have shown antibiotic-loaded bone cement to prevent infection. Gentamicin-containing polymethylmethacrylate was found to prevent infection in 30 femora of dogs undergoing total hip replacement despite direct inoculation of 10^8 bacteria (*S. epidermidis*, *S aureus*, and *Escherichia coli*) (66). This was a statistical improvement against control and against all the other treatment groups, which included saline irrigation, neo-mycin irrigation, and systemic antibiotics (cefazolin).

To preserve the compressive and tensile properties of bone cement, it is important that the antibiotics be added in powder form. Up to 2 g of oxacillin, cefazolin, or gentamicin powder added to a single batch of cement (Simplex, 40 g powder and 20 g liquid) does not significantly affect the compressive or tensile strength of bone cement (67). However, the addition of gentamicin in aqueous solution or 4 mL of water significantly reduces the strength of cement by interfering with the early prepolymerizing process during mixing (67). Doses of gentamicin above 4.5 g per batch of cement caused the compressive strength to drop below 70 MPa, the minimum compressive strength level allowed by ASTM standards (68).

In an in vitro and in vivo animal study in mice antibiotic elution was found to peak rapidly, with most activity appearing within 3 hr and no effective activity after 5 days (69). High doses of antibiotic are sometimes used clinically on a short-term basis to provide sustained effective local concentrations even after a prolonged period (70). Reporting results with the PROSTALAC (prosthesis of antibiotic-loaded acrylic cement) system for staged revision surgery the authors detected levels of tobramycin in fluid from 47 of 48 joints (hip and knee) and vancomycin from 44 of 48 joints at an average of almost 4 months from insertion (118 days). If 3.6 g of tobramycin were used per package of cement, the periprosthetic concentration remained above the breakpoint sensitivity limit for sensitive organisms, but this was not achieved if 2.4 g of tobramycin or less were used. The presence of tobramycin also improved the elution of vancomycin, although vancomycin levels were not above the breakpoint sensitivity limit for sensitive organisms at the time of sampling. The breakpoint sensitivity limit is the level above which bacteria are killed, but below which antibiotic resistance may form.

C. Infecting Organisms, Antibiotic Resistance/Superbugs

A variety of different bacterial species can cause deep periprosthetic hip infections. In most reports of periprosthetic infection, *S. aureus* and *S. epidermidis* are the common infecting organisms, although a wide range of gram-positive and gram-negative organisms as well as anaerobic organisms have also been implicated. The timing of infection varies by species with *S. aureus* dominating early infections and bacteria from the normal skin flora, including aerobes and anaerobes such as *S. epidermidis*, *Propionobacterium acnes*, and peptostreptococci, tending to present later with delayed infections (71). There have also been occasional reports of infection caused by rare organisms including *Mycobacterium tuberculosis*, from a patient with no previous history of skeletal tuberculosis (CP Beauchamp, personal communication, 1992), *Candida paraspilosis*, *Candida albicans*, *Actinomyces israelii*, and *Echinococcus* (72–75).

Table 1 shows the breakdown by species from 34 papers on infected total hip arthroplasty from 1977 to 1999 comprising a total sample size of

Table 1 Breakdown of a Total of 2330 Infecting Organisms from 34 Published Series

Coagulase-negative staphylococci	648	*Aerobacter*	6
Staphylococcus aureus	636	*Clostridium perfringens*	5
Streptococci, not A or D	168	*Haemophilus* spp.	4
Anaerobic + microaerophilic strep	135	*Citrobacter*	3
Pseudomonas	131	*Listeria monocytogenes*	3
E. coli	129	*Gram positive not otherwise*	
Enterococcus	104	*specified*	2
Corynebacteria (anaerobic)	74	*Pasteurella multocida*	2
Proteus	73	*Campylobacter intestinalis*	2
P. acnes	40	*Aeromonas hydrophilia*	2
Klebsiella	31	*Moraxella*	2
Enterobacter cloacae	24	*Micrococcus*	1
Diphtheroid	22	*Mycoplasma hominis*	1
Group A strep	17	*K. oxytoca*	1
Bacteroides fragilis	12	*Alkaligenes*	1
Bacillus species	11	*Actinomyces*	1
Candida	8	*Clostridium bifermentans*	1
Serratia	8	*Neisseria*	1
Salmonella spp.	7	*Rothia*	1
M. tuberculosis	6	*Sarcina*	1
Acinetobacter	6	Total	2330

2330 infected arthroplasties. This shows that coagulase-negative staphylococci and *S. aureus* dominate, accounting for 28% and 27% respectively (18,21,38,50,76–105).

Several authors have drawn attention to the importance of the identified bacterial flora in planning treatment of an infected total hip arthroplasty. It has been suggested that high-virulence organisms such as gram-negative organisms are more difficult to eradicate. The definition of virulence differs from paper to paper. Gram-negative and group D streptococcal organisms generally are considered virulent by most authors. *S. aureus*, both methicillin-sensitive and resistant, other streptococci and enterococci have been considered as both virulent and less virulent (86,94). *S. epidermidis* is generally considered to be of low virulence. Organisms that elaborate a glycocalyx or slime layer in vivo, are less susceptible to eradication regardless of their presumed virulence.

Recurrent infection rates have previously been found to be higher in patients infected with gram-negative and more virulent gram-positive organisms (*S. aureus* and beta-hemolytic streptococcal species) in some studies (82,92). For this reason, many have considered these to be more difficult infections to eradicate, a fact that has been attributed in part to glycocalyx formation. It is now thought that most microorganisms, including the "low-virulence" *S. epidermidis*, can elaborate a glycocalyx given the appropriate conditions (106). In contrast to the concerns raised regarding gram-negative and highly virulent organisms, others have recommended that coagulase-negative staphylococcal species should be treated with caution owing to their tendency toward resistance of multiple antibiotics, and several different multiresistant coagulase-negative staphylococcal species may coexist in a single infected joint (107).

The concern, regarding infection with particular organisms may well have been founded on papers that do not reflect current practice. Hunter and Dandy (90) reviewed 135 cases of infected total hip arthroplasties in a Canadian national survey. They found that 20 out of 30 of these patients had failed reimplantation of a prosthetic joint. Of the successful cases, 9 grew gram-positive organisms from the infected joint and one had sterile cultures, while 4 of the failed cases grew *E. coli*. From this they deduced that eradication of gram-negative organisms presented a particular problem. Importantly, in their report, they noted that none of these cases involved the use of antibiotic-loaded cement or "massive antibiotic regimes." Jupiter et al. (92) reported on reconstruction of 9 infected total hip arthroplasties. Of the 9 procedures, 4 were complicated by recurrent infection, including both of the 2 cases infected with gram-negative organisms. Antibiotic-loaded cement does not appear to have been used in these cases. The numbers in this study are too small to make a firm conclusion about the difference in infection eradication between gram-positive and gram-negative organisms.

Several, more recent papers have explicitly addressed the question of the difficulty in eradicating particular groups of organisms (21,22,76,93,94, 99,108). None of these authors have identified an independent relationship between recurrence of infection and organism type. Only McDonald et al. (94) found a significant increase in recurrent infection, following treatment of gram-negative bacilli or group D streptococcal organisms, but this was only when looking at patients who also had less than 4 weeks of antibiotics and reimplantation at less than a year.

More important than the identity of the organisms is the susceptibility of the organisms to attack by antimicrobial agents and the ability to deliver antibiotics in appropriate doses to the site of infection. For example, most staphylococci with the exception of the strains designated as methicillin- or oxacillin-resistant are susceptible to first- or second-generation cephalosporins. There is substantial regional variation in the sensitivity profile of *S. epidermidis* and *S. aureus*. In our hospital, more than 95% of the *S. aureus* organisms encountered are oxacillin- (and therefore cephalosporin-) sensitive, while less than 70% of the *S. epidermidis* organisms share this sensitivity (64). James et al. (109) reported 67% of their *S. epidermidis* infections to be methicillin-resistant. With increased use of vancomycin, there are now concerns about vancomycin-resistant organisms, including enterococci. As previously mentioned, a range of differing bacterial sensitivities and resistances may be encountered among staphylococci isolated from a single infected joint (110). The authors' practice is to identify the infecting organism or organisms and their antibiotic sensitivities by synovial biopsy and joint aspiration preoperatively. These then guide the antibiotic regimen adopted for antibiotic-loaded cement and intravenous antibiotics in the postoperative period but do not influence the surgical approach or technique.

IV. DIAGNOSIS OF INFECTION

The infected total hip arthroplasty can present as an obvious infection (Figure 1) but can also at times present a diagnostic challenge owing to the lack of consistently sensitive and specific preoperative investigations. The diagnosis begins with a careful interpretation of the history. Risk factors for infection are sought and any problems with persistent drainage or delayed wound healing are recorded. Pain is one feature that is consistently associated with infection (111). Physical examination includes wound inspection for any persistent sinuses and/or drainage, warmth, and localized tenderness.

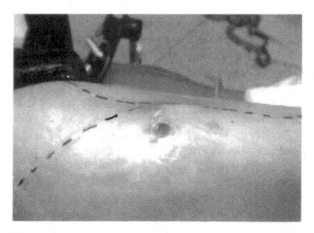

Figure 1 An obvious clinical infection with a draining sinus.

A. Laboratory Investigations

1. Erythrocyte Sedimentation Rate

The erythrocyte sedimentation rate (ESR) is a measure of red blood cells, that have been caused to agglutinate by acute-phase proteins. Our recent prospective study of 202 revision total hip arthroplasties showed the sensitivity of a raised ESR (greater than 30 mm/hr) for the diagnosis of infection to be 82%, the specificity to be 85%, the positive predictive value to be 58%, and the negative predictive value to be 95% (11). It is obviously important to be aware that other factors may elevate the ESR, including concomitant but unrelated infection, inflammatory arthritis, collagen vascular disease, recent surgical intervention, and some malignant diseases. A raised ESR, therefore, may not necessarily indicate infection, and other tests may be required to rule it out. A raised ESR (greater than 30 mm/hr) at 6 months after two-stage revision has a 62% chance of indicating persistent infection (112).

2. C-Reactive Protein

C-reactive protein (CRP) is one of the acute-phase proteins that contribute to elevation in the ESR and is a more sensitive indicator of infection (113). CRP decreases sooner after infection has resolved than the ESR does and is therefore more useful in the follow-up of infection. It also returns to normal after surgery within 3 weeks, whereas the ESR may take 12 months after an uncomplicated procedure to return to normal (114). Our recent prospective study of 202 revision total hip arthroplasties showed the sensitivity of a raised CRP (greater than 10 mg/L) for the diagnosis of infection to be 96%, the specificity to be 92%, the positive predictive value to be 74%, and the negative predictive value to be 99% (11).

3. White Blood Cell Count

The white blood cell (WBC) count is rarely elevated in patients with a chronically infected total hip arthroplasty (80). Our recent prospective study of 202 revision total hip arthroplasties showed the sensitivity of a raised WBC (greater than 11.0×10^9/L) for the diagnosis of infection to be 20%, the specificity to be 96%, the positive predictive value to be 50% and the negative predictive value to be 85% (11).

4. Combinations

Our recent prospective study of 202 revision total hip arthroplasties (11) showed the combination of a normal ESR and C-reactive protein to reliably rule out infection with a probability of infection of 0.00 (0 to 95). When both tests are positive, the probability of infection is 0.83 (20 of 24).

B. Radiographic Investigations Including Radionuclide Scans

1. Plain Radiographs

There are unfortunately no pathognomonic radiographic features of infection. Plain radiographs are indeed often normal in the presence of infection (115). Radiographic features suggestive of infection include periostitis, diffuse lysis, and endosteal scalloping (116). Loosening is not necessarily associated with infection and acute infections usually have solidly fixed components (Figure 2). Good-quality serial radiographs are important so that comparisons can be made and subtle findings detected. A diagnosis of infection is more likely with a rapid onset of osteolysis (Figure 3) or endosteal scalloping in the absence of obvious mechanical causes, such as thin or faulty polyethylene, prostheses with poor design features, excessive polyethylene wear, or incorrect component placement.

2. Magnetic Resonance Imaging

Magnetic resonance imaging can be of help, particularly with preoperative planning. Radiolucent cement, which cannot be seen on plain radiographs, shows up as a signal void within the medullary canal of the femur (117).

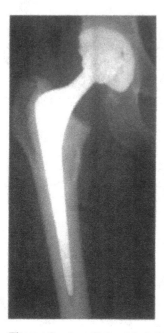

Figure 2 A well-fixed hybrid total hip replacement with a hematogenous strep-tococcal infection following a dental abscess.

Periprosthetic abscesses can be delineated and any intrapelvic extension identified.

3. Ultrasonography

Ultrasonography can be used if infection is suspected, and routine hip aspiration can be improved with ultrasonography, as it may detect any abscesses, so that the needle can be directed to obtain appropriate fluid for culture. It has also been reported as being useful to detect a thickened capsule, suggesting infection (118).

4. Radionuclide Scans

Technetium-99m bone scans are sensitive but not specific (119). A normal scan should rule out the presence of infection or mechanical complications and should weigh against operative intervention (119). Most patients with infection will have an abnormal scan, but so will patients with aseptic loosening, which is the main differential diagnosis. Bone scans remain abnormal for up to 1 year after uncomplicated arthroplasty (120) (Figure 4). Other

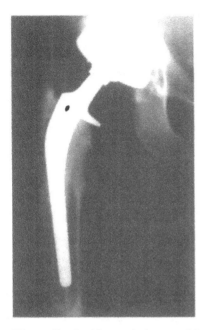

Figure 3   Rapid osteolysis caused by infection 2 years after primary total hip replacement.

conditions that can cause increased uptake on bone scan include heterotopic ossification, inflammatory conditions, fractures, and tumors.

Indium-111–labeled WBC scans are sensitive at diagnosing conditions with increased vascularity and WBC uptake but can be negative in chronic osteomyelitis due to poor uptake. Okerlund showed the predictive value of a positive ^{111}In-WBC scan to be only 63% (121).

The two techniques have been combined into a sequential bone and ^{111}In-WBC scan protocol with improved sensitivity of between 87 and 100% and specificity between 50 and 94% (122–126). These tests are not recommended for routine use but may have a role in difficult situations where there is a high index of suspicion for infection but other results are negative or inconclusive, perhaps due to concomitant antibiotic therapy, making the isolation of viable bacteria difficult.

Immunoglobulin-G scans use radioactive labeled IgG as a tracer. The test is similar to ^{111}In-WBC scans, but immunoglobulins have a more specific affinity for areas of acute inflammation than the crude preparation of the WBC used in ^{111}In scanning. One study using ^{111}In-IgG scans to diagnose infected total hip arthroplasties had a sensitivity of 77.8% and specificity of

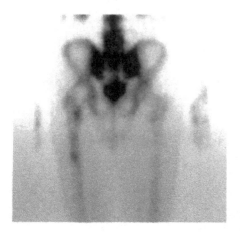

Figure 4   An abnormal bone scan of an uninfected total hip replacement.

95.5% (127). The sensitivity and specificity are therefore no better than those of the C-reactive protein; thus these scans are not recommended for routine use. Indeed, in practice, nuclear scans play a limited role in the diagnosis of infection after total hip arthroplasty.

C.   Invasive Diagnostic Tests

1.   Hip Aspiration and Arthrography

Cultures obtained from draining sinuses are unreliable, as they often grow mixed flora and not necessarily the main pathogen causing the deep peri-prosthetic infection. If infection is suspected, either because of abnormal hematological screening tests or because of suspicious clinical or radio-graphic features, an aspiration of the hip joint is required. This can confirm the presence of infection and identify the organism(s) involved, which will help to determine the antibiotic sensitivity profile not only for intravenous antibiotic therapy but also for the choice of which antibiotic to be added to bone cement. The value of preoperative aspiration has been reviewed, with opinions varying from it being a valuable test to be performed routinely on every revision hip replacement to its having little value (116,128).

By itself, arthrography is rarely useful in the diagnosis of infection, although the accumulation of dye in pockets may suggest abscess formation (129); in the case of a negative aspiration, it may help in redirecting the needle to an abscess in order to obtain a positive aspirate. We recommend that these aspirations be performed by experienced personnel, such as a dedicated musculoskeletal radiologist, with strict aseptic techniques and under fluoroscopic guidance. Blood-culture bottles have previously been recommended, but this practice can increase the false-positive rate to 58% (130) and are not currently recommended. A minimum of three samples should be obtained. If all three samples are negative, infection is unlikely. If all three samples are positive, infection is almost definite. If only one of three samples is positive, the aspiration should be repeated. Any history of antibiotic use should always be elicited prior to proceeding with an aspiration biopsy, and every effort should be made to ensure that the patient is off antibiotics for a minimum of 4 weeks.

In our prospective series of 202 consecutive revision total hip arthroplasties, routine hip joint aspiration was performed to determine the role of hip aspiration, as well as other tests for the diagnosis of infection (11). Two synovial fluid samples and one synovial biopsy were obtained. A Westcot needle (Becton Dickinson and Company, Franklin Lakes, NJ) was used for the synovial biopsy. If no fluid could be aspirated, nonbacteriostatic, sterile normal saline was injected into the joint under fluoroscopic control and was then reaspirated. One out of three positive cultures was arbitrarily defined as false-positive. Two or more positive cultures were arbitrarily defined as indicative of infection. The sensitivity of a preoperative aspiration for the diagnosis of infection, using these criteria, was 86%, the specificity 94%, the predictive value of a positive test 67%, and the predictive value of a negative test 98%. The aspiration of clear synovial fluid with negative cultures can reliably exclude infection in the majority of patients. While a routine preoperative aspiration is not recommended, we agree with the recommendations of Lachiewicz et al. (131) that selective aspiration in suspicious circumstances remains an invaluable tool for the diagnosis of infection.

The value of hip aspiration lies not only in determining whether the culture shows bacterial growth but also in confirming or ruling out a diagnosis of infection via adjuvant tests that may be performed on the aspirate. If enough fluid is aspirated, a complete cell count and differential may give valuable information. If the cell count shows more than 25,000 leukocytes per milliliter and the differential count reveals that more than 25% are polymorphonuclear leukocytes, infection should be suspected. Clearly, the higher the number of polymorphonuclear leukocytes, the greater the possibility of infection. Fluid should also be analyzed for glucose and protein levels. In normal synovial fluid, protein levels are about one-third serum levels, while in infection, they approach serum levels. Glucose values in synovial fluid are similar to those in plasma. In the presence of infection, the synovial glucose levels are lowered, perhaps due to the consumption of glucose by bacterial organisms and inflammatory cells or due to abnormalities in the cellular transport mechanisms. Thus, a higher protein level and a lower glucose level are suggestive of infection.

Elevated lactic acid levels in synovial fluid have been associated with septic arthritis and have been found to be helpful in patients in whom antibiotic therapy was started before joint aspiration. Sequential measurements can be helpful in assessing the response of septic arthritis to treatment. The role of lactic acid levels in the diagnosis of the infected arthroplasty is unknown, although they may play a role in the difficult case.

D. Emerging Molecular Biological Techniques

Immunological and molecular biological techniques for the diagnosis of infection following total joint replacement surgery are currently under investigation. These include measuring levels of various cytokines such as interleukin-2 and gamma interferon. Another new technique using molecular biology principles, which can be used on aspiration samples, is the polymerase chain reaction (PCR). The very small quantities of DNA in the specimen are replicated and increased in volume using the polymerase chain reaction, so that the presence of bacterial DNA or RNA remnants within the tissues may be determined. PCR is used to detect the genetic code of the infecting organism within the patients' periprosthetic tissues, which can then be identified by comparing the obtained DNA sequence to a number of standard sequences (132–134). This test is exquisitely sensitive but unfortunately has a low specificity. Because this test depends on the availability of minuscule amounts of genetic material, DNA from dead microorganisms can be detected, and it is difficult to distinguish an infection that had been successfully treated from a clinically active infection. At present, this technology holds great promise, but is not in widespread clinical use, and it remains to be seen what its role will be in the diagnosis of infection following total hip arthroplasty. One possible application is in the identification of the infecting organism once antibiotic therapy has commenced, as is unfortunately seen is a substantial number of cases.

Rafiq et al. (135) described a serological marker for staphylococcal infection around prostheses using an enzyme-linked immunosorbent assay (ELISA). The serum IgG levels specific to a novel antigen produced by staphylococci were significantly elevated in a group of 15 patients with staphylococcal periprosthetic hip infections compared with a control group. The sensitivity of this test was 93.3%, with a false-positive rate of 3% and specificity of 96.9%. If further studies confirm the value of this test, it should provide an inexpensive serodiagnostic method for the preoperative diagnosis of staphylococcal periprosthetic infection.

Another technique currently being investigated depends on the identification of a DNA sequence common to all bacteria, such as that encoding the major heat-shock proteins (136). This technique has the significant advantage that a sample of aspirated joint fluid, or possibly even serum, could be initially probed for the presence of any bacteria which could subsequently be identified by the fact that there are sufficient nucleotide variations to allow the unique allocation of each amplified sequence to its parental bacterium. Further work on this is ongoing and there are concerns that it may be oversensitive with a low specificity.

E. Intraoperative Tests

Occasionally, despite an extensive and negative preoperative investigation, the surgeon will be faced with intraoperative findings suggestive of infection. The gross appearance of the tissues, however, is not always diagnostic of infection. Feldman and associates correlated the intraoperative surgical opinion with the pathological diagnosis for a sensitivity of 70% and a specificity of 87% (122). Because of the relatively poor sensitivity and specificity of the gross appearance of the tissues at the time of revision total hip arthroplasty, a variety of adjunctive tests can be performed to rule out infection. These include an immediate Gram's stain with subsequent culture of the synovial fluid and frozen section of the inflamed tissues. The synovial fluid should also be sent immediately for a complete cell count and differential as well as glucose and protein level measurements.

1. Intraoperative Gram's Stain

Despite the widespread use of a Gram's stain at the time of revision total hip arthroplasty, there has been questionable support in the literature (137). In our recent prospective study of 202 revision total hip arthroplasties, the sensitivity of intraoperative Gram's staining for the diagnosis of infection was 19%, the specificity 98%, the positive predictive value 63%, and the negative predictive value 89% (11). The false-negative rate of a Gram's stain is so high that it cannot be relied on unless the infection is so overt that a large load of bacteria is present, thus allowing observation of bacteria on the Gram's stain. In less virulent infections, particularly in chronic infections, the bacterial load is not enough to allow reliable visualization on Gram's stain. This is supported by a series of 194 revision total hip and knee arthroplasties (137) in which intraoperative Gram's stains were obtained in all patients. There were no positive Gram's stains despite the presence of infection in 32 cases. Therefore, the sensitivity of an intraoperative Gram's stain in this study was 0%.

2. Intraoperative Frozen Section

Intraoperative frozen section of the periprosthetic tissues has also been used. The surgeon should sample the most inflamed looking tissue at the time of surgery, and the pathologist should examine the microscopic specimen under low power first so that high-power study can be made of the most inflamed portion of the sample. Mirra reported the criteria of more than five polymorphonuclear leukocytes per high-power field as suggestive of infection (138). In a study of 33 consecutive revision total hip and knee arthroplasties by Feldman et al. (122), the sensitivity and specificity of intraoperative frozen sections were 100 and 96%, respectively, when the Mirra criteria of at least five polymorphonuclear leukocytes per high-power field were used. There was 100% correlation between the frozen sections and the permanent section in that study.

In a follow-up study by the same group (139), 175 revision total hip and knee arthroplasties were prospectively evaluated with intraoperative frozen sections and intraoperative cultures. Of the 175 cases, 19 were considered infected based on intraoperative cultures. The frozen sections were assessed according to the numbers of polymorphonuclear neutrophils (PMNs) per high-power field and were stratified into two groups: 5–9 PMNs per high-power field and at least 10 PMNs per high-power field. For the first group, the sensitivity was 84%, the specificity 96%, the predictive value of a positive test 70%; the predictive value of a negative test was 98%. For the second group, the sensitivity and predictive value of a negative test were unchanged, while the specificity and predictive value of a positive test were improved to 99 and 89%, respectively. The authors concluded that with the more stringent criterion of at least 10 PMNs per high-power field, it is less likely to overdiagnose infection.

In our own prospective series of 202 revision total hip arthroplasties (11) using more than 5 PMNs per high-power field as the diagnostic criterion, the sensitivity was 80%, the specificity 94%, the predictive value of a positive test 74%; the predictive value of a negative test was 96%. These values are virtually identical to those obtained by Lonner et al. (139). The application of the stricter criterion of at least 10 PMNs per high-power field to our data raised serious concern that a significant number of infected cases would be missed (reduced sensitivity and negative predictive value).

In another study of 106 revision total hip and knee arthroplasties, Athanasou et al. (140) used frozen sections for the diagnosis of infection with a sensitivity of 90%, specificity of 96%, a predictive value of a positive test of 88%, and a predictive value of a negative test of 98%. Although some authors (141) have refuted intraoperative frozen section in the diagnosis of the infected total hip replacement based on the previously presented data, we believe that it is helpful, but only when an experienced and motivated pathologist examines the samples. It would not be appropriate to send the samples to any pathologist, particularly at a large hospital, where there is increasing subspecialization amongst the pathologists.

The role of intraoperative frozen section at the second stage of a two-stage exchange protocol for the treatment of deep hip and knee periprosthetic infection has recently been reviewed in a series of 64 consecutive cases (142). Using the stricter criteria of a mean of 10 PMNs or more per high-power field (40 times magnification) in the five most cellular fields, they had a sensitivity of 25%, specificity of 98%, positive predictive value of 50%, and a negative predictive value of 95%. They would have had the same results with the Mirra criteria, as no samples had a mean of between 5 and 9 PMNs per high-power field in the five most cellular fields. Thus, although the analysis is not as sensitive as when performed at the time of an initial revision procedure, the specificity is high (98%), with only one false-positive.

3. Intraoperative Cultures

Intraoperative cultures are considered the "gold standard" for the diagnosis of infected arthroplasties. The area that appears to be most inflamed should be sampled, and at least three tissue samples should be sent for culture to improve the yield and to decrease the likelihood of a false-negative culture. All cultures should be incubated for at least 5 days. Unfortunately, errors in culture technique can occur, antibiotics may have been administered pre-operatively without the knowledge of the surgeon, and antibiotics may have been added to the irrigation fluid prior to the harvesting of tissue for culture. Sampling error at the time of surgery may also occur. All these factors can contribute to a false-negative culture (143). Contamination of the tissue samples at the time of transfer to the culture media or in the laboratory may contribute to false-positive results (144). In our prospective series of 202 revision total hip arthroplasties, at least three intraoperative tissue samples were obtained (11). Using the arbitrary criterion that at least two samples had to be positive to be considered a true-positive culture, the sensitivity of this test was 94%, the specificity 97%, the positive predictive value 77% and the negative predictive value 99%. In the same study, the removed implant was swabbed for culture and sensitivity with three culture swabs. The sensitivity of this test was 76%, the specificity 99%, the positive pre-dictive value 93% and the negative predictive value 97%. As the sensitivity of swab cultures was found to be lower than that of tissue cultures, we recommend the sampling of inflamed tissue only at the time of revision total hip arthroplasty.

F. Authors' Preferred Protocol for the Diagnosis of Infection

A high index of suspicion is essential, particularly when the patient presents with a persistently painful arthroplasty despite unremarkable radiographs. A careful history and physical examination should precede any tests for the diagnosis of infection. The patient should be carefully questioned regarding any wound healing complications, early local or distant infections, or prolonged administration of antibiotics after surgery. Delays in discharge from hospital also suggest a significant early complication. Questions regarding recent infections—such as skin infections or ulcerations, urinary tract infections, dental infections, or manipulations—can also be revealing. Radiographs should be obtained and compared to previous ones. In the early postoperative period, ectopic ossification can explain persistent pain.

The next investigation should be an ESR and CRP. If both tests are normal, no further tests are necessary. If the ESR and/or CRP are elevated and the suspicion for infection is high, a hip joint aspiration with the patient off all antibiotics for at least 4 weeks can then be performed. If the aspiration confirms infection, the surgeon may proceed with the most appropriate treatment. If the aspiration is negative and the index of suspicion remains high, the aspiration is repeated with the guidance of arthrography and/or ultrasound. If it remains negative, ancillary tests such as a repeat hip aspiration with arthroscopic means, obtaining tissue culture, or a sequential technetium-indium nuclear scan may be performed. If all these tests are negative, the surgeon may finally have to resort to intraoperative tests such as Gram's stain, cell count, differential, and frozen section at the time of revision arthroplasty to distinguish between aseptic loosening and infection. If the frozen section is negative, we then proceed with a revision total hip arthroplasty. Several intraoperative tissue cultures are obtained in all patients. If unexpected positive intraoperative cultures are obtained, a 6-week course of intravenous antibiotics is administered after the revision.

In summary, the rational use of preoperative investigations in a sequential fashion will allow the correct diagnosis of infection in the majority of cases. This will minimize the complications, increased morbidity, and cost of treatment of the incorrectly diagnosed total hip arthroplasty.

V. TREATMENT

A. For Positive Intraoperative Cultures

How should the positive intraoperative culture be managed in the "aseptic" revision total hip arthroplasty?

The significance of positive intraoperative cultures taken during revision total hip arthroplasty in a case that was not thought to be infected following preoperative investigation remains controversial. Tsukuyama et al. (21) reported their experience of 31 patients in whom intraoperative cultures were positive but infection was not suspected preoperatively. These patients represented 11% of the 275 revision arthroplasties performed over the study period. All were treated with a 6-week course of intravenous antibiotics. In 3 patients, infection was not eradicated at 6 weeks, and 2 had recurrence of infection at a minimum of 2 years; therefore a total of 5 of 31 (16%) were not successfully treated by the antibiotic course. It would seem that in at least some cases, positive cultures represent previously undiagnosed infection and require treatment. It is not, however, known if the treatment with 6 weeks of intravenous antibiotics reduced the rate of recurrence of infection compared to no additional antibiotic treatment, as there was no control group. Dupont (143) had previously shown a 40% (6 of 15) incidence of recurrent infection in revisions with positive cultures which did not receive additional antibiotics. These figures, within the limitations of using historical controls, suggest that the additional 6 weeks of antibiotics are indeed beneficial.

A recent study, using strict anaerobic bacteriological practice and ultrasonication to dislodge bacteria from biofilms, isolated bacteria in 22% of patients (26 out of 120) undergoing revision total hip arthroplasty (145). Infection was suspected in only 6 of the 26 patients. The same authors used immunofluorescent microscopy and reverse transcriptase PCR to amplify the 16S bacterial ribosomal RNA signal and identified bacteria or bacterial RNA in 71 out of 113 patients (63%) and 85 out of 118 patients (72%) sampled with these techniques, respectively (12). Their findings correlated well with histopathology. They did not, unfortunately, give any details on whether the revision surgery was staged or not and, if single-stage surgery was performed, whether cemented or cementless implants were used. They did not describe how they managed the patients with positive cultures and what was the ultimate clinical outcome in terms of reinfection. The significance of these findings are not yet known. If 60–70% of all revisions are truly infected, does this imply that most cases of loosening are caused by low-grade infection, or can bacteria be associated with orthopaedic implants in small enough numbers to be incidental to the clinical outcome but detectable with these sophisticated tests?

The idea of unsuspected infection or colonization of prostheses is not a new one, but the significance is not always clear. Murray (146) reported that 40% (61 out of 151) of culture-positive revision hip arthroplasties were diagnosed only at the time of surgery. To be considered positive, it has been suggested (147) that cultures should be positive from at least two different sites within the operative field. Although it has been recommended (21,147) that all cases of positive intraoperative cultures should be treated with antibiotics, no prospective study has looked at the results of treatment with antibiotics as compared with no additional antibiotic treatment on top of the revision surgery and perioperative antibiotics.

B. Antibiotic Suppression

Coventry (19) suggested that while antibiotic suppression may control the symptoms and delay another operation, it is probably not strictly curative. Goulet (96) followed up 19 patients with infected total hip arthroplasties who were treated with long-term suppressive antibiotics. Most (18 of 19) of these were acute infections. Eleven patients had a surgical debridement. The group was made up of patients who had refused surgery or who were deemed to be unsuitable for an extensive reconstructive procedure. Seven out of 19 patients (37%) eventually required revision within a 2 to 10 (mean 4.1) year follow-up period, and a further two had persistent draining sinuses. They concluded that two-stage reimplantation was preferred, but suppressive antibiotic treatment was an option for an old or frail patient with an early infection caused by bacteria responsive to oral antibiotic therapy or in an otherwise compliant patient who refuses removal of an infected prosthesis.

Zimmerli et al. (148) followed 33 patients, with staphylococcal infection of a variety of orthopaedic implants, including eight total hip arthroplasties. All underwent a surgical debridement and were randomized to take long-term ciprofloxacin with or without rifampicin. All 12 of those who completed the 3- to 6-month course of ciprofloxacin with rifampicin were free of infection at 2 years. This was a significant difference compared with a cure rate of 58% (7 of 12) in the ciprofloxacin-placebo group. The authors did not explicitly outline the results for the total hip replacement patients. Nevertheless, these results are promising for the treatment of patients who are unable to have extensive surgery.

It is recommended that antibiotic suppression be reserved for patients with well-fixed components, without systemic symptoms, in whom there is a contraindication to surgery, or who refuse surgery. The organism must be sensitive to the antibiotics, which should be available in an oral form and well tolerated (64,96).

C. Debridement and Prosthesis Retention

Debridement and prosthesis retention is often used as the initial treatment in cases of acute or acute hematogenous infection. The former practice of closed suction-irrigation has now largely been abandoned owing to the occurrence of superinfection (50). With a chronic periprosthetic infection, debridement and prosthesis retention is uniformly associated with a dismal outcome (20,80,84). Fitzgerald et al. (20) reported that only 1 of 18 patients retained the hardware at a minimum of 2 years. Canner et al. (80), in patients grouped by time from operation rather than chronicity of infection, reported failure in 22 out of 23 cases who were also treated with concomitant antibiotics. Crockarell et al. (84) reported the results of 19 cases with chronic infection. None were successfully treated by debridement and prosthesis retention.

The results of treatment of early postoperative and acute hematogenous infections are better than for chronic infections. Tsukuyama et al. (21) reported 71% (25 of 35) success in treatment of early postoperative infection with debridement and component retention (with 4 weeks of intravenous antibiotics) and 50% success in treatment of acute hematogenous infection with debridement and component retention (with 6 weeks of intravenous antibiotics). In a small series, Hyman et al. (91) treated eight patients with acute hematogenous infections with arthroscopic drainage, irrigation, and debridement, followed by prolonged antibiotic suppression. At a mean follow-up of 70 months, no infection recurred. Even in the selected population of acute and acute hematogenous infections, success rates as low as 26% (6 of 23) have been reported (84).

The duration of symptoms appears to correlate well with the success of treatment. Brandt et al. (149) looking only at patients infected with *S. aureus*, found that 56% (8 of 18) of those treated within 2 days of onset of symptoms still had successful eradication of disease at 2 years, whereas only 13% (2 of 15) debrided after 2 days of symptoms had not had recurrence of infection at 2 years. They did not distinguish between chronic and acute hematogenous infections. Crockarell et al. (84) noted no patient treated by debridement, performed more than 2 weeks after onset of symptoms, had the infection eradicated.

D. Single-Stage Exchange

Direct exchange or single-stage revision hip arthroplasty for infection was popularized in Europe using gentamicin-impregnated bone cement (79,81, 100,150). In 1978 Carlsson et al. (81) reported their work using gentamicin-impregnated bone cement in one- and two-stage exchange arthroplasties performed for infection; an overall success rate of 78% was achieved and no significant difference could be detected between those treated in one versus two stages. These results are strongly supported by the reports of Raut et al., who had an eradication-of-infection rate of 84–86% in spite of a large number of discharging sinuses (98,151,152). A meticulous debridement is critical, and failure to adequately remove infected, necrotic, or devitalized tissue or failure to remove all foreign material can compromise the outcome of the procedure. Moreover, failure to use antibiotic-loaded cement in the reconstruction or to carefully administer intravenous antibiotics for a minimum of 6 weeks may lead to a higher failure rate.

Single-stage revision without the use of antibiotic-loaded cement has been associated with a higher rate of recurrence of infection, which was summarized by Hanssen and Rand (153). They found the cumulative success rate of single-stage exchange to be 83% when antibiotic-loaded cement was used and 60% when it was not used. Single-stage revision for infection therefore demands the use of cemented implants with antibiotic-impregnated cement. In such cases, restriction of the surgical options to a cemented prosthesis may be responsible for the high rates of aseptic loosening that have been reported (100).

Comparisons of studies comparing one- and two-stage revision procedures are complicated by the fact that some studies are performed in selected patient populations rather than on a consecutive series, with certain patients being excluded from the one-stage group. Ure et al. (102) did not recommend direct exchange "for patients who are immunocompromised, for those who have an infection with a known resistant gram-negative or methicillin-resistant organism, or for those who have a major skin, soft-tissue, or osseous defect that makes it impossible to obtain a closed wound or a stable implant." Garvin et al. (86) described the results of one- and two-stage revisions of 123 infected hip arthroplasties as well as a combination of 88 conversion arthroplasties (from infected hardware or a previously septic joint), at-risk primary hip arthroplasties, and revision total knee arthroplasties. They used gentamicin-impregnated polymethylmethacrylate cement. While conceding that "less severe infections" were more likely to be treated in one stage, they found that these procedures carried a higher recurrence risk (10.1 versus 5.6%), though this was not statistically significant. They recommended that one-stage revision should be reserved for elderly—infirm patients, who are ill-suited for 3 weeks of skeletal traction—in the presence of sensitive organisms and an adequately debrided joint.

E. Two-Stage Exchange Arthroplasty

A staged approach can provide a better environment for the eradication of infection. It also means that uncemented reconstruction can be considered. Organisms may be cultured from tissues that are accessible only after removal of the implant, and the interval before reimplantation allows for further microbiological assessment and the appropriate adjustment of antibiotic therapy. This approach minimizes the possibility of attempting a reconstruction in the presence of unresolved sepsis, and allograft augmentation may be performed with more security.

This technique involves two procedures. The first is equivalent to a Girdlestone excisional arthroplasty and the second to reimplantation of a total hip arthroplasty. Between stages, the patient is treated with at least 6 weeks of intravenous antibiotics, and antibiotic loaded cement may be placed in the femur and the acetabulum as a concentrated depot (Figure 5). The response to treatment is carefully assessed between stages, and reimplantation is not performed if there is ongoing evidence of sepsis. If necessary, a second debridement may be performed, although this is rarely necessary. The ESR and CRP are excellent tests for monitoring the effect of treatment; a steady decline in both parameters is suggestive of the eradication of infection, although, to the best of our knowledge, this has not been proven in the peer-reviewed literature. An aspiration biopsy between stages may also help rule out ongoing infection, although this has not specifically been looked at for revision hip surgery. Mont et al. (154) reported it to be beneficial in staged revision knee arthroplasty for infection. In a prospective study comparing two surgeons' protocols, the aspiration between stages revealed persistent infection in 3 of 34 patients (9%), all of whom were suc-

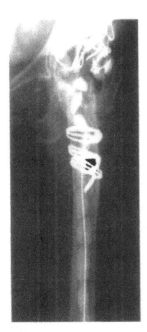

Figure 5   An excisional arthroplasty with antibiotic-loaded beads in-situ.

cessfully managed with repeat debridement. Overall, the group without aspiration between stages had 5 recurrent infections from 35 patients (14%) compared with 1 recurrent infection from 34 patients (3%) in the group with aspiration between stages.

At the time of the second-stage procedure, any temporary spacers, antibiotic-loaded cement beads, or retained foreign body from the first procedure are removed. Multiple tissue samples are obtained for culture and sensitivity. If there is any doubt about the control of infection, a sample is sent to the laboratory for a frozen section, looking for acute inflammatory cells. As discussed earlier, this has a high specificity (98%) but a low sensitivity (25%) when compared with the results of frozen section during the first stage (142).

There are many variable factors even within the two-stage exchange protocols. These include the duration of postoperative systemic antibiotic therapy, timing of reimplantation, use of allograft bone in the reconstruction and, choosing between a cemented and a cementless implant. A further area of controversy is the use of antibiotic-loaded cement in the form of beads or temporary spacer devices between the first and second stages. The ideal duration of antibiotic therapy and route of administration have not been determined. Most reported protocols include 4 to 6 weeks of intravenous antibiotic administration. The measurement of minimal serum bactericidal titers is a convenient method of ensuring adequate antibiotic doses. A minimum bactericidal titer of 1:8 is recommended (120) for optimal infection control; however, with the high concentrations of local antibiotics in the periprosthetic space when antibiotic-loaded cement in the form of beads or temporary spacer devices is used, it may not be as critical to maintain a 1:8 minimum bactericidal titer.

The length of the interval period also generates debate and has considerable economic implications. Early studies of two-stage revision of infected total hip arthroplasty recommended a prolonged interval of approximately 1 year between implant removal and reimplantation (94,155). More recent reports fail to support a lengthy interval. Lieberman et al. reported results from a protocol of reimplantation at 6 weeks after excision arthroplasty (93). These did not differ from the results of patients in whom reimplantation was delayed for over 1 year (94). Colyer and Capello (83) found that 2 out of 9 patients suffered reinfection with reimplantation after 22 weeks compared with 4 out of 28 who were reimplanted within 6 weeks. These investigators pointed out that a shorter interval to reimplantation facilitates the second-stage procedure. Tsukuyama et al. (21) also noted better results (only 1 out of 15 cases reinfected) in those who were reimplanted early. A further report, from Garvin et al. (86), also noted that shortening the duration to reimplantation had improved the success of the reimplantation from 85 to 93%. In summary, recent evidence would point to greater success when reimplantation takes place at around 3 months rather than at greater than 1 year.

The popularity of two-stage exchange programs is also related to somewhat higher rates of infection eradication when compared with one-stage protocols. Hanssen and Rand (153) found the cumulative rate of infection eradication to be 82% when antibiotic-loaded cement was not used. This increased to 90% when antibiotic-loaded cement was used at the second stage, and it increased further to 92% when local antibiotic delivery with beads or spacers was undertaken in the interval period.

F. Two-Stage Revision to an Uncemented Prosthesis

When bone stock in the upper femur is deficient, the use of cemented implants may not be appropriate. This is commonly seen where the quality of the intramedullary cavity of the femur is such that adequate fixation with cement is unlikely. In occasional cases, bone loss or altered anatomy will demand customized implants, although this is now less frequent, with improved inventories of revision implants. Moreover, uncemented fixation avoids the very challenging scenario of the reinfected distally cemented prosthesis (Figure 6). There are a few reports of two-stage revision to uncemented prostheses (77,103,104,108,156–160). Berry et al.. used uncemented prostheses with allograft and reported reinfection in 2 of 11 patients (18%) (77). Nestor et al. (108) published the results of a Mayo Clinic series in which 34 patients were treated with two-stage exchange to a first-generation porous-coated prosthesis. The interval period averaged 8 months. Infection recurred in 6 patients (18%) at an average follow-up of almost 4 years. There was a higher risk of reinfection in patients with rheumatoid arthritis. If these are excluded, infection recurred in only 10% of the remaining patients. Moreover, Lai et al. published the results of two-stage exchange using a variety of cementless implants (159). The interval period averaged 48 weeks. They recorded a recurrent infection rate of 12.5% at a mean follow-up of 4 years and an average Harris hip score of 91 in the remaining noninfected cases. Gustilo and Tsukayama used antibiotic-loaded beads in the interval period and reported reinfection in only 2 of 18 patients (11%) (157). Wang et al. used uncemented femoral prostheses in 16 of 22 cases treated with a two-stage protocol with delayed allograft reconstruction (103). At an average follow-up of 4 years, 2 of the 16 cases were reinfected (12.5%). The acceptable rates of eradication of infection and the good fixation and function obtained in the majority of these studies support the use of uncemented implants in a previously infected bed.

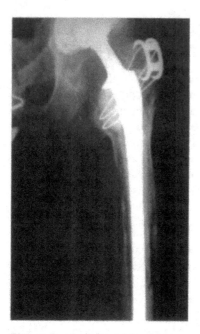

Figure 6   An infected long-stem total hip replacement.

G.   The Use of Allograft

Chronic bone infection around an infected implant frequently results in significant femoral or acetabular bone loss, which must be addressed as part of the treatment plan for managing infection (38). Until recently, severe bone stock deficiency has been considered a contraindication to reimplantation (93,99). There has been concern that the use of bone allograft in reconstruction following infection might be associated with a higher rate of recurrent sepsis by acting as a potential sequestrum. A two-stage reconstruction, allowing infection to be eradicated before inserting large amounts of foreign material, seems rational. Even the advocates of one-stage reconstruction will concede that dealing with extensive bone loss requires a staged treatment plan (102). Use of bone grafting even in primary total hip arthroplasty has been associated with an increased rate of infection despite the use of prophylactic antibiotics, vertical laminar airflow, and use a helmet aspirator suit. In a study of 659 hips, 4 of 125 (3%) who received a structural graft had a subsequent infection, compared with 1 of 534 (0.2%) who had none (161). It is not clear whether this observation relates to increased complexity, prolonged operating time, or disease transmission by the graft.

There are now a few papers looking at the use of allograft bone in revision hip surgery for infection. Berry et al. used various combinations of morcellized and bulk allografts in the second stage of two-stage revisions for infection (77). They reported only 2 recurrent infections out of 18 cases at a mean follow-up of 4.2 years. Alexeef et al. used massive structural allografts in the second stage of a two-stage procedure in 11 patients (162). They reported no further sepsis at a mean follow-up of 4 years. Wang et al. (103) used a combination of morcellized and bulk allograft in 22 cases, with an eradication of infection rate of 91%. It appears from these papers that allograft bone can be used for reconstruction at the second stage of a staged revision without prejudicing the outcome (Figure 7). Although a three-stage protocol has previously been proposed for bone grafting in the presence of infection (108,111,163), this does not appear to be necessary, and three-stage exchange is not currently widely used or recommended.

Segmental bone loss presents a significant technical problem in management of the infected case. When the initial resection arthroplasty is performed, substantial proximal bone loss may result in considerable shortening of the limb unless a spacer is used (129). This shortening may make the

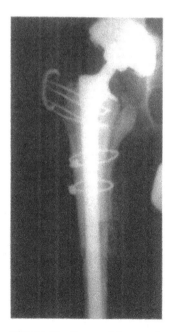

Figure 7 Successful second-stage reconstruction after infection with a proximal femoral allograft in situ.

subsequent reimplantation procedure more difficult (88). The experience from Vancouver using a prosthesis coated with antibiotic-loaded acrylic cement (PROSTALAC) shows that function may be maintained in the interval between resection and reimplantation while creating an infection-free bed for subsequent reconstruction using massive allografts or megaprostheses (38).

H. Articulated Spacers (PROSTALAC)

Because of the advantages of antibiotic-loaded bone cement as an antibiotic depot, it has become very popular to insert such beads within the hip joint between stages in two-stage exchange arthroplasty of the hip. The use of antibiotic beads, however, does not change the functional status of the patient between stages. The patient still has to endure a period of poor function and relatively increased morbidity between stages and may develop soft tissue contractures that render reimplantation difficult. If the bone loss is very severe, the limb may be unstable between stages, and traction, with its attendant cost and morbidity may be necessary (129,164). Most health care systems cannot afford the additional cost of inpatient hospital traction. The complications of bed rest are well known, and, if the leg length is not

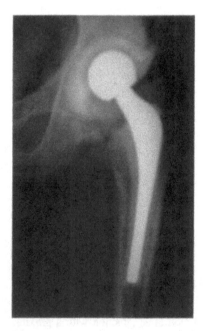

Figure 8   Radiograph to show a PROSTALAC in situ.

maintained during the interval period, it may not be regained at the time of the second-stage procedure, compromising the final outcome.

These difficulties may be overcome with the use of articulated antibiotic-loaded spacers inserted between stages. These allow the patient some function, keep the soft tissues out to length, and decrease scarring within the periprosthetic tissues. Since 1986, we have abandoned the standard two-stage exchange arthroplasty in favor of a system where a facsimile of a total hip replacement prosthesis is inserted between stages. This is the PROSTALAC prosthesis (38,85,165–168) (Figure 8). This interval arthroplasty initially had a cement-on-cement articulation but has now been developed further and refined into a system using a metal on polyethylene bearing, available with a variety of stem sizes and lengths (Figure 9). This system provides a highly antibiotic-loaded reservoir that increases the periprosthetic antibiotic levels above and beyond those achieved by parenteral therapy alone and maintains these high levels until the second-stage procedure (70). The greatest advantages are that a stable reconstruction is achieved, so that mobilization is possible, and this greatly facilitates the definitive reconstruction by maintaining the soft tissues at near normal tension.

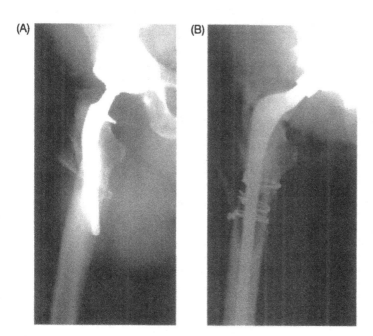

(A)   (B)

Figure 9   A. An infected periprosthetic fracture. B. Staged treatment with a long-stem PROSTALAC was required.

The PROSTALAC system currently consists of a constrained cemented acetabular component and a modular femoral component that is made intraoperatively with antibiotic-loaded cement surrounding a stainless steel endoskeleton using a series of moulds (Figure 10). Following thorough debridement and removal of all dead and foreign material, the acetabular

(A)

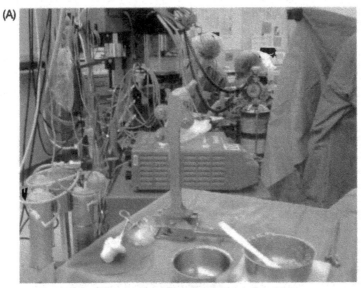

(B)

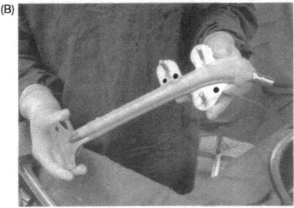

Figure 10 A. The PROSTALAC is manufactured intraoperatively on a back table using customized molds. B. When the cement has set, the mold is opened to reveal the temporary prosthesis. C. The finished long-stem PROSTALAC is now ready for implantation.

(C)

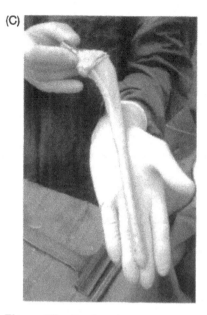

Figure 10   Continued

component is loosely cemented and the femoral component is press-fitted into the medullary canal, so that both are easily removed at the second stage without damaging bone stock. Our most commonly used antibiotic combination is 3.6 g of tobramycin (Nebcin, Eli Lilly Canada Inc., Scarborough, Ontario) and 1.5 g of vancomycin (Vancocin, Eli Lilly Canada Inc., Scarborough, Ontario) per package of Palacos bone cement (Biomet, Warsaw, IN). We avoid the use of wound suction drains so as to encourage high levels of antibiotic within the infected tissues. Postoperatively, the patient is allowed to mobilize partial weight bearing with crutches until the time of the second-stage procedure. Parenteral antibiotic therapy is continued for 6 weeks. We proceed with definitive reconstruction if the culture of a hip aspirate performed 4 weeks following discontinuation of antibiotics is negative and the ESR and CRP show a steady decline over the 12-week interval between stages. At the second stage, the femoral component is removed without difficulty using a stem extractor. The acetabular component easily debonds from the cement mantle. The underlying cement mantle is then fragmented and removed piecemeal, without sacrificing acetabular bone stock. Appropriate implants are then reimplanted. At the second stage, the operation is performed similarly to any revision procedure, with no special treatment because of the previous infection. If cement is used, it is impregnated with antibiotics, usually 0.6–1.2 g of tobramycin per package of bone cement.

In combination with our initial series of high-friction first-generation prostheses, we have now reviewed a total of 81 procedures with a minimum 2-year follow up. The infection eradication rate for the total group is 95% (4 failures in 81 cases). In our initial series of 48 patients using the metal on polyethylene PROSTALAC articulated spacer, 94% (45 patients) were infection-free over 2 years after the reconstruction. The mean Harris hip score at presentation was 33.5 points, improving to 55.2 between stages and to 75.17 at the latest review. Eighty percent of patients had a Harris hip score of greater than 80 or greater than a 30-point improvement (168).

In addition to the control of infection, the PROSTALAC system offers social and economic advantages. With earlier mobilization out of bed and out of hospital, rehabilitation is accelerated and discharge from hospital between stages is feasible, even in the face of substantial loss of bone stock. Our results suggest that the mobility of the patient with a two-stage exchange arthroplasty for infection can be improved using the PROSTALAC prosthesis without compromising the rate of eradication of infection. Our figures support an infection eradication rate of 94–96%, an outcome comparable to other two-stage exchange procedures reported in the literature (94,99,110,169).

I. Excision Arthroplasty

As recently as 1984 (80), it was reported that "only excisional arthroplasty consistently eliminated infection and resulted in a clinically satisfactory result." Removal of all cement and infected tissue, production of a dry surgical wound, and adherence to Girdlestone's procedure: excision of infected muscle, superior acetabular rim, femoral neck, and portion of greater trochanter (170) have been said to enhance the eradication of infection (80). In their study, they found that adherence to these principles resulted in a good, infection-free outcome in 10 out of 10 patients thus treated, while only 10 out of 23 patients, who underwent a less radical excisional arthroplasty, had a similar result. Bourne et al. (78) reported only one reinfection in a group of 33 patients, who had undergone a resection arthroplasty. They did, however, comment that an additional 5 patients had prolonged wound discharges. Unfortunately, while excisional arthroplasty may be a reasonably successful means of eradicating infection in the majority of patients, the functional outcome often leaves much to be desired. Six patients who underwent excision arthroplasty were found to have pain scores similar to those of patients with a reimplanted prosthesis, but functional scores were comparable to their preoperative, infected status (82). Although resection arthroplasty can provide some pain relief and help to control infection, the poor functional outcome means that, in the present day, this procedure is rarely indicated as a primary procedure. Its place is as a salvage procedure in patients unsuitable for a more exacting reconstructive program or after failure of exchange arthroplasty.

J. Arthrodesis

Arthrodesis has been suggested as a treatment option in selected young patients with an infected prosthesis. Kostuik and Alexander (171) reported on 7 patients treated for infection with a hip arthrodesis. Of these, 4 were performed in one stage and three in two stages. There were no recurrent infections and 5 patients returned to their former work. This technique does not appear to have been used by others.

VI. RESULTS OF REINFECTION

Reinfection after reconstruction of an infected total hip arthroplasty has a poor outlook, particularly if a further reconstruction is envisaged. Pagnano et al. (97) reported on 34 patients who became reinfected after reimplantation. Most were treated by long-term antibiotics with or without debridement or by resection arthroplasty. Of the 8 patients who underwent a further reconstruction (3 one-stage, 5 two-stage), 3 (38%) became reinfected, and these patients had the worst functional outcome of all. At present, the authors recommend excision arthroplasty instead of a repeat two-stage exchange arthroplasty, for patients in whom two-stage exchange arthroplasty fails.

VII. SUMMARY

The infected total hip replacement continues to be a challenging problem. Its management remains expensive and places an increasing burden on the health care system. It also leads to a long and difficult course for the patient and frequently a suboptimal functional outcome. The choice of a particular treatment program will be influenced by a number of factors. These include the acuteness or chronicity of the infection; the infecting organism, its antibiotic sensitivity profile, and its ability to manufacture glycocalyx; the health of the patient; the fixation of the prosthesis; the available bone stock;

and the particular philosophy and training of the surgeon. For most patients, antibiotics alone are not an acceptable method of treatment.

The authors use a variety of treatment modalities, tailored to the individual case. In early postoperative or acute hematogenous infection, with a well-documented brief history and a well-fixed prosthesis, we prefer a thorough, open debridement after establishing the diagnosis by erythrocyte sedimentation rate, C-reactive protein estimation, and aspiration and Gram's stain of the affected hip if required. At debridement, copious lavage is used. In the case of an uncemented cup, we will, where appropriate, exchange the polyethylene liner. Postoperatively, 4 to 6 weeks of intravenous antibiotics are used under the supervision and guidance of infectious diseases personnel.

For chronic infections we use a staged approach with the PROSTALAC interval arthroplasty. This is a modular, custom-made, immediate fit, antibiotic-selective, temporary hip replacement system. It affords patients rapid pain relief and allows rapid mobilization and an early discharge home. This reduces the cost of care while successfully eradicating infection and setting an appropriate soft tissue environment for a relatively straightforward second-stage procedure. With the increasing cost of delivery of health care, this has economic advantages; it also combines the benefits of two-stage exchange— including a thorough debridement and high local antibiotic concentrations— with flexibility with regard to the duration of the interval period and the type of fixation used, and the potential for allograft reconstruction.

For patients with positive intraoperative cultures from revision for presumed aseptic loosening, we recommend a 6-week course of intravenous antibiotics, in agreement with the recommendations of Tsukuyama et al. (21).

We reserve the use of resection arthroplasty for patients who are considered medically unfit for further reconstruction, for those who are mentally impaired and would be unable to cooperate with postoperative restrictions and rehabilitation. We also advocate it for patients who are taking major immunosuppression, particularly following solid organ transplantation, and in those who have an active history of intravenous drug abuse, because such patients have a tendency to be poorly compliant with postoperative instructions and a high risk of reinfection (GD Paiement, personal communication, 1997). We also recommend this option for patients with a failed two-stage exchange arthroplasty.

ACKNOWLEDGMENTS

We would like to acknowledge the help of Professor A. Chow and Mr. M. G. McAlinden FRCS (Tr & Orth) for their help in compiling the data shown in Table 1.

REFERENCES

1. Laupacis A, Bourne R, Rorabeck C, Feeny D, Wong C, Tugwell P, Leslie K, Bullas R. The effect of elective total hip replacement on health-related quality of life. J Bone Joint Surg Am 1993; 75:1619–1626.
2. Sculco TP. The economic impact of infected total joint arthroplasty. Instr Course Lect 1993; 42:349–351.
3. Charnley J, Eftekhar N. Postoperative infection in total prosthetic replacement arthroplasty of the hip-joint. With special reference to the bacterial content of the air of the operating room. Br J Surg 1969; 56:641–649.
4. Charnley J. Postoperative infection after total hip replacement with special reference to air contamination in the operating room. Clin Orthop 1972; 87:167–187.
5. Hanssen AD, Osmon DR, Nelson CL. Prevention of deep periprosthetic joint infection. J Bone Joint Surg Am 1996; 78:458–471.
6. Garvin KL, Hanssen AD. Infection after total hip arthroplasty. J Bone Joint Surg Am 1995; 77:1576–1588.
7. Kreder HJ, Deyo RA, Koepsell T, Swiontkowski MF, Kreuter W. Relationship between the volume of total hip replacements performed by providers and the rates of postoperative complications in the State of Washington. J Bone Joint Surg Am 1997; 79-A:485–494.
8. Fender D, Harper WM, Gregg PJ. Outcome of Charnley total hip replacement across a single health region in England: The results at five years from a regional hip register. J Bone Joint Surg Br 1999; 81:577–581.
9. Lidwell OM. Clean air at operation and subsequent sepsis in the joint. Clin Orthop 1986; 211:91–102.
10. Madhavan P, Blom A, Karagkevrkis B, Pradeep M, Huma H, Newman JH. Deterioration of theatre discipline during total joint replacement—have theatre protocols been abandoned? Ann R Coll Surg Engl 1999; 81:262–265.
11. Spangehl MJ, Masri BA, O'Connell JX, Duncan CP. Prospective analysis of preoperative and intraoperative investigations for the diagnosis of infection at the sites of two hundred and two revision total hip arthroplasties. J Bone Joint Surg Am 1999; 81:672–683.
12. Tunney MM, Patrick S, Curran MD, Ramage G, Hanna D, Nixon JR, Gorman SP, Davis RI, Anderson N. Detection of prosthetic hip infection at revision arthroplasty by immunofluorescent microscopy and PCR amplification of the bacterial 16S rRNA gene. J Clin Microbiol 1999; 37:3281–3290.
13. Lidwell OM, Elson RA, Lowbury EJL, Whyte W, Blowers R, Stanley S, Lowe D. Ultraclean air and antibiotics for prevention of postoperative infection. Acta Orthop Scand 1987; 58:4–13.
14. Salvati EA, Robinson RP, Zeno SM, Koslin BL, Brause BD, Wilson PD Jr. Infection rates after 3175 total hip and total knee replacements performed with and without a horizontal unidirectional filtered air-flow system. J Bone Joint Surg Am 1982; 64:525–535.
15. Schmatzried TP, Amstutz HC, Au MK, Dorey FJ. Etiology of deep sepsis in total hip arthroplasty. The significance of haematogenous and recurrent infections. Clin Orthop 1992; 280:200–207.

16. Surin VV, Sundholm K, Backman, L. Infection after total hip replacement, with special reference to a discharge from the wound. J Bone Joint Surg Br 1983; 65:412–418.

17. Gaine WJ, Ramamohan NA, Hussein NA, Hullin MG, McCreath SW. Wound infection in hip and knee arthroplasty. J Bone Joint Surg Br 1999; 82:561–565.

18. Maderazo EG, Judson S, Pasternak H. Late infections of total joint prostheses: A review and recommendations for prevention. Clin Orthop 1988; 229:131–142.

19. Coventry MB. Treatment of infections occurring in total hip surgery. Orthop Clin North Am 1975; 6:991–1003.

20. Fitzgerald RH, Nolan DR, Ilstrup DM, Van Scoy RE, Washington JA II, Coventry MB. Deep wound sepsis following total hip surgery. J Bone Joint Surg Am 1977; 59:847–855.

21. Tsukayama DT, Estrada R, Gustilo RB. Infection after total hip arthroplasty. A study of the treatment of one hundred and six infections. J Bone Joint Surg Am 1996; 78:512–523.

22. Poss R, Thornhill TS, Ewald FC, Thomas WH, Batte NJ, Sledge CB. Factors influencing the incidence and outcome of infection following total joint arthroplasty. Clin Orthop 1984; 182:117–126.

23. Espehaug B, Havelin LI, Engesaeter LB, Langelang N, Vollset SE. Patient-related risk factors for early revision of total hip replacements. Acta Orthop Scand 1997; 68:207–215.

24. Tannenbaum DA, Matthews LS, Grady-Benson JC. Infection around joint replacements in patients who have a renal or liver transplant. J Bone Joint Surg Am 1997; 79:36–43.

25. Sakalkale DP, Hozack WJ, Rothman RH. Total hip arthroplasty in patients on long-term renal dialysis. J Arthroplasty 1999; 14:571–575.

26. Bishop AR, Roberson JR, Eckman JR, Fleming LL. Total hip arthroplasty in patients who have sickle-cell hemoglobinopathy. J Bone Joint Surg Am 1988; 70:853–855.

27. Clarke HJ, Jinnah RH, Brooker AF, Michaelson JD. Total replacement of the hip for avascular necrosis in sickle cell disease. J Bone Joint Surg Br 1989; 71:465–470.

28. Acurio MT, Friedman RJ. Hip arthroplasty in patients with sickle-cell haemoglobinopathy. J Bone Joint Surg Br 1992; 74:367–371.

29. Gherini S, Vaughn BK, Lombardi AV Jr, Mallory TH. Delayed wound healing and nutritional deficiencies after total hip arthroplasty. Clin Orthop 1993; 293: 188–195.

30. Ritter MA, Eitzen HE, Hart JB, French MLV. The surgeon's garb. Clin Orthop 1980; 153:204–209.

31. Lidwell OM, Lowbury EJ, Whyte W, Blowers R, Stanley SJ, Lowe D. Effect of ultraclean air in operating rooms on deep sepsis in the joint after total hip or knee replacement. A randomized study. Br Med J 1982; 285:10–14.

32. Berg M, Bergman BR, Hoborn J. Shortwave ultraviolet radiation in operating rooms. J Bone Joint Surg Br 1989; 71:483–485.

33. Berg M, Bergman BR, Hoborn J. Ultraviolet radiation compared to an ultra-clean air enclosure. J Bone Joint Surg Br 1991; 73:811–815.

34. Lowell JD. The ultraviolet environment in a nutshell. Am J Surg 1984; 148: 575–577.

35. Brown AR, Taylor GJS, Gregg PJ. Air contamination during skin preparation and draping in joint replacement surgery. J Bone Joint Surg Br 1996; 78:92–94.

36. Davis N, Curry A, Gambhir AK, Panigrahi H, Walker CRC, Wilkins EGL, Worsley MA, Kay PR. Intraoperative bacterial contamination in operations for joint replacement. J Bone Joint Surg Br 1999; 81:886–889.

37. James ETR, Hunter GA, Cameron HU. Total hip revision arthroplasty. Does sepsis influence the results? Clin Orthop 1982; 170:88–94.

38. Younger ASE, Duncan CP, Masri BA. Treatment of infection associated with segmental bone loss in the proximal part of the femur in two stages with use of an antibiotic-loaded interval prosthesis. J Bone Joint Surg Am 1998; 80: 60–69.

39. Katz RP, Callaghan JJ, Sullivan PM, Johnston RC. Long-term results of re-vision total hip arthroplasty. J Bone Joint Surg Br 1997; 79:322–326.

40. Haddad FS, Garbuz DS, Masri BA, Duncan CP. Structural proximal femoral allografts for failed total hip replacements: a minimum review of five years. J Bone Joint Surg Br 2000; 82:830–836.

41. Schafer D, Dick W, Morscher E. Total hip arthroplasty after arthrodesis of the hip joint. Arch Orthop Trauma Surg 2000; 120:176–178.

42. Kreder HJ, Williams JI, Jaglal S, Axcell T, Stephen D. A population study in the Province of Ontario of the complications after conversion of hip or knee arthrodesis to total joint replacement. Can J Surg 1999; 42:433–439.

43. Proctor RA, Hamill RJ, Mosher DF, Textor JA, Olbrantz PJ. Effects of sub-inhibitory concentration of antibiotics on Staphylococcus aureus interactions with fibronectin. J Antimicrob Ther 1983; 12:85–95.

44. Josefsson G, Kolmert L. Prophylaxis with systematic antibiotics versus gen-tamicin bone cement in total hip arthroplasty. A ten-year survey of 1,688 hips. Clin Orthop 1993; 292:210–214.

45. Espehaug B, Engesaeter LB, Vollset SE, Havelin LI, Langeland N. Antibiotic prophylaxis in total hip arthroplasty. J Bone Joint Surg Br 1997; 79:590–595.

46. Malchau H, Herberts P. Prognosis of total hip replacement: Revision and re-revision rate in total hip replacement: A revision–re-revision study of 148,359 primary operations. American Academy of Orthopaedic Surgeons, New Or-leans, LA, March 19–23, 1998.

47. Lynch M, Esser MP, Shelley P, Wroblewski BM. Deep infection in Charnley low-friction arthroplasty. Comparison of plain and gentamicin-loaded cement. J Bone Joint Surg Br 1987; 69:355–360.

48. Bowers WH, Wilson FC, Greene WB. Antibiotic prophylaxis in experimental bone infections. J Bone Joint Surg Am 1973; 55:795–807.

49. Hill C, Mazas C, Mazas F, Flamant R. Prophylactic cefazolin versus placebo in total hip replacement. Lancet 1981; 1:795–797.

50. Nelson CL, Evarts CM, Andrish J, Marks K. Results of infected total hip arthroplasty. Clin Orthop 1980; 147:258–261.

51. Beer KJ, Lombardi AV, Mallory TH, Vaughn BK. The efficacy of suction drains after routine total joint arthroplasty. J Bone Joint Surg Am 1991; 73: 584–587.

52. Willett KM, Simmons CD, Bentley G. The effect of suction drains after total hip replacement. J Bone Joint Surg Br 1988; 70:607–610.

53. Kim YH, Cho SH, Kim RS. Drainage versus nondrainage in simultaneous bilateral total hip arthroplasties. J Arthrop 1998; 13:156–161.

54. Wroblewski BM, Del Sel HJ. Urethral instrumentation and deep sepsis in total hip replacement. Clin Orthop 1980; 146:209–212.

55. Michelsen JD, Lotke PA, Steinberg ME. Urinary-bladder management after total joint replacement surgery. N Engl J Med 1988; 319:321–326.

56. Ritter MA, Faris PM, Keating EM. Urinary tract catheterisation protocols following total joint arthroplasty. Orthopaedics 1989; 12:1085–1087.

57. Gristina AG, Kolkin J. Current concepts review. Total joint replacement and sepsis. J Bone Joint Surg Am 1983; 65:128–134.

58. Petty W. The effect of methylmethacrylate on chemotaxis of polymorphonuclear leukocytes. J Bone Joint Surg Am 1978; 60:492–498.

59. Petty W. The effect of methylmethacrylate on bacterial phagocytosis and killing by human polymorphonuclear leukocytes. J Bone Joint Surg Am 1978; 60:752–757.

60. Rae T. A study on the effects of particulate metals of orthopaedic interest on murine macrophages in vitro. J Bone Joint Surg Br 1975; 57:444–450.

61. Cordero J, Munuera L, Folgueira MD. Influence of metal implants on infection. An experimental study in rabbits. J Bone Joint Surg Br 1994; 76:717–720.

62. Santavirta S, Konttinen YT, Bergroth V, Eskola A, Tallroth K, Lindholm TS. Aggressive granulomatous lesions associated with hip arthroplasty. Immunological studies. J Bone Joint Surg Am 1990; 72:252–258.

63. Santavirta S, Hoikka V, Eskola A, Konttinen YT, Paavilainen T, Tallroth K. Aggressive granulomatous lesions in cementless total hip arthroplasty. J Bone Joint Surg Br 1990; 72:980–984.

64. Masterson EL, Masri BA, Duncan CP. Treatment of infection at the site of total hip replacement. J Bone Joint Surg Am 1997; 79:1740–1749.

65. Gristina AG, Costerton JW. Bacterial adherence to biomaterials and tissue. The significance of its role in clinical sepsis. J Bone Joint Surg Am 1985; 67:264–273.

66. Petty W, Spanier S, Shuster JJ. Prevention of infection after total joint replacement. Experiments with a canine model. J Bone Joint Surg Am 1988; 70:536–539.

67. Lautenschlager EP, Marshall GW, Marks KE, Schwarz J, Nelson CL. Mechanical strength of acrylic bone cements impregnated with antibiotics. J Biomed Mater Res 1976; 10:837–845.

68. Lautenschlager EP, Jacobs JJ, Marshall GW, Meyer PR Jr. Mechanical properties of bone cements containing large doses of antibiotic powders. J Biomed Mater Res 1976; 10:929–938.

69. Picknell B, Mizen L, Sutherland R. Antibacterial activity of antibiotics in acrylic bone cement. J Bone Joint Surg Br 1977; 59:302–307.

70. Masri BA, Duncan CP, Beauchamp CP. Long-term elution of antibiotics from bone-cement. J Arthrop 1998; 13:331–338.

71. Kamme C, Lindberg L. Aerobic and anaerobic bacteria in deep infections after total hip arthroplasty. Clin Orthop 1981; 154:201–207.

72. Evans RP, Nelson CL. Staged reimplantation of a total hip prosthesis after infection with Candida albicans: A report of two cases. J Bone Joint Surg Am 1990; 72:1551–1553.

73. Strazzeri JC, Anzel S. Infected total hip arthroplasty due to Actinomyces israelii after dental extraction: A case report. Clin Orthop 1986; 210:128–131.

74. Voutsinas S, Sayakos S, Smyrnis P: Echinococcus infestation complicating total hip replacement: A case report. J Bone Joint Surg Am 1987; 69:1456–1458.

75. Younkin S, Evarts CMcC, Steigbigel RT: Candida paraspilosis infection of a total hip-joint replacement: Successful reimplantation after treatment with amphotericin B and 5-fluorocytosine: A case report. J Bone Joint Surg Am 1984; 66:142–143.

76. Balderson RA, Hiller WDB, Ianotti JP, Pickens GT, Booth RE, Gluckman SJ, Buckley RM, Rothman RH. Treatment of the septic hip with total hip arthroplasty. Clin Orthop 1987; 221:231–237.

77. Berry DJ, Chandler HP, Reilly DT. The use of bone allografts in two-stage reconstruction after failure of hip replacements due to infection. J Bone Joint Surg Am 1991; 73:1460–1468.

78. Bourne RB, Hunter GA, Rorabeck CH, Macnab JJ. A six-year follow-up of infected total hip replacements managed by Girdlestone's arthroplasty. J Bone Joint Surg Br 1984; 66:340–343.

79. Buchholz HW, Elson RA, Engelbrecht E, Lodenkamper H, Rottger J, Siegel A. Management of deep infection of total hip arthroplasty. J Bone Joint Surg Br 1981; 63:342–353.

80. Canner GC, Steinberg ME, Heppenstall RB, Balderston R. The infected hip after total hip arthroplasty. J Bone Joint Surg Am 1984; 66:1393–1399.

81. Carlsson AS, Joseffson G, Lindberg L. Revision with gentamicin-impregnated cement for deep infections in total hip arthroplasty. J Bone Joint Surg Am 1978; 60:1059–1064.

82. Cherney DL, Amstutz HC. Total hip replacement in the previously septic hip. J Bone Joint Surg Am 1983; 65:1256–1265.

83. Colyer RA, Capello WN. Surgical treatment of the infected hip implant. Two-stage reimplantation with a one-month interval. Clin Orthop 1994; 298:75–79.

84. Crockarell JR, Hanssen AD, Osmon DR, Morrey BF. Treatment of infection with debridement and retention of the components following hip arthroplasty. J Bone Joint Surg Am 1998; 80:1306–1313.

85. Duncan CP, Beauchamp C. A temporary antibiotic-loaded joint replacement system for management of complex infections involving the hip. Orthop Clin North Am 1993; 24:751–759.

86. Garvin KL, Fitzgerald RH, Salvati EA, Brause BD, Nercissian OA, Wallrichs SL, Ilstrup DM. Reconstruction of the infected total hip and knee arthroplasty with gentamicin-impregnated palacos bone cement. Instr Course Lect 1993; 42:293–302.

87. Goodman SB, Schurman DJ. Outcome of infected total hip arthroplasty. An inclusive, consecutive series. J Arthrop 1988; 3:97–102.

88. Grauer JD, Amstutz HC, O'Carroll PF, Dorey FJ. Resection arthroplasty of the hip. J Bone Joint Surg Am 1989; 71:669–678.

89. Hughes PW, Salvati EA, Wilson PD, Blumenfeld EL. Treatment of subacute sepsis of the hip by antibiotics and joint replacement: Criteria for diagnosis with evaluation of twenty-six cases. Clin Orthop 1979; 141:143–157.

90. Hunter GA, Dandy D. The natural history of the patient with an infected total hip replacement. J Bone Joint Surg Br 1977; 59:293–297.

91. Hyman JL, Salvati EA, Laurencin CT, Rogers DE, Maynard M, Brause BD. The arthroscopic drainage, irrigation and debridement of late, acute total hip arthroplasty infections. J Arthrop 1999; 14:903–910.

92. Jupiter JB, Karchmer AW, Lowell JD, Harris WH. Total hip arthroplasty in the treatment of adult hips with current or quiescent sepsis. J Bone Joint Surg Am 1981; 63:194–200.

93. Lieberman JR, Callaway GH, Salvati EA, Pellicci PM, Brause BD. Treatment of the infected total hip arthroplasty with a two-stage reimplantation protocol. Clin Orthop 1994; 301:205–212.

94. McDonald DJ, Fitzgerald RHJ, Ilstrup DM. Two-stage reconstruction of a total hip arthroplasty because of infection. J Bone Joint Surg Am 1989; 71: 828–834.

95. Miley GB, Scheller AD, Turner RH. Medical and surgical treatment of the septic hip with one-stage revision arthroplasty. Clin Orthop 1982; 170:76–82.

96. Goulet JA, Pellicci PM, Brause BD, Salvati EM. Prolonged suppression of infection in total hip arthroplasty. J Arthroplasty 1988; 3:109–116.

97. Pagnano MW, Trousdale RT, Hanssen AD. Outcome after reinfection following reimplantation hip arthroplasty. Clin Orthop 1997; 338:192–204.

98. Raut VV, Siney PD, Wroblewski BM. One-stage revision of infected total hip replacements with discharging sinuses. J Bone Joint Surg 1994; 76:721–724.

99. Salvati EA, Chekofsky KM, Brause BD, Wilson, PD Jr. Reimplantation in infection. A 12-year experience. Clin Orthop 1982; 170:62–75.

100. Sanzén L, Carlsson AS, Josefsson G, Lindberg LT. Revision operations on infected total hip arthroplasties: two-to nine year follow-up study. Clin Orthop 1988; 229:165–172.

101. Stinchfield FE, Bigliani LU, Neu HC, Goss TP, Foster CR. Late hematogenous infection of total joint replacement. J Bone Joint Surg Am 1980; 62: 1345–1350.

102. Ure KJ, Amstutz HC, Nasser S, Schmalzried TP. Direct-exchange arthroplasty for the treatment of infection after total hip replacement. An average ten-year follow-up. J Bone Joint Surg Am 1998; 80:961–968.

103. Wang J-W, Chen C-E. Reimplantation of infected hip arthroplasties using bone allografts. Clin Orthop 1997; 335:202–210.

104. Wilson MG, Dorr LD. Reimplantation of infected total hip arthroplasties in the absence of antibiotic cement. J Arthroplasty 1989; 4:263–269.

105. Wroblewski BM. One-stage revision of infected cemented total hip arthroplasty. Clin Orthop 1986; 211:103–107.

106. Zavasky DM, Sande MA. Reconsideration of rifampicin: A unique drug for a unique infection. JAMA 1998; 279:1575–1577.

107. Elson R. Sepsis: One-stage exchange. In: JJ Callaghan, AG Rosenberg, HE Rubash, eds. The Adult Hip. Philadelphia: Lippincott-Raven, 1998:1307–1315.

108. Nestor BJ, Hanssen AD, Ferrer-Gonzalez R, Fitzgerald RH. The use of porous prostheses in delayed reconstruction of total hip replacements that have failed because of infection. J Bone Joint Surg Am 1994; 76:349–358.

109. James PJ, Butcher IA, Gardner ER, Hamblen DL. Methicillin-resistant Staphylococcus epidermidis in infection of hip arthroplasties. J Bone Joint Surg Br 1994; 76:725–727.

110. Hope PG, Kristinsson KG, Norman P, Elson RA. Deep infection of cemented total hip arthroplasties caused by coagulase-negative staphylococci. J Bone Joint Surg Br 1989; 71:851–855.

111. Fitzgerald RH Jr, Jones DR. Hip implant infection. Treatment with resection arthroplasty and late total hip arthroplasty. Am J Med 1985; 78:225–228.

112. Sanzén L. The erythrocyte sedimentation rate following exchange of infected total hips. Acta Orthop Scand 1988; 59:148–150.

113. Sanzén L, Carlsson ÅS. The diagnostic value of C-reactive protein in infected total hip arthroplasties. J Bone Joint Surg Br 1989; 71:638–641.

114. Shih L-Y, Wu J-J, Yang D-J. Erythrocyte sedimentation rate and C-reactive protein values in patients with total hip arthroplasty. Clin Orthop 1987; 225:238–246.

115. Tigges S, Stiles RG, Robertson JR. Appearance of septic hip prostheses on plain radiographs. AJR 1994; 163:377–380.

116. Barrack RL, Harris WH. The value of aspiration of the hip joint before revision total hip arthroplasty. J Bone Joint Surg Am 1993; 75:66–76.

117. Fehrman DA, McBeath AA, DeSmet AA, Tuite MJ: Imaging barium-free bone cement. Am J Orthop 1996; 25:172–174.

118. Graif M, Schwartz E, Strauss S, Mouallem M, Schecter M, Morag B. Occult infection of hip prosthesis: Sonographic evaluation. J Am Geriatr Soc 1991; 39:203–204.

119. Reing CM, Richin PF, Kenmore PI. Differential bone-scanning in the evaluation of a painful total joint replacement. J Bone Joint Surg Am 1979; 61:933–936.

120. Brause BD. Infections associated with prosthetic joints. Clin Rheum Dis 1986; 12:523–536.

121. Okerlund M, Chehabi H, Huberty J, Rosen-Levin E, Murray W, Hattner R. Indium-111 granulocyte studies in the evaluation of complicated post-operative prostheses (abstr). J Nucl Med 1988; 29:883.

122. Feldman DS, Lonner JH, Desai P, Zuckerman JD. The role of intraoperative frozen sections in revision total joint arthroplasty. J Bone Joint Surg Am 1995; 77:1807–1813.

123. Glithero PR, Grigoris P, Harding LK, Hesslewood SR, McMinn DJ. White cell scans and infected joint replacements. Failure to detect chronic infection. J Bone Joint Surg Br 1993; 75:371–374.

124. Johnson JA, Christie MJ, Sandler MP, Parks PF Jr, Homra L, Kaye JJ. Detection of occult infection following total joint arthroplasty using sequential technetium 99m HDP bone scintigraphy and indium 111 WBC imaging. J Nucl Med 1988; 29:1347–1353.

125. Wukich DK, Abreu SH, Callaghan JJ, Van Nostrand D, Savory CG, Eggli DF, Garcia JE, Berrey BH. Diagnosis of infection by preoperative scintigraphy with indium-labeled white blood cells. J Bone Joint Surg Am 1987; 69: 1353–1360.

126. Palestro CJ, Kim CK, Swyer AJ, Capozzi JD, Solomon RW, Goldsmith S. Total hip arthroplasty: Periprosthetic indium-111—labeled leukocyte activity and complementary technetium-99m-sulfur colloid imaging in suspected infection. J Nucl Med 1990; 31:1951–1955.

127. Oyen WJG, Claessens RAMJ, van der Meer JWM, Corstens FHM. Detection of subacute infectious foci with indium 111–labeled autologous leukocytes and indium 111–labeled human nonspecific imunoglobulin G: A prospective comparative study. J Nucl Med 1991; 32:1854–1860.

128. Mulcahy DM, Fenelon GCC, McInerney DP. Aspiration arthrography of the hip joint: its uses and limitations in revision hip surgery. J Arthrop 1996; 11: 64–68.

129. Fitzgerald RH Jr. Infected total hip arthroplasty: Diagnosis and treatment. J Am Acad Orthop Surg 1995; 3:249–262.

130. Baker S, Fraise AP. Use of sentinel blood culture system for analysis of specimens from potentially infected prosthetic joints. J Clin Pathol 1994; 47: 475–476.

131. Lachiewicz PF, Rogers GD, Thomason HC: Aspiration of the hip joint before revision total hip arthroplasty. J Bone Joint Surg Am 1996; 78:749–754.

132. Levine MJ, Mariani BA, Tuan RS, Booth RE Jr. Molecular genetic diagnosis of infected total joint arthroplasty. J Arthrop 1995; 10:93–94.

133. Nayeri F, Cameron R, Chryssanthou E, Johansson L, Soderstrom C. Candida glabrata prosthesis infection following pyelonephritis and septicaemia. Scand J Infect Dis 1997; 29:635–638.

134. Roggenkamp A, Sing A, Hornef M, Brunner U, Autenrieth IB, Heesemann J. Chronic prosthetic hip infection caused by a small-colony variant of Escherichia coli. J Clin Microbiol 1998; 36:2530–2534.

135. Rafiq M, Worthington T, Tebbs SE, Treacy RBC, Dias R, Lambert PA, TSJ Elliott. Serological detection of gram-positive bacterial infection around prostheses J Bone Joint Surg Br 2000; 82:1156–1161.

136. Francis KP, Stewart GS. Detection and speciation of bacteria through PCR using universal major cold-shock protein primer oligomers. J Ind Microbiol Biotechnol 1977; 19:286–293.

137. Chimento GF, Finger S, Barrack RL. Gram stain detection of infection during revision arthroplasty. J Bone Joint Surg Br 1996; 78:838–839.

138. Mirra JM, Amstutz HC, Matos M, Gold R. The pathology of the joint tissues and its clinical relevance in prosthesis failure. Clin Orthop 1976; 117:221–240.

139. Lonner JH, Desai P, DiCesare PE, Steiner G, Zuckerman JD. The reliability of analysis of intraoperative frozen sections for identifying active infection during revision hip or knee arthroplasty. J Bone Joint Surg Am 1996; 78:1553–1558.

140. Athanasou NA, Pandey R, De Steiger R, Crook D, McLardy Smith P. Diagnosis of infection by frozen section during revision arthroplasty. J Bone Joint Surg Br 1995; 77:28–33.

141. Fehring TK, McAlister JA Jr. Frozen histologic section as a guide to sepsis in revision joint arthroplasty. Clin Orthop 1994; 304:229–237.

142. Della Valle CJ, Bogner E, Desai P, Lonner JH, Adler E, Zuckerman J, Cesare PE. Analysis of frozen sections of intraoperative specimens obtained at the time of reoperation after hip or knee resection arthroplasty for the treatment of infection. J Bone Joint Surg Am 1999; 81:684–689.

143. Dupont JA. Significance of operative cultures in total hip arthroplasty. Clin Orthop 1986; 211:122–127.

144. Padgett DE, Silverman A, Sachjowicz F, Simpson RB, Rosenberg AG, Galanter JO: Efficacy of intraoperative cultures obtained during revision total hip arthroplasty. J Arthrop 1995; 10:420–426.

145. Tunney MM, Patrick S, Curran MD, Ramage G, Hanna D, Nixon JR, Gorman SP, Davis RI, Anderson, N. Improved detection of infection in hip replacements. A currently underestimated problem. J Bone Joint Surg Br 1998; 80:568–572.

146. Murray WR. Use of antibiotic-containing bone cement. Clin Orthop 1984; 190:89–95.

147. Graziani AL, Hines JM, Morgan AS, MacGregor RR, Esterhai JL Jr. Infecting organisms and antibiotics. In: Steinberg ME, Garino JP, eds. Revision Total Hip Arthroplasty. Philadelphia: Lippincott, Williams & Wilkins, 1999:407–417.

148. Zimmerli W, Widmer AF, Blatter M, Frei R, Oschner PE. Role of rifampicin for treatment of orthopaedic implant-related staphylococcal infections. JAMA 1998; 279:1539–1541.

149. Brandt CM, Sistrunk WW, Duffy MC, Hanssen AD, Steckelberg JM, Ilstrup DM, Osmon DR. Staphylococcus aureus prosthetic joint infection treated with debridement and prosthesis retention. Clin Infect Dis 1997; 24:914–919.

150. Buchholz HW, Elson RA, Heinert K. Antibiotic-loaded acrylic cement: Current concepts. Clin Orthop 1984; 190:96–108.

151. Raut VV, Siney PD, Wroblewski BM. One-stage revision of total hip arthroplasty for deep infection. Long-term follow-up. Clin Orthop 1995; 321:202–207.

152. Raut VV, Siney PD, Wroblewski BM. One-stage revision arthroplasty of the hip for deep gram negative infection. Int Orthop 1996; 20:12–14.

153. Hanssen AD, Rand JA. Evaluation and treatment of infection at the site of a total hip or knee arthroplasty. Instr Course Lect 1999; 48:111–122.

154. Mont MA, Waldman BJ, Hungerford DS. Evaluation of preoperative cultures before second-stage reimplantation of a total knee prosthesis complicated by infection. J Bone Joint Surg Am 2000; 82:1552–1557.
155. Hunter GA. The results of reinsertion of a total hip prosthesis after sepsis. J Bone Joint Surg Br 1979; 61:422–423.
156. Gustilo RB, Pasternak HS. Revision total hip arthroplasty with titanium ingrowth prosthesis and bone grafting for failed cemented femoral component loosening. Clin Orthop 1988; 235:111–119.
157. Gustilo RB, Tsukayama D. Treatment of infected cemented total hip arthroplasty with tobramycin beads and delayed revision with a cementless prosthesis and bone grafting. Orthop Trans 1988; 12:739.
158. Haddad FS, Manktelow ARJ, Bacarese-Hamilton I, Muirhead-Allwood SK. Two-stage uncemented revision hip arthroplasty for infection. J Bone Joint Surg Br 2000; 82:689–694.
159. Lai KA, Shen WJ, Yang CY, Lin RM, Lin CJ, Jou IM. Two-stage cementless revision THR after infection. 5 recurrences in 40 cases followed 2.5–7 years. Acta Orthop Scand 1996; 67:325–328.
160. Morscher E, Babst R, Jenny H. Treatment of infected joint arthroplasty. Int Orthop 1990; 14:161–165.
161. Schutzer SF, Harris WH. Deep-wound infection after total hip replacement under contemporary aseptic conditions. J Bone Joint Surg 1988; 70:724–727.
162. Alexeeff M, Mahomed N, Morsi E, Garbuz D, Gross A. Structural allograft in two-stage revisions for failed septic hip arthroplasty. J Bone Joint Surg Br 1996; 78:213–216.
163. Jasty M, Harris WH. Salvage total hip reconstruction in patients with major acetabular bone deficiency using structural femoral head allografts. J Bone Joint Surg Br 1990; 72:63–67.
164. Nasser S. Prevention and treatment of sepsis in total hip replacement surgery. Orthop Clin North Am 1992; 23:265–277.
165. Duncan CP, Masri BA. Antibiotic depots. J Bone Joint Surg Br 1993; 75:349–350.
166. Duncan CP, Masri BA. The role of antibiotic-loaded cement in the treatment of an infection after hip replacement. J Bone Joint Surg Am 1994; 76:1742–1751.
167. Kendall RW, Masri BA, Duncan CP, Beauchamp CP, McGraw RW, Bora B. Temporary antibiotic loaded acrylic hip replacement: A novel method for management of the infected THA. Semin Arthrop 1994; 5:171–177.
168. Younger ASE, Duncan CP, Masri BA, McGraw RW. The outcome of two-stage arthroplasty using a custom-made interval spacer to treat the infected hip. J Arthrop 1997; 12:615–623.
169. Garvin KL, Evans BG, Salvati EA, Brause BD. Palacos gentamicin for the treatment of deep periprosthetic infections. Clin Orthop 1994; 298:97–105.
170. Girdlestone GR. Acute pyogenic arthritis of the hip. Lancet 1943; 1:419–421.
171. Kostuick J, Alexander D. Arthrodesis for failed arthroplasty of the hip. Clin Orthop 1984; 188:173–182.

11
Hip Arthroscopy

James T. Ninomiya
Medical College of Wisconsin, Milwaukee, Wisconsin

I. INTRODUCTION

The use of arthroscopy for the evaluation and treatment of hip pathology is an exciting and growing area of interest for all hip surgeons. It offers the advantages of other arthroscopic procedures, including minimal incisions and decreased morbidity and hospitalization. Although offering huge potential, hip arthroscopy has remained a relatively unpopular procedure, particularly when compared with arthroscopy of the knee, shoulder, elbow, and wrist. The deep location of the hip, the extensive surrounding musculature, the close proximity of major neurovascular structures, and the anatomic nature of the hip joint itself all make arthroscopic exposure difficult. The insertion of instruments and their maneuverability are all more difficult because of these anatomic limitations.

The first report of arthroscopy of the hip was that of Burman in 1931 (7,19,49); many reports have subsequently appeared (10,19). As the popularity of hip arthroscopy has grown, multiple indications for the procedure have been suggested, including assessment of the painful hip following failure of conservative measures or use as an aid to diagnosis when other investigations are unhelpful. Other applications include evaluation of idiopathic hip pain, removal of retained projectiles, treatment of a septic hip (4,5,14,83), or even as an adjunct in core decompression performed for osteonecrosis (16,28,37,67,70). Some authors have even advocated the use of hip arthroscopy for an assessment of the osteoarthritic hip in order to plan further, more invasive surgery. Other indications include debridement of the arthritic hip for pain relief in osteoarthritis, the removal of loose or foreign bodies, synovectomy, or excision of a torn acetabular labrum (9,10, 12,46,47,81).

II. EVALUATION OF PATIENTS WITH HIP PAIN

The diagnosis of patients with labral pathology has remained an enigmatic problem. Frequently, patients with symptoms of catching or locking of the hip have seen several orthopaedic surgeons and have had multiple imaging studies, including plain films, computed tomography (CT) scans, bone scans, and magnetic resonance imaging (MRI). Physical examination findings for patients with symptoms of catching or locking of the hips have been described by Fitzgerald and others, where the hip was brought into acute flexion, external rotation, and full abduction and was then extended with internal rotation and adduction (20,40,61). At our institution we have examined over 100 patients with clinical histories or symptoms suggestive of a torn acetabular labrum, and in all cases we have found pain elicited on this provocative maneuver. However, it is also important to compare the results from examination of both hips, since the circumduction motion can elicit tenderness in normal invididuals. We consider the results of the circumduction test positive when there is a notable difference as compared with the asymptomatic limb.

Although plain films are a requisite starting point for the evaluation of any patient with hip pain, they are unlikely to confirm the presence of labral pathology. The only suggestive finding from plain radiographs is the presence of a perilabral cyst at the superolateral rim of the acetabulum, indicative of possible undermining of the labrum. This may be particularly true in patients with associated hip dysplasia, where cysts in the lateral aspect of the acetabulum have been associated with torn acetabular labra (20).

A variety of methods have been described for determining the presence of labral pathology, and MRI is the study of choice. Some reports have suggested that noncontrast MRI scans were effective in evaluating the labrum, and an investigation of 35 dysplastic hips in 28 patients demonstrated labral tears in 24 (41). However, most studies now support MRI arthrography as having superior sensitivity and specificity compared to conventional MRI (80). In a comparison study, Czerny and coworkers evaluated a series of 56 hips before and after the intra-articular injection of gadopentate demeglumine. Of these, 22 underwent surgical intervention, and 35 were treated conservatively. Following surgical confirmation, it was determined that the sensitivity and specificity of MRI arthrography were 90 and 91%, while the sensitivity of nonenhanced MRI was 30%, with an accuracy of only 36% (18).

Other studies also support the use of MRI arthrograpy as the imaging study of choice in the evaluation of labral pathology (31,32,38,48,52,53,60, 64,68,69,71). Using this method, Petersilge and coworkers reported a series of 22 patients, of whom 10 went on to surgery. Eight had confirmation of the radiographic findings. The authors concluded that MRI arthrography appeared to be a promising imaging modality for accurate diagnosis of acetabular labral tears (68). A further 23 patients were evaluated by MRI arthrography for symptoms and signs of abnormality of the acetabular labrum. Of these, 18 had confirmation at surgery, while in 2 patients MRI arthrography erroneously suggested an intact labrum (57,58). A cadaver evaluation investigated the effectiveness of conventional MRI versus MRI arthrography in assessing labral pathology and concluded that the addition of contrast media increased both the sensitivity and specificity of MRI in the evaluation of the labrum (6,42). In contrast, plain MRI scans were not efficient in demonstrating labral pathology, suggesting the need for strict radiographic criteria in making the diagnosis of tears, detachments, and degeneration of the labrum (1,17,56).

At our institution, we have prospectively evaluated 21 patients with clinical symptoms of labral tears by MRI arthrography and CT arthrography. MRI arthrograms were performed with the use of saline injections and T2-weighted imaging using hip surface coils (62,63). All of the scans were randomized and read independently by three musculoskeletal radiologists. MRI arthrography revealed tears in 19 of 21 patients (90%), while CT arthrograms were positive in only 9 of 21 (43%). However, two patients who had negative MRI arthrograms had positive findings on CT arthrograms, which were subsequently confirmed at hip arthroscopy. Therefore we advocate the use of MRI arthrography for the evaluation of patients with suspected labral pathology. However, a CT arthrogram is warranted if clinical symptoms of a labral tear exist in the presence of a negative or equivocal MRI arthrogram.

Viewing a hip through the arthroscope provides a perspective with which most surgeons are unfamiliar, and several reports have described the anatomy and pathology as seen through the arthroscope (Figure 1). Classifications of labral pathology have been proposed based upon their appearance and etiology (10,15,66,67,72,75). In general, labral pathology is most common in the anterior and superior location, possibly reflecting an area of greatest weight bearing or possible impingement by the femoral neck (15,27).

III. INDICATIONS FOR HIP ARTHROSCOPY

A number of studies have described the results following hip arthroscopy. However, many of these reports have notable shortcomings, including mul-

(A)

(B)

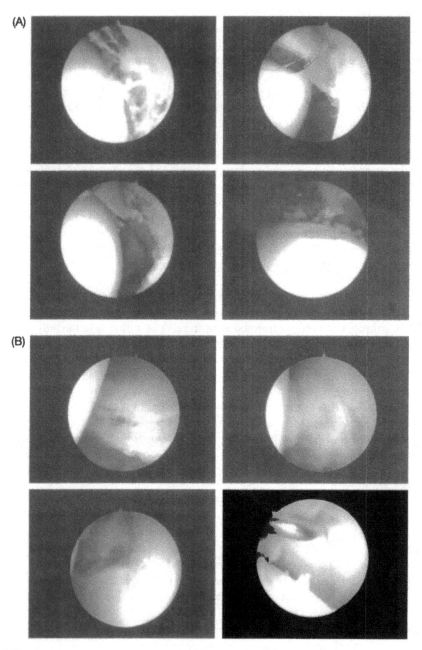

Figure 1 A. Example of a torn acetabular labrum as viewed through the arthroscope. B. Appearance of labral edge after resection by a thermal probe.

tiple diagnoses, small numbers of patients, or reporting of short-term results. For example, a prospective study of 35 patients with a minimum follow-up of 2 years described the results of arthroscopy for multiple diagnoses, including arthritis, sepsis, loose bodies, and others (12). The indications for the original surgery were not described, and it was not clear whether the diagnosis was made at the time of the procedure or prior to surgery. Of the 35 patients, 10 had no improvement in their hip scores and went on to further surgeries. Additionally, 10 of the patients dropped out of the study and did not meet the criteria for a minimum of a 2-year follow-up despite the title of the paper. Therefore the conclusions regarding the results of hip arthroscopy for multiple diagnoses suffered from insufficient numbers, and no statistical conclusions were offered. Recurrent dislocation of the hip has also been ascribed to labral pathology in a patient who had previously suffered a traumatic posterior dislocation (84). At the time of surgery, the acetabular labrum was found to be torn, with a Bankart-type lesion. This was successfully treated with an open arthrotomy and placement of a bone block on the postero-superior wall of the acetabulum. Other studies have described avulsion of the acetabular labrum with intra-articular displacement and subsequent treatment via open arthrotomy (61).

The relationship between labral pathology and osteoarthritis remains unclear. One report suggested that an inverted and intra-articular acetabular labrum might be a possible etiological factor in osteoarthritis of the hip. Harris described a series of eight patients with early degenerative arthritis of the hip where at surgery the labrum was found to lie within the articulation between the femoral head and the acetabulum (39). None of these patients had a history of trauma, and the authors postulated that an intra-articular labrum was a developmental abnormality that had caused the early degenerative arthritis. Another study reported the results of 64 pelvic osteotomies performed for early arthritis and demonstrated superior surgical results in patients with normal or torn acetabular labra, with less satisfactory outcomes in patients with detached labra (65). Altenberg reported on two patients who had disabling hip pain as the result of torn acetabular labra (2). At the time of surgery, large erosions of the articular surfaces of the femoral head and acetabulum were noted, corresponding to the location of the displaced torn labrum. The authors postulated that a torn labrum could be the cause of degenerative hip disease where no pre-existing condition was present.

The role of the labrum in the hip has been evaluated experimentally. A biomechanical study on cadavers did not produce any significant changes with regard to contact area, load, mean pressure, or maximum pressure when the labrum was removed (51). These results imply that removal of all or part of the labrum would not predispose a patient to abnormal weight bearing in the acetabulum or in early osteoarthritis (51). It is therefore possible that the hip may be analogous to the knee, where torn cartilage may predispose an individual to abnormal wear and the generation of early osteoarthritis. Unlike the case with the knee, however, removal of the labrum may not lead to early arthritis.

In contrast, finite element modeling studies suggested that during normal gait, the femoroacetabular forces might increase by as much as 92%, using the assumptions in the evaluations (24,25). Only long-term follow up studies will validate either the mathematical or experimental models regarding the role of the labrum in the hip and the effect of its removal on the genesis of arthritis.

Acetabular rim syndrome has been described as a pathological entity that was felt to be a precursor of osteoarthritis secondary to acetabular dysplasia. The symptoms were pain and impaired function. Twenty-nine patients were treated by periacetabular osteotomy and arthrotomy of the hip. In all cases the labrum was found to be detached from the bony rim of the acetabulum (50). The authors postulated that the acetabular rim was subject to abnormal stresses in acetabular dysplasia, which might result in rupture of the labrum and subsequent arthritis. Cystic deformation of the labrum has also been reported as a cause of hip pain, as described in a case study of two patients who were investigated by open arthrotomy (79). In a similar study, femoroacetabular impingement and a cam effect may result in labral damage as the result of repetitive impingement in nondysplastic hips, a possible mechanism for labral injury and subsequent osteoarthritis (45).

Unfortunately, most studies reported in the literature describe either multiple diagnoses or comprise only small numbers of patients. In general, it appears that hip arthroscopy is most beneficial for patients with tears of the acetabular labrum that have been diagnosed preoperatively by MRI arthrography. Removal of loose or foreign bodies is another obvious application, while there is little convincing evidence to support the use of arthroscopy for the treatment or evaluation of arthritis.

IV. RESULTS OF HIP ARTHROSCOPY

The results following hip arthroscopy clearly depend upon the underlying clinical diagnosis. Glick reported a small series of 18 hips that were debrided for osteoarthritis; 9 showed some improvement, while the remainder did not obtain any relief from pain (28,33–35,49). A later study by the same authors found that only 21% of patients who had undergone arthroscopy for osteoarthritis derived any long-term relief. Our results mirror those of Glick, where a small subset of patients with osteoarthritis and a concomitant labral tear were evaluated arthroscopically and none of the patients achieved any long lasting results. They generally reported a lessening of their catching and locking phenomena, but the underlying aching associated with osteoarthritis was not improved.

Conversely, other authors have suggested that up to 60% of patients may derive benefit following arthroscopic debridement for osteoarthritis (82). In a report of 40 consecutive patients undergoing arthroscopic debridement of the hip for osteoarthritis, Villar reported that patients felt 60% better 6 months following surgery compared to their preoperative state. The mean Harris hip score was 43 (range 2–73), while at 6 months, the postoperative score was 64 (range 11–91). However, no statistical analysis of these results was offered.

For patients with a diagnosis of an acetabular labral tear, results following arthroscopy were more positive (10,15,23,26,40,44,55). In a small series of 10 patients, 8 patients who underwent arthroscopic debridement experienced prompt pain relief, while 2 patients who were treated conservatively did not achieve any decrease in their symptoms (40). In general, most studies support the concept that hip arthroscopy is very effective in the treatment of patients with tears of the acetabular labrum.

Several authors have advocated the use of hip arthroscopy as a diagnostic procedure (3,19,21,67,81,82). In one series of 59 patients with hip pain, evaluation by hip arthroscopy revealed that 69% had synovitis, while 59% had a torn labrum (59). Likewise, Ikeda reported a series of 7 patients who were diagnosed with a torn acetabular labrum through hip arthroscopy (44). Only one patient subsequently underwent open arthrotomy, and had a satisfactory outcome. A smaller series described the findings in 8 patients with inexplicable hip pain who subsequently underwent hip arthroscopy (77). Five of the 8 had ruptures of the posterior or posterosuperior labrum that was not visualized by arthrography. No treatment outcomes from arthroscopic debridement were described in either of these reports.

A larger series of 58 patients with a mean follow-up of 3.5 years was evaluated following arthroscopy, where labral pathology was identified at the time of surgery. Over half of the patients had moderate chondral damage of the hip, consisting of softening or fibrillation of the acetabulum or femoral head (Figure 2). Of the total, 67% were pleased with the results of their surgery while 33% were not. The authors were not able to establish any statistical relationship between the location of the tear and the clinical outcome of the surgery.

Villar has suggested that MRI has limitations in diagnosing pathology in the hip, particularly regarding the assessment of early chondral changes, and has advocated the use of arthroscopy for the diagnosis and treatment of chondral abnormalities, labral tears, and loose bodies (21) (Figure 3). He

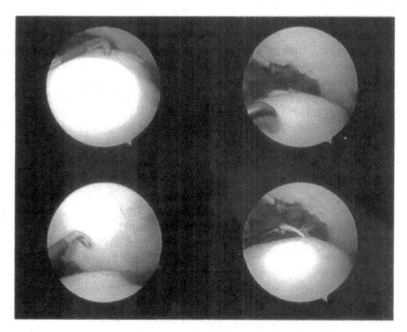

Figure 2 Appearance of soft femoral head cartilage in an area of underlying osteonecrosis. Note adjacent hemorrhage and indentation of cartilage by probe.

has also reported on a group of 20 patients with pathology associated with the ligamentum teres, including ruptures or degeneration (36). It was not clear whether this pathology was known prior to surgery or was a finding during a diagnostic procedure. A later report by the same authors advocated the use of hip arthroscopy as a diagnostic tool, stating that the preoperative diagnoses were altered following arthroscopy in 30% of the patients (3). These included the revised diagnoses of arthritis, osteochondral defects, torn labra, synovitis, and loose bodies. Of note is that the majority of the patients did not undergo evaluation of their hips by MR arthrography prior to surgery, suggesting that the diagnoses might have been established prior to surgery if further imaging studies had been performed.

Hip arthroscopy may also have special applications for the pediatric population (78). An early report on 13 patients with rheumatoid arthritis suggested that arthroscopy could visualize joint erosions with more sensitivity than plain radiographs (43). However, the authors did not report on the outcome of the surgery or describe any improvement in the patients' symptoms. A later case report described the use of hip arthroscopy in Legg-Calve-Perthes (LCP) disease (54). A 7-year-old male with LCP had a prom-

(A)

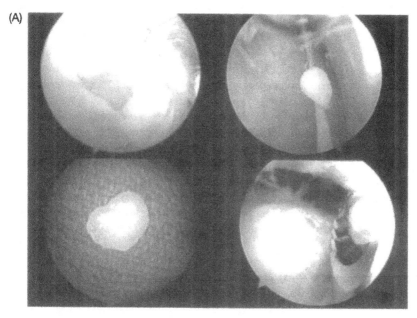

(B)

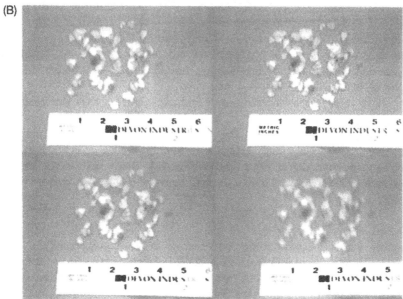

Figure 3 A. Loose body within hip joint in a patient with synovial osteochondromatosis. B. Loose bodies removed via hip arthroscopy.

inent island of superficial epiphyseal ossification in his right femoral head, which were successfully identified and treated by hip arthroscopy. The patient had a reduction in pain and an increase in range of motion following the procedure. The authors suggested that hip arthroscopy was a useful procedure for the treatment of this unusual sequela of Legg-Calve-Perthes disease.

Hip dysplasia may also represent a unique indication for hip arthroscopy (66). An evaluation of 20 patients with an average CE angle of Wiberg of 23 degrees (range 19–27) revealed the presence of a labral tear in 18 patients (59). Following surgery, 85% of the patients had resolution of their preoperative pain. All had associated chondral lesions adjacent to the labral pathology, suggesting a relationship between the development of arthritis and the abnormal labrum and joint forces resulting from a dysplastic hip.

In another study, the results of diagnostic and therapeutic arthroscopy of the hip in children and adolescents were evaluated. In a series of 24 hips, arthroscopy confirmed the presumptive diagnosis in 13 (54%), while 11 had no correlation (46%) (73). Based upon these findings, the authors concluded that hip arthroscopy was not helpful as a confirmatory diagnostic tool. They did acknowledge that hip arthroscopy might be useful for obtaining synovial biopsies, treatment of the complications of hip dislocation, or possibly the removal of osteochondral loose bodies. Likewise, a series of five hips with slipped capital femoral epiphysis (SCFE) were evaluated prior to pinning in situ. Arthroscopy revealed erosion of the acetabular cartilage and damage to the posterolateral labrum, suggesting a traumatic pathomechanism for the cause of SCFE (30).

Two reports describe the use of arthroscopic lavage for the treatment of septic hip arthritis (14,49). In one study, nine cases were successfully treated by arthroscopic lavage. The treatment, combined with standard medical therapy, was completely effective in treating the hip infections and offered an attractive alternative to open arthrotomy. There was a lower surgical morbidity, effective joint lavage through large-bore cannulae, and early return of joint mobility.

Most studies suggest that arthroscopic debridement is an effective method of treatment for tears of the acetabular labrum. In a series of 42 patients who underwent either an open or arthroscopic procedure, 89% showed improvement following surgery (26). An early case report described the diagnosis and treatment of two patients with rupture of the acetabular labrum who achieved pain relief following hip arthroscopy (79).

We prospectively reviewed the results of 85 patients who underwent hip arthroscopy for a diagnosis of an acetabular labral tear, with a minimum follow-up of 2 years after surgery. There were 45 female and 40 male patients (average age 36; range 15–72). Before and after surgery each patient filled out a database form that consisted of questions based upon the Harris hip score. For all patients, the pain on initial presentation was generally described as sharp, along with an underlying dull aching. Frequently, there were associated sharp, snapping, or locking sensations. Over half of the patients (55%) recalled a traumatic event that initiated their symptoms. The pain was localized to the groin region in 51%, the buttock in 7%, and both locations in 40%. MRI arthrography revealed the presence of an antero-superior tear in 26%, superior alone in 18%, posterior in 9%, and postero-superior in 10%. Prior to surgery, 85% of the patients described their pain as being moderate to severe and nearly constant. Following arthroscopy, all patients had decreases in pain severity (100%, $p < 0.0001$) and symptom frequency ($p < 0.0001$). All patients also improved at least one grade in their hip scores for function ($p < 0.0001$). Eight patients experienced transient numbness in the groin or foot secondary to traction. Three patients with radiographic findings of hip arthritis and a labral tear had resolution of their snapping and catching symptoms but had persistent pain due to their arthritic symptoms. Our results suggest that hip arthroscopy is a very effective technique for treating acetabular labral tears but is not as effective in relieving symptoms of osteoarthritis.

V. TECHNIQUES OF HIP ARTHROSCOPY

Hip arthroscopy can be performed using either the lateral decubitus or supine position. Glick described a series of 11 patients who underwent arthroscopy in the lateral position, with traction applied through a series of pulleys and weights (33). A portal was made over the superior edge of the greater trochanter, and specialized instruments were used for visualization of the hip. Two other portals were utilized, with one incision being anterior and the other about 3–4 cm posterior to the original incision (35). In his follow-up report, the use of a standard fracture table was recommended, again using the lateral approach with skin traction. Due to the limitations of the two portal technique, other options include the use of a limited anterior exposure, which used a modified 4-cm Smith-Peterson anterior approach. No complications were described through the use of this incision, although procedures were performed with this technique. The potential advantages include easier introduction of the arthroscope, and easier visualization for placement of instruments and the removal of loose bodies (74).

Other positioning techniques are also possible, and several studies have described the use of a fracture table in the supine position (8,22). Successful surgical visualization was possible with 300–500 n (newtons) of force applied to the hip, but the authors also reported one case of skin necrosis of the scrotum and one transection of the lateral femoral cutaneous nerve in their series of 30 patients (22). The use of traction plus joint distension with fluid may aid in arthroscopic visualization (11). Regardless of the position or location of the arthroscopic portals, a thorough understanding of the anatomy is critical to avoid complications.

At our institution we have now performed over 100 hip arthroscopies, with the majority of patients having a diagnosis of acetabular labral tears. We have also treated patients with irreducible traumatic hip dislocations and have successfully removed intact bullets from the hip joint without needing to resort to open arthrotomy. In all of these cases we have had successful visualization of the hip joint using a standard fracture table with skin traction and image intensification in the lateral position. No special traction apparatus was required other than a traction post that enabled the patient to be placed in the lateral decubitus position. We also favor abduction of the hip to relieve tension on the overlying iliotibial band, and internal rotation to neutralize the native anteversion of the femoral neck. The hip is also placed in extension, to minimize the chance of traction injuries to the sciatic nerve.

VI. COMPLICATIONS OF HIP ARTHROSCOPY

Complications from hip arthroscopy are rare and are generally related to either the traction or inadvertent damage from arthroscopic instruments (29). Injury to the neurovascular structures surrounding the hip remains a significant challenge during hip arthroscopy. The femoral artery, vein, and nerve can be punctured or lacerated if care is not used in placing the anterior portal, while the sciatic nerve and superior gluteal structures can be injured with the posterior approach. Erkisson reported a case of scrotal skin necrosis as a result of the traction, as well as a transection of the lateral femoral cutaneous nerve from an arthroscopic shaver (22). Glick described 3 patients out of 29 who sustained transient neuropraxias as a result of traction (35). All of these resolved within a few days.

In a retrospective review of 19 patients, another study reported three patients with complications: 1 had a pudendal nerve neuropraxia, 1 a hematoma of the labia majora, and 1 had the onset of acute abdominal pain forcing the early termination of the procedure (29). The authors emphasized the importance of understanding the anatomy of portal placement as well as the need to adequately pad the traction post. In a large series of over 640 procedures, Villar reported an overall complication rate of 1.6%, none of which were major or long-term. These included transient palsy of the sciatic and femoral nerves, perineal injury, bleeding from the arthroscopic portals, trochanteric bursitis, and intra-articular instrument breakage. They concluded that the risks associated with the procedure are generally low.

In a laboratory investigation, Byrd and coworkers placed Steinmann pins into the hip under fluoroscopic control, and the relationships between the lateral femoral cutaneous nerve, femoral nerve, ascending branch of the lateral femoral circumflex artery, superior gluteal nerve, and sciatic nerve were investigated (13). They found that the lateral femoral cutaneous nerve was in close proximity to the Steinmann pin inserted through the anterior arthroscopic portal, with an average distance of only 0.3 cm (range 0.2–1.0 cm) between the pin and branches of the nerve. They also cautioned that injury to nerve branches could result in the formation of a painful neuroma. Despite the proximity to the nerve, they advocated the use of a sharp trocar through the anterior portal. As a result of this potential risk, one report suggested the use of a sheathed knife versus a sharp trochar for entry of instrumentation through the hip capsule (76). However, the authors also stated that they had tried this technique on only four patients, so the true efficacy of this method remains to be established.

At our institution, we have performed over 100 hip arthroscopies and have seen one wound infection at the portal sites in an immunocompromised patient which required an open irrigation and debridement. This patient subsequently healed without the need for further intervention. Two patients had instrument breakage of the arthroscopic guide wire used for instrument insertion. Both of these had the wire fragments successfully removed arthroscopically at the time of the original surgery. Ten percent of the patients reported transient numbness of the dorsum of their foot or the perineal region lasting less than 3 days, while one patient described penile numbness that persisted for over 3 weeks but resolved completely.

VII. SUMMARY

In summary, hip arthroscopy is a new and growing field, with the potential for the evaluation and treatment of a wide variety of hip abnormalities. The main limitations remain the technical demands associated with performing the surgery due to decreased ability to manipulate the arthroscope and associated instruments. It appears that the complication rate is low, and the morbidity associated with the procedure is minimal. In most applications, an arthroscopic procedure is likely to be less invasive than an open arthrotomy. As our knowledge base increases, larger clinical series and longer-term results will be required to establish the validity and indications for hip arthroscopy, but the future of the procedure remains very promising.

REFERENCES

1. Abe, I., Harada, Y., Oinuma, K., Kamikawa, K., Kitahara, H., Morita, F., and Moriya, H. Acetabular labrum: abnormal findings at MR imaging in asymptomatic hips. Radiology 216:576–581, 2000.
2. Altenberg, A. R. Acetabular labrum tears: a cause of hip pain and degenerative arthritis. South Med J 70:174–175, 1977.
3. Baber, Y. F., Robinson, A. H., and Villar, R. N. Is diagnostic arthroscopy of the hip worthwhile? A prospective review of 328 adults investigated for hip pain. J Bone Joint Surg (Br) 81:600–603, 1999.
4. Blitzer, C. M. Arthroscopic management of septic arthritis of the hip. Arthroscopy 9:414–416, 1993.
5. Bould, M., Edwards, D., and Villar, R. N. Arthroscopic diagnosis and treatment of septic arthritis of the hip joint. Arthroscopy 9:707–708, 1993.
6. Brossmann, J., Plotz, G. M., Steffens, J. C., Hassenpflug, J., and Heller, M. [MR arthrography of the labrum acetabulare—a radiological-anatomical correlation in 20 cadaveric hips]. Fortschr Geb Rontgenstrahlen Neuen Bildgeb Verfahr Erganzungsbd 171:143–148, 1999.
7. Burman, M. Arthroscopy or the direct visualization of joints. J Bone Joint Surg 13:669–695, 1931.
8. Byrd, J. W. Hip arthroscopy utilizing the supine position. Arthroscopy 10:275–280, 1994.
9. Byrd, J. W. Hip arthroscopy for posttraumatic loose fragments in the young active adult: three case reports. Clin J Sports Med 6:129–133; discussion 133–134, 1996.
10. Byrd, J. W. Labral lesions: an elusive source of hip pain case reports and literature review. Arthroscopy 12:603–612, 1996.
11. Byrd, J. W., and Chern, K. Y.: Traction versus distension for distraction of the joint during hip arthroscopy. Arthroscopy 13:346–349, 1997.
12. Byrd, J. W., and Jones, K. S. Prospective analysis of hip arthroscopy with 2-year follow-up. Arthroscopy (Online) 16:578–587, 2000.
13. Byrd, J. W., Pappas, J. N., and Pedley, M. J. Hip arthroscopy: an anatomic study of portal placement and relationship to the extra-articular structures. Arthroscopy 11:418–423, 1995.
14. Chung, W. K., Slater, G. L., and Bates, E. H.: Treatment of septic arthritis of the hip by arthroscopic lavage. J Pediatr Orthop 13:444–446, 1993.
15. Conn, K. S., and Villar, R. N. [Labrum lesions from the viewpoint of arthroscopic hip surgery]. Orthopade 27:699–703, 1998.
16. Cory, J. W., and Ruch, D. S. Arthroscopic removal of a .44 caliber bullet from the hip. Arthroscopy 14:624–626, 1998.
17. Cotten, A., Boutry, N., Demondion, X., Paret, C., Dewatre, F., Liesse, A., Chastanet, P., and Fontaine, C. Acetabular labrum: MRI in asymptomatic volunteers. J Comput Assist Tomogr 22:1–7, 1998.
18. Czerny, C., Hofmann, S., Neuhold, A., Tschauner, C., Engel, A., Recht, M. P., and Kramer, J. Lesions of the acetabular labrum: accuracy of MR imaging and MR arthrography in detection and staging. Radiology 200:225–230, 1996.

19. Dorfmann, H., and Boyer, T. Arthroscopy of the hip: 12 years of experience. Arthroscopy. 15:67–72, 1999.
20. Dorrell, J. H., and Catterall, A. The torn acetabular labrum. J Bone Joint Surg 68B:400–403, 1986.
21. Edwards, D. J., Lomas, D., and Villar, R. N. Diagnosis of the painful hip by magnetic resonance imaging and arthroscopy. J Bone Joint Surg (Br) 77:374–376, 1995.
22. Eriksson, E., Arvidsson, I., and Arvidsson, H. Diagnostic and operative arthroscopy of the hip. Orthopedics (Thorofare, NJ) 9:169–176, 1986.
23. Farjo, L. A., Glick, J. M., and Sampson, T. G. Hip arthroscopy for acetabular labral tears. Arthroscopy 15:132–137, 1999.
24. Ferguson, S. J., Bryant, J. T., Ganz, R., and Ito, K. The acetabular labrum seal: a poroelastic finite element model. Clin Biomech 15:463–468, 2000.
25. Ferguson, S. J., Bryant, J. T., Ganz, R., and Ito, K. The influence of the acetabular labrum on hip joint cartilage consolidation: a poroelastic finite element model. J Biomech 33:953–960, 2000.
26. Fitzgerald, R. H. Acetabular labrum tears. Clin Orthop Rel Res 311:60–68, 1995.
27. Fitzgerald, R. H., Jr. Acetabular labrum tears. Diagnosis and treatment. Clin Orthop Rel Res 113:60–68, 1995.
28. Frich, L. H., Lauritzen, J., and Juhl, M. Arthroscopy in diagnosis and treatment of hip disorders. Orthopedics (Thorofare, NJ). 12:389–392, 1989.
29. Funke, E. L., and Munzinger, U. Complications in hip arthroscopy. Arthroscopy 12:156–159, 1996.
30. Futami, T., Kasahara, Y., Suzuki, S., Seto, Y., and Ushikubo, S. Arthroscopy for slipped capital femoral epiphysis. J Pediatr Orthop 12:592–597, 1992.
31. Garcia, J. [MR arthrography]. J Radiol 81:945–952, 2000.
32. Ghebontni, L., Roger, B., El-khoury, J., Brasseur, J. L., and Grenier, P. A. MR arthrography of the hip: normal intra-articular structures and common disorders. Eur Radiol 10:83–88, 2000.
33. Glick, J. M. Hip arthroscopy using the lateral approach. Instr Course Lect 19:169–178, 1988.
34. Glick, J. M. Hip Arthroscopy. In: J. B. McGinty (ed.) Operative Arthroscopy. New York: Raven Press, 1991, pp. 663–676.
35. Glick, J. M., Sampson, T. G., Gordon, R. B., Behr, J. T., and Schmidt, E. Hip arthroscopy by the lateral approach. Arthroscopy 3:4, 1987.
36. Gray, A. J., and Villar, R. N. The ligamentum teres of the hip: an arthroscopic classification of its pathology. Arthroscopy 13:575–578, 1997.
37. Grontvedt, T., and Engebretsen, L. Arthroscopy of the hip. Scand J Med Sci Sports 5:7–9, 1995.
38. Haims, A., Katz, L. D., and Busconi, B. MR arthrography of the hip. Radiol Clin North Am 36:691–702, 1998.
39. Harris, W. H., Bourne, R. B., and Oh, I: Intra-articular acetabular labrum: a possiblem etiological factor in certain cases of osteoarthitis of the hip. J Bone Joint Surg 61A:510–514, 1979.

40. Hase, T., and Ueo, T.: Acetabular labral tear: arthroscopic diagnosis and treatment. Arthroscopy 15:138–141, 1999.
41. Hasegawa, Y., Fukatsu, H., Matsuda, T., Iwase, T., and Iwata, H. Magnetic resonance imaging in osteoarthritis of the dysplastic hip. Arch Orthop Trauma Surg 115:243–248, 1996.
42. Hodler, J., Yu, J. S., Goodwin, D., Haghighi, P., Trudell, D., and Resnick, D. MR arthrography of the hip: improved imaging of the acetabular labrum with histologic correlation in cadavers. AJR 165:887–891, 1995.
43. Holgersson, S., Brattstrom, H., Mogensen, B., and Lidgen, L. Arthroscopy of the hip in juvenile chronic arthritis. J Pediatr Orthop 1:273–278, 1981.
44. Ikeda, T., Awaya, G., Suzuki, S., Okada, Y., and Tada, H. Torn acetabular labrum in young patients. Arthroscopic diagnosis and management. J Bone Joint Surg (Br) 70:13–16, 1988.
45. Ito, K., Minka, M. A. II, Leunig, M., Werlen, S., and Ganz, R. Femoroacetabular impingement and the cam-effect. A MRI-based quantitative anatomical study of the femoral head-neck offset. J Bone Joint Surg (Br) 83:171–176, 2001.
46. Keene, G. S., and Villar, R. N. Arthroscopic anatomy of the hip: an in vivo study. Arthroscopy 10:392–399, 1994.
47. Keene, G. S., and Villar, R. N. Arthroscopic loose body retrieval following traumatic hip dislocation. Injury 25:507–510, 1994.
48. Kelley, B., Anderson, R., and Miles, K. Acetabular labrum tear in a 15-year-old male: diagnosis with correlative imaging. Australas Radiol 41:157–159, 1997.
49. Kim, S. J., Choi, N. H., and Kim, H. J. Operative hip arthroscopy. Clin Orthop Rel Res 353:156–165, 1998.
50. Klaue, K., Durnin, C. W., and Ganz, R. The acetabular rim syndrome. A clinical presentation of dysplasia of the hip. J Bone Joint Surg (Br) 73:423–429, 1991.
51. Konrath, G. A., Hamel, A. J., Olson, S. A., Bary, B., and Sharkey, N. A. The role of the acetabular labrum and the transverse acetabular ligament in load transmission in the hip. J Bone Joint Surg 80:1781–1788, 1998.
52. Kubo, T., Horii, M., Harada, Y., Noguchi, Y., Yutani, Y., Ohashi, H., Hachiya, Y., Miyaoka, H., Naruse, S., and Hirasawa, Y. Radial-sequence magnetic resonance imaging in evaluation of acetabular labrum. J Orthop Sci 4:328–332, 1999.
53. Kubo, T., Horii, M., Yamaguchi, J., Inoue, S., Fujioka, M., Ueshima, K., and Hirasawa, Y. Acetabular labrum in hip dysplasia evaluated by radial magnetic resonance imaging. J Rheumatol 27:1955–1960, 2000.
54. Kuklo, T. R., Mackenzie, W. G., and Keeler, K. A.: Hip arthroscopy in Legg-Calve-Perthes disease. Arthroscopy 15:88–92, 1999.
55. Lage, L. A., Patel, J. V., and Villar, R. N. The acetabular labral tear: an arthroscopic classification. Arthroscopy 12:269–272, 1996.
56. Lecouvet, F. E., Vande Berg, B. C., Malghem, J., Lebon, C. J., Moysan, P., Jamart, J., and Maldague, B. E. MR imaging of the acetabular labrum: variations in 200 asymptomatic hips. AJR 167:1025–1028, 1996.

57. Leunig, M., Werlen, S., Ungersbock, A., Ito, K., and Ganz, R. Evaluation of the acetabular labrum by MR arthrography. J Bone Joint Surg (Br) 79:230–234, 1997.

58. Leunig, M., Werlen, S., Ungersbock, A., Ito, K., and Ganz, R. Evaulation of the acetabular labrum by MR arthrography [published erratum appears in J Bone Joint Surg Br 1997 Jul;79(4):693]. J Bone Joint Surg (Br) 79:230–234, 1997.

59. McCarthy, J. C., and Busconi, B.: The role of hip arthroscopy in the diagnosis and treatment of hip disease. Orthopedics 18:753–756, 1995.

60. Miller, T. T. MR arthrography of the shoulder and hip after fluoroscopic landmarking. Skel Radiol 29:81–84, 2000.

61. Nelson, M. C., Lauerman, W. C., Brower, A. C., and Wells, J. R. Avulsion of the acetabular labrum with intraarticular displacement. Orthopedics 13:889–891, 1990.

62. Niitsu, M., Mishima, H., and Itai, Y. [High resolution MR imaging of the hip using pelvic phased-array coil]. Nippon Igaku Hoshasen Gakkai Zasshi 57:58–60, 1997.

63. Niitsu, M., Mishima, H., Miyakawa, S., and Itai, Y. High resolution MR imaging of the bilateral hips with dual phased-array coil. J Magn Reson Imaging 6:950–953, 1996.

64. Nishii, T., Nakanishi, K., Sugano, N., Naito, H., Tamura, S., and Ochi, T. Acetabular labral tears: contrast-enhanced MR imaging under continuous leg traction. Skel Radiol 25:349–356, 1996.

65. Nishina, T., Saito, S., Ohzono, K., Shimizu, N., Hosoya, T., and Ono, K. Chiari pelvic osteotomy for osteoarthritis. The influence of the torn and detached acetabular labrum. J Bone Joint Surg (Br) 72:765–769, 1990.

66. Noguchi, Y., Miura, H., Takasugi, S., and Iwamoto, Y. Cartilage and labrum degeneration in the dysplastic hip generally originates in the anterosuperior weight-bearing area: an arthroscopic observation. Arthroscopy 15:496–506, 1999.

67. Norman-Taylor, F. H., and Villar, R. N. Arthroscopic surgery of the hip: current status. Knee Surg Sports Traumatol Arthrosc 2:255–258, 1994.

68. Petersilge, C. A. Current concepts of MR arthrography of the hip. Semin Ultrasound CT MR 18:291–301, 1997.

69. Plotz, G. M., Brossmann, J., Schunke, M., Heller, M., Kurz, B., and Hassenpflug. J. Magnetic resonance arthrography of the acetabular labrum. Macroscopic and histological correlation in 20 cadavers. J Bone Joint Surg (Br) 82:426–432, 2000.

70. Ruch, D. S., and Satterfield, W. The use of arthroscopy to document accurate position of core decompression of the hip. Arthroscopy 14:617–619, 1998.

71. Sadro, C. Current concepts in magnetic resonance imaging of the adult hip and pelvis. Semin Roentgenol 35:231–248, 2000.

72. Santori, N., and Villar, R. N. Acetabular labral tears: result of arthroscopic partial limbectomy. Arthroscopy 16:11–15, 2000.

73. Schindler, A., Lechevallier, J. J., Rao, N. S., and Bowen, J. R. Diagnostic and therapeutic arthroscopy of the hip in children and adolescents: evaluation of results. J Pediatr Orthop 15:317–321, 1995.

74. Sekiya, J. K., Wojtys, E. M., Loder, R. T., and Hensinger, R. N. Hip arthroscopy using a limited anterior exposure: an alternative approach for arthroscopic access. Arthroscopy 16:16–20, 2000.
75. Seldes, R. M., Tan, V., Hunt, J., Katz, M., Winiarsky, R., and Fitzgerald, R. H., Jr. Anatomy, histologic features, and vascularity of the adult acetabular labrum. Clin Orthop Rel Res 232–240, 2001.
76. Skaggs, D. L., and Grelsamer, R. P. Use of a sheathed knife in hip arthroscopy. Orthop Rev 22:1171–1172, 1993.
77. Suzuki, S., Awaya, G., Okada, Y., Maekawa, M., Ikeda, T., and Tada, H. Arthroscopic diagnosis of ruptured acetabular labrum. Acta Orthop Scand 57: 513–515, 1986.
78. Suzuki, S., Kasahara, Y., Seto, Y., Futami, T., Furukawa, K., and Nishino, Y. Arthroscopy in 19 children with Perthes' disease. Pathologic changes of the synovium and the joint surface [see comments]. Acta Orthop Scand 65:581–584, 1994.
79. Ueo, T., and Hamabuchi, M. Hip pain caused by cystic deformation of the labrum acetabulare. Arthritis Rheum 27:947–950, 1984.
80. Vahlensieck, M., Peterfy, C. G., Wischer, T., Sommer, T., Lang, P., Schlippert, U., Genant, H. K., and Schild, H. H. Indirect MR arthrography: optimization and clinical applications. Radiology 200:249–254, 1996.
81. Villar, R. Hip arthroscopy. J Bone Joint Surg (Br) 77:517–518, 1995.
82. Villar, R. Hip arthroscopy [editorial]. J Bone Joint Surg (Br) 77:517–518, 1995.
83. Williams, M. S., Hutcheson, R. L., and Miller, A. R. A new technique for removal of intraarticular bullet fragments from the femoral head. Bull Hosp Joint Dis 56:107–110, 1997.
84. Rashleigh-Belcher, H. J., and Cannon, S. R. Recurrent dislocation of the hip with a "Bankert-type" lesion. J Bone Joint Surg 75B:183–185, 1986.

12
Computer-Assisted Orthopaedic Surgery for the Hip

Anthony M. DiGioia III, Frederic Picard, Branislav Jaramaz, James Moody, and Anton Plakseychuk
The Western Pennsylvania Hospital and Carnegie Mellon University, Pittsburgh, Pennsylvania

I. INTRODUCTION AND BACKGROUND

Neurosurgeons and craniofacial surgeons were among the first surgical specialists to research and develop technology for computer-assisted surgery (58). Accuracy requirements and potential major complications in many procedures led surgeons and computer scientists to work together in order to implement new surgical devices designed to improve reliability and consistency of difficult surgical procedures.

Orthopaedic surgeons performing spinal instrumentation were the first orthopaedic specialists to look into computer assisted technology (34,47). Computer-assisted orthopedic surgery (CAOS) refers to an expanding list of computer-enabled technologies that are known by many different names, including robotic assistive tools, computer-assisted surgery, computer-integrated surgery, image-guided surgery, surgical navigation, computer-integrated advanced orthopaedics, stereotactic guidance, and computer-assisted medical interventions.

Derived from CAD/CAM (computer assisted design/computer assisted machining) technology developed in the eighties, a spectrum of computer-assisted surgical approaches were developed in hip replacement surgery: the robotics assistive concept for femoral canal milling and navigation for cup orientation. Total hip replacement was one of the first computer-assisted orthopaedic surgical applications.

Avoiding or at least minimizing the number of complications was the goal for implementing computer-assisted hip systems. The ultimate goals of computer-assisted orthopaedic technology are to improve the accuracy of surgical procedures, to reduce variation from optimal solutions, to enable less invasive surgical techniques, and to "close the loop" in outcomes studies (16).

These technologies have already undergone several cycles of testing, improvement, and validation in other surgical domains. Orthopaedics surgery is especially well suited for the use of these technologies because of the rigidity of human bone. Unlike many soft tissues, bone can be precisely imaged noninvasively, drilled and cut by conventional hand tools; and predictably manipulated without significant deformation.

A growing number of operating rooms around the world are now equipped with CAOS tools, and numerous orthopaedic surgeons are being assisted by computers and computer-enabled technologies. These synergistic partnerships of humans and machines benefit patients by increasing the accuracy of surgical execution as well as the amount of surgically relevant information available to the physician before, during, and after surgery.

Although computer-enabled technologies may use sophisticated tools, the methodology underlying all CAOS technologies is simple: synergistic combinations of surgeons and machines that combine the best human abilities and the advantageous characteristics of machines to produce results that are better than would be possible otherwise. Humans and machines have several complementary advantages that are useful in surgical scenarios.

A. Early Developments

In 1979, two clinical research groups introduced methods by which computed tomography (CT) image data were used to manufacture models of patient anatomy. Tonner (59) and coworkers recommended the use of CT to construct an actual-sized three-dimensional model for the conservative resection of malignant lesions of the pelvis. In a coincident effort, Burri (11) in Germany also reported a similar approach for total hemipelvectomies. The custom prostheses were then designed using the CT and three-dimensional reconstruction data.

In 1982, Nerubay reported a technique of building hemipelvic prostheses using CT. This prosthesis had to be accurately constructed, matching the size and shape of the original bone. A CT scan and three-dimensional reconstruction model was used to design and machine perfectly fitting implants (39).

Several teams have worked on computer-aided interactive surgical simulation systems. In the early eighties, Fujioka and collaborators were among the first to introduce such computer-assisted system planning. In 1989, they presented a three-dimensional surface-reconstruction CT imaging system used for orthopaedic surgery for various procedures, such as osteotomy simulation (20).

Murphy was one of the first authors to describe computer-aided simulation and design in orthopaedic surgery (37,38). Preoperative three-dimensional computer reconstruction of the hip enabled the authors to adjust a stem for a 28-year-old woman with congenital dislocation of the hip. Using three-dimensional models, the surgeon chose the ideal implant, which was then designed and machined using a computer-controlled milling machine.

Aldinger was also a pioneer of CAD/CAM/CAO in orthopaedic surgery (2). the authors described an algorithm allowing them to extract the intrafemoral and canal from CT scan images and deductively design an adapted implant that was subsequently machined. In 1984, Woolson and coworkers described three-dimensional image processing from CT and emphasized the accuracy of the 3D model with respect to the normal anatomy. This work was useful for pursuing 3D model reconstruction using CAD/CAM technology (64).

In 1986, Bechtold presented an overview of computer graphics in the design of custom orthopaedic implant. He reported the preliminary works of Giliberty et al. in the use of CAD/CAM techniques to custom design a femoral stem (23). Garg and Walker, the Muller Institute for Biomechanics in Bern (Switzerland), and the Hospital for Special Surgery in New York had all developed CAD/CAM systems for joint implant or model designs. At the end of the 1980s, numerous teams were working in this field, such as Herman, Vannier, Brand, and Rhodes (7,10,18,25,40,51,62). Some commercial firms also used CAD/CAM for prosthesis design, especially for implant sizing and quality control.

Sutherland wrote an article on computer-aided orthopaedic surgery in 1986, and he concluded that "real time operative rehearsal, precision surgical planning and execution, and interactive teaching programs will be widely used once the costs associated with this technology come within the reach of clinical and teaching budgets" (56). Three areas were subsequently enhanced: research tools, 3D planning, and custom-made implants. At the same time, due to increasing power and decreasing cost of computer, researchers used this technology as a measurement tool for gait analysis (46) and spinal deformity evaluation (12).

In 1988, Haralson (24), and 2 years later, Pho (44) did an overview on computer applications in orthopaedics. Pho described four main applications: computerized medical information retrieval (as Haraldson did 2 years before), application in rehabilitation, applications in prosthetics, and computer graphics. He explained the importance of the work of Vannier and collaborators in producing 3D surface reconstructions of complex anatomical structures from CT scans (62). Actually, as mentioned previously, some other teams (29,54,60) also developed computational methods for 3D reconstructions. However, Michael Vannier and collaborators implemented a computer program that was more efficient in computation times and storage requirements and that could be added with modest effort to virtually any modern CT scanner. The work of Vannier et al. had already been used in craniofacial surgical planning and had also been evaluated but not developed in orthopaedic surgery. Whereas Hounsfield and coworkers first described CT in 1973 (1), 3D model visualization appeared almost 10 years later, owing to the need for advanced computers and new algorithms.

B. Robotic Technology

Using CAD/CAM technology to fit hip implants precisely gives rise to the concept of improving not just the machining of anatomic implants but also enhancing the quality of bone milling. Mittelstadt and Paul were the pioneers in using CAD technology and the patient's anatomy to machine the femoral canal for precise fitting of the femoral stem. In 1993, Mittelstadt and Paul described the development of a surgical robot for cementless total hip replacement (35,36). Mittelstadt, an engineer from the University of California at Davis, worked with IBM's Automation Research Division at Yorktown Heights and researched CT-guided total hip replacement. As a result of his research and collaborative work with other engineers and surgeons, such as H.A. Paul, the first robotic assistive system, called Robodoc, was introduced (43). Bargar from Sacramento, California, Borner from Frankfurt, Germany, and Bauer from Marbella, Spain, reported the different phases of the Robodoc project in 1998 (5). The European teams were more focused on knee robotic applications (32,33).

More recently, Orto Maquet of Rastatt, Germany, introduced another commercial orthopaedic robotic system called Computer Assisted Surgical Planning and Robotics (CASPAR), which was very similar to the Robodoc system. It was designed to assist the surgeons in total hip replacement (THR) (femoral stem implant) and more recently in knee surgery [total knee replacement (TKR) and anterior cruciate ligament (ACL) surgery] (31,61).

C. Navigation Technology

Soon after the introduction of the first robotic tools, navigation systems were developed and introduced into surgical practice. In 1995, Hans Reinhart, one of the pioneers in neurosurgery navigation technology, concluded that "compared with the automobile industry, computer-assisted surgery is now in about the year 1910" (48). Neurosurgeons and craniofacial surgeons were once again pioneers in this field of navigation. In 1995, only two interactive image assisted systems were known. The most advanced was the device of Kelly (27).

Using new processing of medical images, mathematicians, engineers, and physicians worked together to implement computer-assisted navigation systems (22,57). As mentioned previously, tremendous efforts were spent in the area of enhancement methods and methods for segmentation and filtering (17). Most important, the basic work on 3D registration enabled the surgeon to use preoperative images intraoperatively. Our purpose is not to describe in detail the accomplishments achieved in this field but to highlight the seminal advances.

Spine surgeons were the first to use the navigation technologies in orthopaedics, and Grenoble University in France had one of the leading teams in this approach (28). Their primary goal was to be able to place vertebral pedicle screws to avoid cord and nerve damage during trauma reconstruction or scoliosis surgery (34,47). Concomitantly, the groups at the Muller Institute in Bern, Switzerland, and the Center for Medical Robotics and Computer Assisted Surgery in Pittsburgh developed orthopaedic applications around the hip joint. This technology was used at Bern University in a system able to guide the very difficult periacetabular osteotomy procedure (30). Pelvic and surgical tools were tracked simultaneously during surgery and depicted on a computer screen that showed real-time updated information issuing directly from the CT patient's data. The HipNav was developed at the Center for Medical Robotics and Computer Assisted Surgery. A 3D reconstruction and simulation software also enabled surgeons to plan implant placement preoperatively and to predict postoperative range of motion and impingement. These data and preoperative plans were then transferred to a computer station in the operating room for interactive surgical navigation. This was the first hip navigation concept to be developed and used clinically (15). Later, several teams followed similar principles for other applications in the hip and knee, namely in Osaka, Japan and in Europe (Muller Institute, Bern, Switzerland) (22,53).

In the preoperative model approach, the 3D anatomy of the patient and surgical plans may be preoperatively generated from CT or MRI scans. Another approach recently developed, called intraoperative model navigation system, uses anatomic or kinematic information without the need for preoperative imaging. Using basic concepts developed for knee applications, some teams try to use data collected intraoperatively to orient the cup (14,50,52). However this non-image-based approach is still at the very first stage of development.

Computer-assisted image navigation technology (the preoperative model) is divided into two steps: (a) preoperative planning and simulation and (b) intraoperative surgical navigation, each of which is further broken down. The preoperative planner allows the surgeon to adjust and test the performance of the hip implants and optimize the outcomes before the surgery. The intraoperative guidance system allows the surgeon to measure and assist in accurate placement of acetabular cup and femoral stem. The intraoperative navigation requires additional steps to relate the position of the patient's pelvis to the CT scan and preoperative plan. This procedure, called registration, is a keystone of computer-assisted navigation technology. Bainville in 1999 explained the main principles of registration, tracking, and calibration (4).

1. Registration

Registration by definition consists of establishing a relationship between coordinate systems that are not in the same spatial or time domain. In other words, registration attempts to match anatomic data with the preoperative model images (Figure 1).

Taylor and Lavallee in 1995 reviewed the methodology and the state of the art in registration. Although several teams developed and adapted algorithms for intraoperative registration, we would like to emphasize the work from Sautot and Lavallee, of Grenoble, France, who developed one of the first efficient spine registration algorithms and Simon, of Pittsburgh, who defined the algorithm's principles for anatomic hip registration. Numerous teams followed these principles and thus improved the quality and efficiency of the registration (22,28,55).

2. Tracking

Tracking consists of following the motions and deformations of structures over time. In other words, all tracker systems (such as electromagnetic ones) can follow the position of tracked objects in real time with a localizer and provide continuous updates to the computer-assisted system (15,26). Navigation systems typically use optical or magnetic markers to track tools and the patient's bony anatomy (Figure 2).

3. Calibration

Calibration consists of establishing a relationship between coordinate systems that are in the same spatial and time domain. In other words, by using this procedure, all surgical tools equipped with a marker can be followed in real time and simultaneously tracked with the registered bones (Figure 3).

Surgical navigation systems permit intraoperative tracking and guidance of tools. Benefits of this approach include the facts that navigational

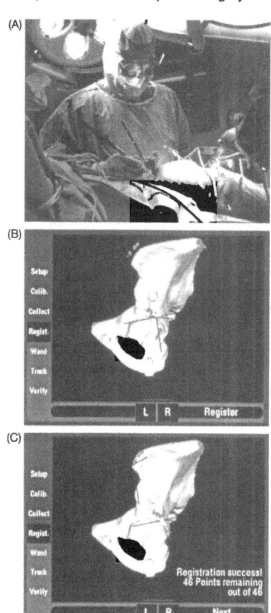

Figure 1 Registration of the pelvis. A. Point collection using a calibrated probe. B. Computer begins to match data sets. C. Computer found the solution matching points collected and preoperative model medical images.

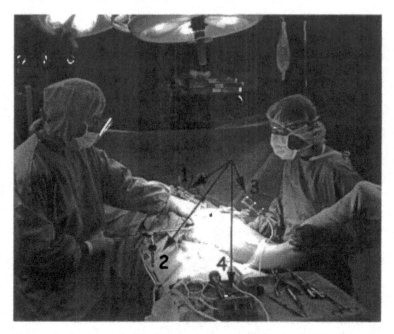

Figure 2 Trackers rigidly fixed on bones (1,3,4) and tool (2) and simultaneously followed in real time by an optical camera (see Figure 3).

tools do not require the rigid fixation of bones as typically used in robotics and that they permit surgeons to update plans intraoperatively. Several adult reconstruction surgical navigation systems for the hip are currently being used clinically. Computer-assisted total hip replacement is growing very fast and will affect the way surgery is done.

II. CLASSIFICATION SYSTEMS FOR CAOS TOOLS

Based on our survey of existing and developing computer-assisted ortho-paedic technologies, we proposed a broad classification system according to the following two basic categories: (a) robotic assistive tools and (b) surgical navigation systems (45).

A. Robotic Assistive Tools

These tools use robotic devices to perform or assist in performing surgical tasks. Three subclassifications of robotic systems have already been defined in the literature.

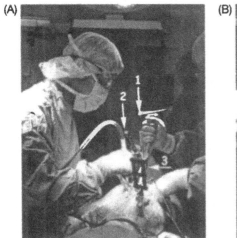 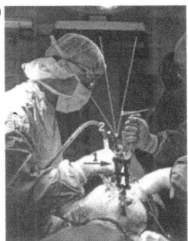

Figure 3 Traditional tools are preoperatively calibrated. A. Traditional tools (1) are equipped with an optical tracking (2) and calibrated. (3 = tracker on the bone). B. Optical camera is following the trackers rigidly fixed on the calibrated tools (2) and spatially localized with respect to the bone (tracker 1).

Active robotic systems perform some surgical task directly and autonomously, such as drilling or milling, without the direct intervention of the surgeon. The surgeon still works out the planning and approach and has the ability to stop or pause the robot during surgery. Robodoc and CASPAR robots belong to this category.

Semiactive robotic systems augment the surgeon's control of the tool. Such a system may not, for example, directly control a saw during a resection but may limit the depth or alignment of cut or milling. Most systems in this category restrict a task within a predetermined envelope by enforcing constraints. The concept was developed and tested for total knee arthroplasty, but is not yet used for THR.

Passive robotic tools assist in some part of the surgical procedure; they perform under the continuous and direct control of the surgeon. For example, a passive robot may be used to position a template or cutting guide block. Again, this concept was developed and tested for total knee arthroplasty, but is not yet used for THR.

B. Surgical Navigation Systems

Surgical navigation systems (SNS) are computer-assisted devices that display information for orientation and guidance during the surgical procedure.

They may present planar or 3D anatomical images based on CT or MRI scans, preoperative plans, simple graphics, or a combination of images (for example, icons superimposed on radiographic data). SNS can be loosely classified into two groups depending on whether the system is based on preoperative imaging or the collection of data intraoperatively.

1. Preoperative Model Systems

Preoperative model systems rely on preoperatively generated anatomic models, usually from CT (or MRI) data sets. This approach can provide a wealth of detailed information typically but not exclusively is used in conjunction with a planning system that includes surgical simulations. Preoperative imaging systems can be either patient-specific or non-patient-specific.

> *Patient-specific* means that a preoperative model of the patient's anatomy is created from the specific data of the particular patient. For example, the preoperative plan can be based on CT images of the patient, and these data will be used for reference and guidance during the surgical procedure. HipNav belongs to this category.
>
> *Non-patient-specific* means that the preoperative model is based on a generic shape or model of the anatomy. A homothetic model resulting from a generic model derived from images or digitized cadaver bones can be used during the surgical procedure. Typically, there is scaling and fitting of data to individual geometry information that is available. The concept has emerged for ACL reconstruction surgery (19).

2. Intraoperative Model Systems

Intraoperative model systems develop partial or complete anatomical models through intraoperative data collection. Those intraoperative model systems can be divided in two categories depending on their use of imaging.

> *Image based systems* provide intraoperative images (such as a set of coordinated fluoroscopic images) that are generated during the surgical procedure and used as a frame of reference and for guidance. Numerous trauma applications, as for femoral neck and intertrochanteric fractures, are in clinical trial investigation.
>
> *Non-image-based* systems provide all the information required for the navigation tool. This is determined from the direct measurement of the bone surface (using, for instance, a calibrated and tracked probe) or from direct measurement of limb kinematics (e.g., computing rotational centers from relative bone movement). Prototypes are in clinical evaluation (50).

This classification scheme relies upon clinical rather than technical criteria and is based on clinical requirements and functionality.

III. SURGICAL TECHNIQUE

Two computer-assisted systems are routinely used clinically: an active robotic assistive (for femoral milling) and a surgical navigation system (for cup placement).

A. Robotic Assistive Surgery

1. Preoperative Phase

a. Fiducial Fixation. Before the patient undergoes the CT scan of the pelvis and femur, the surgeon anchors three pin reference fiducials in the femoral bone under local anesthesia. These reference fiducials are typically titanium screws and are fixed in the greater trochanter and the two femur condyles. These fiducials must be placed carefully in order to avoid any secondary complications (such as a screw in the knee joint). These screws have to be easily accessible during surgery as well so the robotic arm can reach them for registration. (A method without preoperative fiducial fixation has been developed and is currently being tested in Europe) (5,6). The patient then undergoes at CT scan.

b. Planning. Using planning software, the surgeon fits the model of the hip implant in the patient's pelvic model. Frontal, sagittal, and transverse planes and 3D views are displayed. The surgeon ends the planning session by storing all the information regarding implant type, orientation, and size. This step adds approximately 10 to 15 min to the overall procedure. Hip revision can also be planned using the same procedure; the surgeon defines the ideal path for removing cement around implants (5).

c. Preparation of the Robot. The robot is then calibrated. The goal of robot calibration is to provide spatial orientation to the robot.

2. Surgical Steps

a. Surgical Approach and Preparation of the Acetabulum. The surgical approach is identical to a traditional technique. After cutting the femoral neck, the acetabulum is prepared according to conventional procedure.

b. Robot Calibration and Preparation of the Femur. A special arm of the robot is equipped with a clamp that is firmly fixed on the upper aspect of the femur. Fiducials preoperatively anchored in the femoral bone are then surgically exposed. The tip of the robot is then equipped with a probe, which precisely fits to each metallic fiducial. The computer determines the spatial position of these fiducials with respect to the femur, which is firmly stabilized with a clamp (Figure 4). At the end of the registration procedure, the robot has accurately located the fiducials and matched the preoperative plan to the actual patient anatomy.

c. *Milling the Femur.* Once the verification steps are done, the probe is removed from the robotic arm and is replaced by a milling burr. Afterwards, active milling begins under constant irrigation. The milling path follows the path planned preoperatively. During this procedure, the surgeon monitors the robot's progress, which is displayed continuously on a computer screen. Femoral pathway images are permanently updated and the surgeon can stop the robot arm at any time in case of abnormal event. In addition to this control, the robot stops by itself if the bone is dense or if

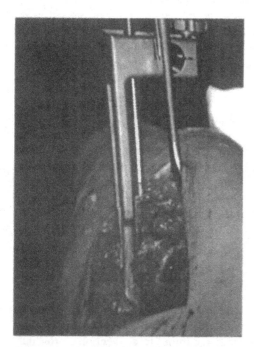

Figure 4 Femoral clamp secured on the upper femur during a robotic assistive procedure. (Courtesy of Dr. Andre Bauer, Marbella High Care Orthopaedic Center, Marbella, Spain.)

the bone fixture is becoming too slack. In case of interruption, the milling procedure can then be restarted (Figure 5).

   d. Implant Fitting.   The robot is then removed from the OR site and the final uncemented implant is secured. The surgeon must also remove all the fiducial screws.

B.   Computer-Assisted Navigation Surgery

We have chosen to describe the first computer assisted hip system (HipNav for Hip Navigation), which has already undergone several cycles of testing. HipNav has three components. The first is a preoperative planner. The second is a range-of-motion simulator that displays and animates the range of motion of the hip to predict impingement conditions for any position of the patient's leg. The third component is the intraoperative navigational system, which enables the surgeon to measure and accurately place the implant in the planned position. Here, we emphasize the intraoperative phase.

   Intraoperative navigation guidance uses a tracking system that senses the location and orientation of markers attached to the tools and the patient's bones. The basic intraoperative components are as follows:

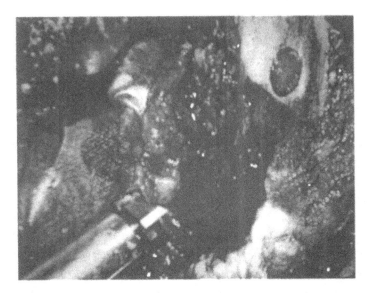

Figure 5   Milling of the femur. (Courtesy of Dr. Andre Bauer, Marbella High Care Orthopaedic Center, Spain.)

1. Computer

At the heart of any surgical navigation system is a computer to run to the application. The various inputs include patient data, surgeon control, and measurements from the position measurement system. The output includes instruction and measurement feedback to the surgeon.

2. Localizer

The localizer measures the position and orientation of targets within the operative volume. Two technologies are currently in use: optical and electromagnetic. Optical systems can use active and/or passive targets but require direct line of sight between the detector and targets. Electromagnetic systems do not require line of sight but can have difficulty in the presence of metal, and they tend to have a smaller working volume (Figure 6).

3. Targets

Any rigid object (tool or bone) to be tracked by a localizer must be equipped with suitable targets. Optical systems may use active or passive (reflective)

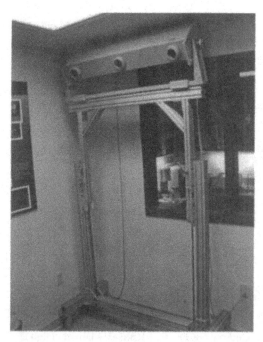

Figure 6   Optical position sensor (Optotrak, Northern Digital, Waterloo, Canada.)

targets. Electromagnetic targets are typically active transmitters and/or receivers.

In order to measure intraoperative bone and mechanical jig positions an association must be established between each object and its attached tracker. Once the association has been established, the object's position and orientation can be inferred from the motion of the attached target. Thus intraoperative measurements between bone and tools can be measured. To establish the relationship two options are possible. The first is to calibrate the traditional surgical device equipped with a tracker. Once the tool calibration is performed, the localizer can follow the jig assembly in real time. This option is used by several image guided systems such as HipNav. The surgical device is equipped with a marker and is calibrated for orienting throughout the surgical procedure (15,26). The second option is to use traditional untracked instruments and then use a specific tracked tool to measure their orientation. This option has not been chosen in any hip navigation systems yet but has been described for knee application. Actually, the traditional jigs are secured as usual and a calibrated removable device is adjusted enabling the computer assisted system to measure the jig orientation (Figure 7).

Based on the preoperatively determined implant size and alignment, the surgeon uses the navigation system to ensure the proper implant place-

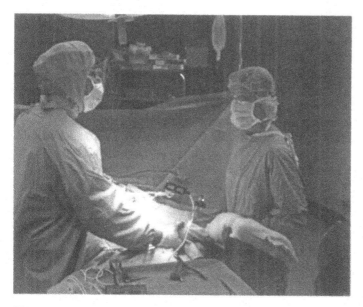

Figure 7 ROM (range of motion) control.

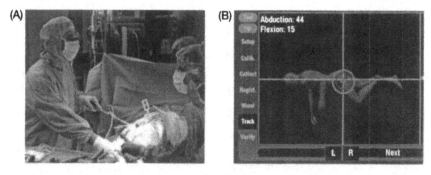

Figure 8 Improvement of the surgical control. A. Intraoperative view of HipNav/ Cup orientation. B. Graphical interface allowing the surgeon to navigate the cup.

ment. First, the preoperative plan is registered to the position of the patient on the operating room table. A surface-based registration method using pre- and intraoperative data is used, where the surgeon uses a digitizing probe to select a series of points along the surfaces of the pelvis and femur (see Figure 1). These data are used to accurately align the intraoperative position of the patient to the images used for preoperative planning without the use of metal pins or other invasive procedures. Once the positions of the pelvis and femur are known, they can be tracked at all times during surgery, thus eliminating the need for rigid fixation. The bones and tools are tracked in space using optical tracking technology. Infrared LED targets are attached to the patient's bones and to conventional surgical tools to allow accurate (0.1 mm) and high-speed (100 Hz) tracking of these objects with an optical tracking camera throughout the surgery. Based upon these continuous measurements, the location of the implant or any tools used to prepare the bone can be reliably determined, measured, and followed.

Since the location of the implant is tracked relative to the bone, navigational feedback can be provided to the surgeon on a computer monitor. Using a simple interface and aligning the crosshairs on the monitor, the surgeon is able to achieve the desired position and orientation of the implants as specified in the preoperative planner and to incorporate necessary adjustments during surgery (Figure 8).

IV. CLINICAL CHALLENGES AND POTENTIAL SOLUTIONS

The surgical techniques can be distinctly different for robotic-assisted versus navigation systems. It is important for surgeons to understand each step and to also understand potential pitfalls in order to avoid clinical problems. Two types of systems for THR are currently in routine use in the OR: (1) robotic assistive systems for stem positioning and (2) navigation systems for cup placement. Robotic assistive surgery and surgical navigation for total hip replacement initially was conceived to improve stem fit and alignment. Acetabular and femoral component placement is critical for outcomes in THR and reduction of short- and long-term complications. The current design of mechanical alignment guides for the stem and especially the cup requires that the patient's bony anatomy to be stabilized in a predetermined orientation. Several practical problems make it impossible to set and maintain the pelvis or femur in a known orientation. These include uncertainty due to limited surgical visibility, compliance of soft tissue (especially in large patients) and inability to rigidly secure internal anatomic structures. Conventional guides cannot compensate for any deviation from the required positions. Both types of systems have the following four goals:

Improving planning and simulation
Improving surgical control (less variation from optimal goal)
Achieving less invasive and more accurate surgery
Documenting surgical techniques (closing the loop for outcomes studies)

A. Improving Planning and Simulation

We have chosen to describe the HipNav planner as a representative and the most comprehensive total hip replacement planner. Conventional planning relies upon planar radiological information. Traditionally, the surgeon overlays acetate templates of implants over the damaged hip in the AP pelvic view. According to additional geometric line constructions drawn directly on the x-ray, the surgeon determines the best fit, implant size, and leg-length evaluation. However, this type of planning only permits the surgeon to roughly approximate the implant size and orientation. Actual intraoperative measurements such as intramedullary canal identification are often necessary for stem alignment.

Using the patient's CT scan and 3D models of the pelvis and the femur derived from the scan, an interactive and intuitive planner has been developed to determine implant size and orientation of the prosthetic components (15,26,49). The planner is subdivided into three steps: (a) an acetabular plan, (b) a femoral plan, and (c) a combined ROM simulation and final implant adjustments.

The first step is the acetabular plan and consists of identifying anatomical landmarks in order to define the pelvic reference coordinate system.

Four bony landmarks define the pelvic frame of reference: the right and the
left anterior iliac spine and the pubic tubercles. Acetabular component angles
are expressed with respect to this anterior pelvic plane. In the HipNav planner, an automatic identification of these four landmarks is used. The surgeon
can verify the proper position of the anterior plane. The size and orientation
of the native acetabulum is calculated from the surface model of the pelvis
by fitting a sphere into the acetabulum. Then a full 3D model of the acetabular component is positioned by the surgeon using three orthogonal cross
sections of the CT scan and the 3D pelvic model. The exact model and size
are selected from the implant database and the surgeon selects the orientation
(Figure 9).

The second step is femoral component placement. Following identical
principles described for the acetabulum, the surgeon identifies the femoral
anatomical landmarks that serve for reference coordinate system. Three
points are actually used to build the femoral frame plane: two on the posterior femoral condyles and one on the lesser trochanter and the femoral
axis parallel to that plane passing through the center of the femoral head
and midcondyles. A sphere is fitted to the native femoral head in three

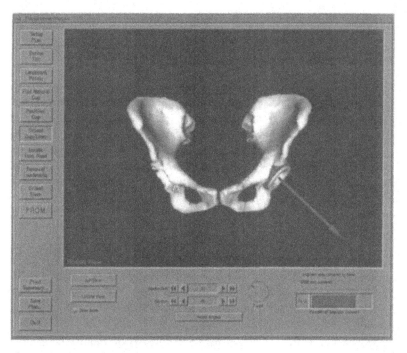

Figure 9 Cup orientation.

orthogonal cross sections of the CT scan and the 3D femoral femur model. An automatic software procedure overlays an implant of ideal size and orientation within the bony landmarks. The surgeon can interactively reorient and resize both components as necessary. The planner also permits the surgeon to modify neck lengths and different types of acetabular liners. All changes are continuously updated in real time (Figure 10).

The third component of the planner is the range-of-motion (ROM) simulation that is interactively performed for any number of leg motion paths, which is typically used to check anterior and posterior instability. After defining size and orientation, the surgeon can in real time verify bone and implant impingements by using the simulator. The surgeon can test and simulate any arbitrary ROM path, or modify cup, liner, and stem orientation in order to locate the ideal orientation of components with regard to ROM limits (Figure 11).

Once the surgeon has optimized implant orientation and size parameters, the information is stored for use either for navigation or robotic assistive systems.

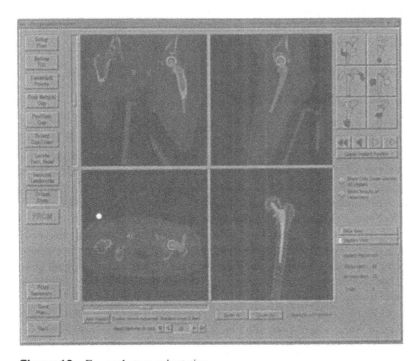

Figure 10 Femoral stem orientation.

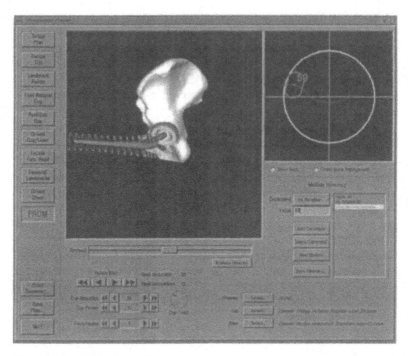

Figure 11   ROM simulation.

B.   Improving Surgical Control

In 2000, as the presidential guest lecturer in the journal *Clinical Orthopaedics and Related Research*, Peter Walker wrote about innovation in total hip
replacement and most specifically on the topic "When is new better?" In a
comprehensive report Walker presented major issues in THR. He also re-
minded us of the conclusions (from Swedish Joint Registry studies) showing
major variations in results and techniques between different centers (63).

Robotic and navigation technologies fulfill the requirements of precision and reproducibility and will likely represent important advancement in
the long term. Navigation systems like HipNav enable the surgeon to reliably
and accurately position the cup and the stem permitting online implant alignment, leg lengths, and patient-specific ROM simulations before and during
surgery.

A clinical trial using HipNav began in April 1997. The clinical information that was collected provided measurements that had never before been
available to surgeons. One of the most important contributions of HipNav
and other computer-assisted systems is to provide the surgeons with an ac-

curate intraoperative measurement tool that can improve interactive surgical control. For instance, HipNav can intraoperatively track movements of the patient's bony anatomy in real time during all phases of surgery and also simultaneously track the surgical tools (Figure 12).

Furthermore, the final position of the implants can also be measured. These measurements and immediate data will permit surgical technique to be related directly to patient outcomes.

HipNav was first used as a measurement tool. Using traditional cup placement instrumentation, more than 130 cups were monitored. Following the manufacturer's instructions, the goal of the surgery was to place the cup in 45 degrees of abduction and 20 degrees of anteversion. With respect to the anterior pelvic plane, final cup positions were tracked, measured, and stored. This first clinical trial showed that 75% of the cups were outside of Lewinnek's "safe" zone (Figure 13).

These systems have the potential to measure every step of the surgical procedure, determine the ideal position and relationships between femoral and acetabular implants, and—most importantly—to evaluate leg length and ROM intraoperatively.

Regarding the robotic assistive technology, the robot can significantly improve the accuracy of femoral preparation. In 1998, Bargar et al. published a study in which expert independent radiographic reviewers found statistically significant differences between the Robodoc group and traditional femoral preparation groups. The authors concluded that "these improved radiologic results for patients in the Robodoc group represent surrogate variables that indicate probable improvement in long term clinical performance" (5).

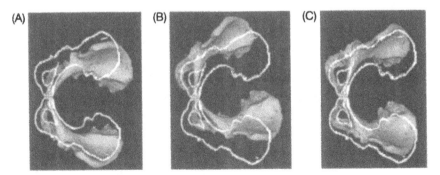

Figure 12 Pelvic motion during THR surgery (pelvic outlines = fixed pelvic on the surgical table and pelvic bone = several real pelvic positions during the surgical procedure).

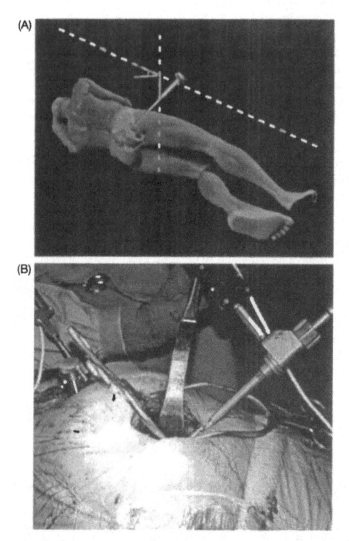

Figure 13 Computer assisted measurement of final cup orientation. A. Manufacturer's instruction for cup placement. B. Intraoperative view of HipNav/Cup orientation. C. Cup orientation using a mechanical traditional guide and measured with the computer-assisted system. Green surface is the "safe zone" of Lewinnek et al.; gray dots are cup orientations.

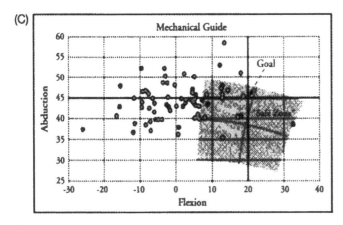

Figure 13 Continued

C. Less Invasive Surgery

All surgeons early in training are taught that wide "surgical exposure" is amoung the most important factors in total hip arthroplasty. Traditionally, it was impossible to achieve accurate fixation and orientation of the implant without complete visualization of the landmarks. Little attention was paid to complications related to the exposure. The Norwegian Arthroplasty Register reported 0.8% mortality rate in 39,543 patients during the first 60 post-operative days after total hip replacement. Also, despite the good overall results of THA, this procedure requires lengthy recovery time. Knutsson and Engberg reported significant difference in patients' total, physical, and psychosocial quality of life 6 months postoperatively compared to the situation prior to the operation, but not between the situation before and 6 weeks after the total hip replacement (27a).

Access to surgical navigation technologies and computer-assisted tools creates opportunity to develop less invasive surgical techniques for total hip replacement. Use of surgical navigation helps to achieve accurate fixation and orientation of the implant without complete visualization of the landmarks.

Using computer-assisted hip navigation technology (HipNav), surgeons developed minimal incision techniques for total hip replacement based on the posterior approach and compared results to traditional posterior approach in patients with similar HHS (Harris hip score) and age. The average length of skin incisions for the mini-incision group was on average 11.7 cm; it was 20.2 cm for traditional incision group.

Improvement in HHS was significantly better in the mini-incision group at 3 and 6 months. There was no significant difference in HHS between groups at 1-year follow-up. At 3 months follow-up, patients in the mini-incision group had significant improvement in limp ($p < 0.05$) and stair-climbing ($p < 0.01$) compared to the traditional incision group. At 6 months follow-up, the mini-incision group was significantly better in terms of limp ($p < 0.05$), distance walked ($p < 0.001$), and stair-climbing ($p < 0.001$). There was no difference between groups in pain, function, and range of motion at 1-year follow-up. The conclusion of the study was that less invasive THA result in less soft tissue disruption, which reduces pain, speeds healing and recovery, and potentially reduces complications (Figure 14).

D. Documenting Surgery

CAOS technologies integrate advanced sensors and high-resolution graphics to acquire and present information to the surgeon in an intuitive, easy-to-use manner. Preoperative images such as those provided by CT (and MRI, which is not currently used in hip surgery) offer patient-specific 3D images of musculoskeletal anatomy. Intraoperative sensors, such as optical trackers, measure a multitude of variables, including bone, implant, and tool positions and orientations. These preoperative and intraoperative data represent an immense source of information enabling the surgeon to document each case in detail. CAOS information systems are capable of measuring the variation from optimal surgical practice and to directly relate patient outcomes to

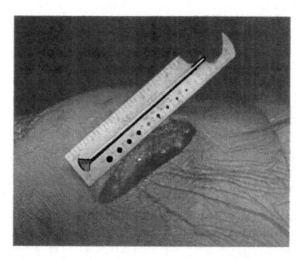

Figure 14   Mini-incision after using computer-assisted navigation.

surgical technique. Tightly coupled and integrated preoperative planning and imaging, quantifying surgical techniques and directly relating patient's outcomes to surgical practice, define what we have called "closing the loop in surgical practice" (16).

V. BENEFITS OF COMPUTER-ASSISTED ORTHOPAEDIC SURGERY

Computer-guided surgical robotic and navigation systems have the potential to become standard operating room tools for many commonly performed surgical procedures. These "smart" tools and computer assisted technologies are being developed to enable surgeons to more accurately achieve their objectives. These new devices and approaches to surgery will promote improved clinical outcomes and are a critical step towards the development of minimally invasive surgical techniques.

A. Measuring Current Surgical Technique

The primary goals driving the adoption of CAOS technologies are optimization of surgical performance and the patient's biological response. Computer-assisted orthopaedic systems enhance progress toward these goals by increasing both the timeliness and accuracy of information (navigation) and the precision of (robotic) surgical performance.

CAOS systems are capable of registering patient-specific preoperative images, models, and surgical plans with the actual patient on the operating table with greater accuracy than when the surgeon operates with conventional means. Surgical accuracy is also improved by the use of computer-controlled sensor and graphics systems that provide real-time feedback on the relative positions of bones, tools, and implants. Improved implant alignment, implant fit and joint function should lead to less wear, less loosening, fewer revisions, and less invasive approaches (21).

Computer-assisted navigation technologies integrate advanced sensors and high-resolution graphics to acquire and present information to the surgeon in an intuitive, easy-to-use manner. Preoperative images such as those from CT and MRI provide patient-specific 3D images of musculoskeletal anatomy and measure a multitude of variables, including bone, implant, and tool positions and orientations.

All CAOS systems involve a registration process to determine the geometrical correspondence between the surgical plan and the patient. Registration can also introduce errors and is the least reliable element—and least understood by clinicians—of most CAOS systems (13). While some surgeons see the use of preoperative CT scans and imaging as an advantage, others see this as an additional and costly requirement. However, the image-guided hip navigation technology still remains the only validated system for cup navigation. The other systems in development, such as non-image-based systems—still must go through the entire validation process.

Most importantly, we need to validate these systems clinically by demonstrating improvements in patient outcomes. For instance, improved femoral machining to achieve a near-perfect stem fit does not necessarily translate into better long-term survivorship. Long-term follow-up is necessary to demonstrate the relationship between surgical technique and outcomes. In the same way, using computer-assisted technology for improving the cup positioning must decrease complications such as dislocations and implant impingement. However, long-term follow-up is necessary to derive a final conclusion.

Long-term studies of computer-assisted hip robotic and navigation tools will be the only way to prove real benefit of computer assisted technology. Three decades ago, orthopaedic surgeons had similar concerns about the cost-effectiveness of hip arthroplasty. One of the major questions was then to prove that arthroplasty was cost-effective and represented a good investment by society despite the high cost. Numerous studies proved that hip arthroplasty was more cost-effective than any other medical treatment in osteoarthritis (3). These studies were conducted more than 30 years after total hip replacement became a regular surgery. Computer-assisted technology must go through all these hurdles before becoming a universally accepted technology.

Although the total hip replacement is a routine surgery with an excellent survivorship after 15 years, failures can occur that adversely affect patient outcomes. In order to reduce these issues, computer-assisted technology should control the factors potentially involved in THR failures. Better knowledge of hip kinematics and causes of failure enabled the building of computer-assisted systems able to control factors responsible for failures. Computer-assisted navigation systems are indeed capable of measuring the variation from optimal surgical practice and directly relate patient outcomes to surgical technique. Future clinical trials and long-term studies should give us a part of the final answer as to whether computer assisted technology will improve patient outcomes. In the meantime, clinical researchers can also use CAOS technologies to measure and document surgical technique for the very first time.

B. Improving the Current Surgical Technique

Many more CAOS technologies are being investigated today than are being clinically applied. The path from concept to clinical practice can be long and arduous. Innovations in this area require the collaborative efforts of multidisciplinary research groups with representation from medicine, engineering, computer science, and robotics. Technologies need to be successfully adapted for orthopaedic application and to address real clinical problems. Then, testing, technical and clinical verification, and outcome studies are required. Tests often begin on artificial anatomic models, such as "sawbones." Clinical trials on animals or humans may be required as part of the regulatory approval process. In the United States, approval from the U.S. Food and Drug Administration (FDA) is required to market the tools, although clinical trials can move forward with an Investigational Device Exception (IDE). The European community requires a CE Mark certification. Any trials conducted with human subjects also require the signed consent of patients and formal approval by the internal review board of the participating hospital. Finally, surgeon, patient, and insurer must accept the technology before it becomes a part of routine clinical practice.

Beyond the benefits that accrue directly to the patient, CAOS technologies as well as robotic and navigation systems may have great impact on surgical practice. With more surgically relevant information available to the surgeon, both intra- and intersurgical adjustments of technique are possible and outcome studies will be facilitated. The result and changes in surgical technique will be more easily observed, efforts to improve on technique will become more systematic, and better techniques will be disseminated through publications and adopted by surgeons. In this way, the entire orthopedic surgical community will benefit from research in CAOS even before access to CAOS technologies becomes ubiquitous. Physicians in training will benefit immensely from CAOS technologies in a manner analogous to the training airplane pilots receive from flight simulators. Instructors will be able to introduce unforeseen circumstances in surgical simulators and observe students' ability to handle them, and surgeons in training

Table 1 Adoption of the Technology and Improvement in Patient Outcomes

Short-term
    Measure and reduce the variability in clinical practice
    Improve precision and accuracy and reduce complications in commonly
        performed procedures
Long term
    Develop techniques to make procedures minimally or less invasive
    Develop the next generation of surgical tools and techniques using computer
        vision to supplement direct and videoscopic images

will be able to perfect their skills before operating on an actual patient (Table 1).

Over the long term, CAOS technologies will allow procedures to be performed less invasively and with increased accuracy. Although the invasiveness of many current orthopaedic procedures cannot be reduced owing to the minimum required by template and implant geometries, future techniques that do not rely on conventional templates and implants, such as tissue-engineered implants, will be conducive to minimally invasive surgical (MIS) procedures. The many benefits of MIS include fewer complications, less risk of infection, less disruption of the blood supply, less bleeding, less damage to soft tissue, reduced pain, accelerated healing and recovery, shorter hospital stay, less time away from work, and improved cosmesis.

VI. FUTURE OF COMPUTER-ASSISTED TECHNOLOGY

Many promising technologies that are not yet in clinical use are being investigated in research laboratories. Semiactive surgical devices are being designed that can assist the surgeon to accurately drill, cut, and machine the patient's bone according to a preoperative plan and combined with a navigation system. The surgeon and the semiactive device together guide the tool, the surgeon controlling the advancement of the tool, and the device constraining the cut to the precise line or surface determined in the preoperative plan.

Surgical simulators that allow physicians in training to see and feel the virtual anatomical structures just as if they were actually performing a procedure are under development (42). Telesurgical systems are under development in other surgical specialities; these may allow a surgeon to operate on a patient at a remote location (9). Augmented reality devices are being investigated that will enable a surgeon to see a 3D model of the patient's internal anatomy in correct registration with the patient's external anatomy even while the patient and the surgeon have freedom of motion (8). Noninvasive ultrasonic sensor technologies are being adapted for use in visualizing internal bone for both real-time registration and tracking during surgery.

In addition to the measurement tool, computer-assisted images can be used with new augmented reality systems. For instance, an image overlay system developed in Pittsburgh permits the display of medical images on the patient during surgery; in essence, this gives the surgeon "x-ray vision" (41) (Figure 15).

(A)

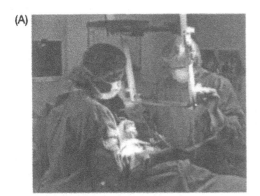

(B)

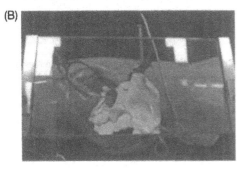

Figure 15 Image overlay. A. Image overlay visualization system, giving the surgeon "x-ray vision." B. Image overlay system displays medical images and preoperative plans overlaid on the patient. In this case, the surgeon can "see through" the patient, permitting display of a pelvic CT and planned acetabular implant orientation.

ACKNOWLEDGMENT

The authors would like to thank Dr. Andre Bauer for providing us with pictures of the Robodoc system.

REFERENCES

1. Ambrose J., Hounsfield G.N. Computed transverse axial tomography. Br J Radiol 1973; 46:148–149.
2. Aldinger G., Fischer A., Kurtz B. Computer aided manufacturing of individual endoprostheses. Arch Orthop Trauma Surg 1983; 102:31–35.
3. Ayers D.C., Berman A.T., Duncan C.P., et al. Economic Aspects of Total Joint Replacement. AAOS Committee on Hip and Knee Arthritis, 1997.

4. Bainville E., Bricault I., Cinquin P., Lavallee S. Concepts and methods of registration for computer integrated surgery. In: Nolte L.P., Ganz R., eds. Computer Assisted Orthopedic Surgery (CAOS). Part I. Bern: Hogrefe & Huber Publishers, 1999:15–34.

5. Bargar W., Bauer A., Borner M. Primary and revision total hip replacement using the Robodoc system. Clin Orthop Rel Res 1998; 354:82–91.

6. Bauer A. Robot assisted total hip replacement in primary and revision cases. Op Tech Orthop 2000; 10:9–13.

7. Bechtold J.E. Application of computer graphics in the design of custom orthopaedic implants. Clin Orthop Am 1986; 17(4):605–612.

8. Blackwell M., Morgan F., DiGioia A.M. Augmented reality and its future in orthopaedics. Clin Orthop 1998; 354(5):111–122.

9. Bowersox J.C. Telesurgery: Transitioning from development to clinical applications. In: DiGioia A.M., ed. Proceeding of the Third Annual North American Program on Computer Assisted Orthopaedic Surgery. Shadyside Hospital, 1999:237–328.

10. Brand R., Pedersen D. Computer modeling of surgery and a consideration of the mechanical effects of proximal femoral osteotomies. The hip. Proceeding of the Twelfth Open Scientific Meeting of the Hip Society. St. Louis: Mosby, 1984.

11. Burri C., Claes L., Gerngross H., Mathys J.R. Total internal hemipelvectomy. Arch Orthop Trauma Surg 1979; 94:219–226.

12. Daruwalla J., Balasubramaniam P. Moire topography in scoliosis—Its accuracy in detecting the site and size of the curve. J Bone Joint Surg (Br) 1985; 67(2):211–213.

13. Delp S.L., Stulberg S., Davies B., Picard F., Leitner F. Computer assisted knee replacement. Clin Orthop Rel Res 1998; 354:49–56.

14. Dessenne V., Lavallee S., Julliard R., Orti R., Martelli S., Cinquin P. Computer-assisted knee anterior cruciate ligament reconstruction. First clinical tests. In: Nolte L.P., Ganz R., eds. Computer Assisted Orthopedic Surgery (CAOS). Part IV. Bern: Hogrefe & Huber Publishers, 1999:190–197.

15. DiGioia A., Jaramaz B., Blackwell M., Simon D., Morgan F., Moody J.E., Nikou C., Colgan B., Aston C., Labarca R., Kischell E., Kanade T. Image guided navigation system to measure intraoperatively acetabular implant alignment. Clin Orthop Rel Res. 1998; 355:8–22.

16. DiGioia A., Jaramaz B. Computer assisted tools and interventional technologies. Lancet 1999:354.

17. Duncan J.S., Ayache N. Medical Image analysis: Progress over two decades and the challenges ahead. IEEE Transactions on Pattern analysis and machine intelligence. 2000; 22(1):85–106.

18. Essinger J.R., Rhodes M.L., Robertson D.D., Aubaniac J.M. Computer assisted prostheses selection. Proceedings of CAR'89:369–370.

19. Fleute M., Lavallee S., Julliard R. Incorporating a statistically-based shape model into a system for computer-assisted anterior cruciate ligament surgery. Medical Image Analysis. Vol. 3. New York: Oxford University Press, 1999: 209–222.

20. Fujioka M., Yokoi S., Yasuda T., Toriwaki J. Computer aided interactive surgical simulation system. Its clinical application. Proceedings of CAR'89:409–412.

21. Galante J.O. Overview of total hip arthroplasty. The Adult Hip. Vol II. Philadelphia: Lippincott Raven Publishers, 1998:829–838.

22. Gerig G., Szekely G. Visualization and image processing of medical image data. In: Nolte L.P., Ganz R., eds. Computer Assisted Orthopedic Surgery (CAOS). Bern: Hogrefe & Huber Publishers, 1999:1–14.

23. Giliberty R.P., Epstein H.Y., Faegenburg D. A prototype femoral stem using CAT and CAD/CAM. Orthop Rev 1983; 12(8):59–63.

24. Haralson R. Current concepts review. Computerized information retrieval and medical education for orthopaedics. J Bone Joint Surg 1998; 70A(4):624–629.

24a. Havelin L.I., Engesaeter L.B., Espehaug B., Furnes O., Lie S.A., Vollset S.E. The Norwegian Arthroplasty Register: 11 years and 73,000 arthroplasties. Acta Orthop Scand 2000; 71:337–353.

25. Herman G.T., Liu H.K. Three-dimensional display of human organs from computed tomograms. Comp Graphics Image Proc 1978; 7:130.

26. Jaramaz B., DiGioia A., Blackwell M., Nikou C. Computer assisted measurement of cup placement in total hip replacement. Clin Orthop Rel Res 1998; 354:70–81.

27. Kelly P.J., Alker G.J., Goerss S. Computer assisted stereostatic laser microsurgery for the treatment of intracranial neoplasms. Neurosurgery 1982; 14:172–177.

27a. Knutsson S., Engelberg I.B. An evaluation of patients' quality of life before, 6 weeks and 6 months after total hip replacement surgery. J Adv Nurs 1999; 30:1349–1359.

28. Lavallee S. Registration for computer-integrated surgery: Methodology, State of the art. In: Taylor, Lavallee, Burdea, Mosges, eds. Computer Integrated Surgery, Technology and Clinical Applications. Cambridge, MA: MIT Press, 1995:77–98

29. Latamore G.B. Creating 3D models for medical research. Comput Graphics World 1983; 7:31–28.

30. Langlotz F., Bachler R., Berlemann U., Nolte L.P., Ganz R. Computer assistance for pelvic osteotomies. Clin Orthop Rel Res 1998; 345:92–102.

31. Mai S., Lorke C., Siebert W. Motivation, realization and first results of robot assisted total knee arthroplasty. CAOS 2001. Davos, Switzerland, February 7–10.

32. Martelli S., Fadda P., Dario M., Marcacci M., Marcenaro G.P., Visani A. A laser scanner system for investigating noninvasive matching strategies in computer assisted orthopedic surgery. Proc Ann Inter Conf IEEE EMBS 1991; 13:1757–1758.

33. Martelli S., Beltrame F., Dario P., Fadda M. A system for computer and robot assisted knee implantation. Proceedings of the 14th IEEE Medicine and Biology Conference. Paris: 1992.

34. Merloz Ph., Tonetti J., Eid A. Computer assisted spine surgery. Clin Orthop Rel Res 1996; 337:86–96.

35. Mittelstadt B.D. Integrated surgical systems. Personal communication, June 1996.

36. Mittelstadt B.D., Kazanzides P., Zuhars J., Williamson B., Cain P., Smith F., Bargar W.L. The evolution of a surgical robot from prototype to human clinical use. First International Symposium on MRCAS. Vol. I. Pittsburgh: 1994: 397–407.

37. Murphy S.B., Kijewski P.K., Walker P.S., Scott R.D. Computer assisted preoperative planning of orthopaedic reconstructive surgery. Proceedings of CAR'93. Berlin: Springer-Verlag, 1993:413–418.

38. Murphy S.B., Kijewski P.K., Millis M.B., Harless A. Simulation of osteotomy surgery about the hip joint. Proceedings of CAR'87. Berlin: Springer Verlag, 1987:413–418.

39. Nerubay J., Robinstein Z., Katznelson A.M. Technique of building hemipelvic prosthesis using computer tomography. Proc Clin Biol 1981; 147–152.

40. Nelson P.C., Robertson D.D., Walker P.S., Granholm J.W. A computerized femoral intramedullary implant design package utilizing computed tomography data. Proceedings of CAR'93. Berlin: Springer-Verlag 1993:419–420.

41. Nikou C., DiGioia A., Blackwell M., Jaramaz B., Kanade T. Augmented reality imaging technology for orthopaedic surgery. Op Tech Orthop 2000; 10: 82–86.

42. O'Toole R.V., Playter R.R. Virtual reality surgical simulators and trainers. In: DiGioia A., ed. Proceedings of the Third Annual North American Program on Computer Assisted Orthopaedics Surgery. Pittsburgh: Shadyside Hospital, 1999:60–61.

43. Paul H.A. Surgical robot for total hip replacement surgery. Proceedings of the IEEE International Conference on Robotics and Automation, Nice, France: 1992. 1992:606–611.

44. Pho H., Lim S.Y.E. Pereira B. Computer applications in orthopaedics. Ann Acad Med 1990; 19(5):691–697.

45. Picard F., Moody J., Jaramaz B., DiGioia A., Nikou C., LaBarca S. A Classification proposal for Computer Assisted Knee Systems. Medical Image Computing and Computer Assisted Intervention, MICCAI 2000, 3rd International Conference, Pittsburgh. New York: Springer-Verlag, 2000:1145–1151.

46. Prodromos C., Andriacchi T., Galante J. A relationship between gait and clinical changes following high tibial osteotomy. J Bone Joint Surg 1985; 67A(8): 1188–1194.

47. Rampersaud Y.R., Foley K.T. Image-guided spinal surgery. Operative Techniques in Orthopaedics. Vol. 10. 2000:64–68.

48. Reinhardt H. Neuronavigation: A ten-year review. In: Taylor, Lavallee, Burdea, Mosges, eds. Computer Integrated Surgery. Technology and Clinical Applications. Cambridge, MA: MIT Press, 1995:329–341.

49. Richolt J.A., Teschner M., Everett P.C., Millis M.B., Kikinis R. Impingement

simulation of the hip in SCFE using 3D models. Comput Aid Surg 1999;4: 144–151.

50. Richolt J.A., Reu G., Graichen H., Froehling M., Leitner F. A simplified navigation system for hip cup implantation—System description and report of first cases. CAOS 2001: Davos, Switzerland, February 7–10.
51. Rhodes M.L. An algorithmic approach to controlling search in 3D image data. ACM SIGGRAPH'79, Proceedings 1979:134–142.
52. Sati M., Staubli H., Bourquin Y., Kunz M., Kasermann S., Nolte L.P. Clinical integration of computer-assisted technology for arthroscopic anterior cruciate ligament reconstruction. Op Tech Orthop 2000; 10:40–49.
53. Sato Y., Sasama T., Sugano N., Nakahodo K., Nishii T., Ozono K., Yonenobu K., Takahiro O., Tamura S. Intraoperative simulation and planning using a combined acetabular and femoral (CAF) navigation system for total hip replacement. Medical Image Computing and Computer-Assisted Intervention. MICCAI, Pittsburgh. New York: Springer-Verlag, 2000:14–25.
54. Schlegel W., Scharfenberg H., Doll J., Pasyr O., Sturm V., Netzeband G., Lorenz W. CT images as the basis of operation planning in stereotactic neurosurgery. Proceedings of the International Symposium Medical Imaging and Interpretation. 1982:172–177.
55. Simon D.A., Lavallee S. Medical Imaging and registration in computer assisted surgery. Clin Orthop Rel Res 1998; 354:17–27.
56. Sutherland C.J. Practical applications of computer generated three dimensional reconstruction in orthopedics surgery. Orthop Clin North Am 1986; 17(4):651–656.
57. Szeliski R., Lavallee S. Matching 3D anatomical surfaces with non rigid deformations using octree-splines. J Comput Vision 1996; 18(2):171–186.
58. Taylor R.H., Brendt D., Mittelstadt B.D., Paul H., Hanson W., Kazanzides P., Williamson B., Musits B., Glassman E., Bargar W. An image directed robotic system for precise orthopaedic surgery. In: Taylor, Lavallee, Burdea, Mosges, eds. Computer Integrated Surgery, Technology and Clinical Applications. Cambridge, MA: MIT Press, 1995:379–391.
59. Tonner H.D., Engelbrecht H. Ein neues Verfahren zur Herstellung alloplastischer Spezialimplantate fur den Beckenteilersatz. Fortschr Med 1979; 97: 781–783.
60. Udupa J.K. Display of 3D information in discrete 3D scenes produced by computerized tomography. Proc IEEE 1983; 71(3):420.
61. Van Ham G., Denis K., Vander Sloten J., Van Audekerche R., Van Der Perre G., De Schutter J., Aertbelien E., Demey S., Bellemans J Machining and accuracy studies for a tibial knee implant using a force controlled robot. Comput Aid Surg 1998; 3:123–133.
62. Vannier M.W., Marsh J.L., Warren J.O. 3-D CT reconstruction images for craniofacial surgical planning and evaluation. Radiology 1984; 150(1):179–184.
63. Walker P. Innovation in total hip replacement—When is new better? Clin Orthop Rel. Res 2000; 381:9–25.
64. Woolson S.T., Dev P., Fellingham L.L., Vassiliadis A. Three dimensional imaging of bone from computerized tomography. Clin Orthop 1986; 202:239–248.

13

A Five-Step Approach to Preoperative Planning in Total Hip Arthroplasty

Rajit Saluja and Rohit R. Dhir
St. Luke's Hospital Medical Center, Milwaukee, Wisconsin

William L. Bargar
Sutter Orthopedic Center, Sacramento, California

I. INTRODUCTION

Total hip arthroplasty (THA) provides excellent pain relief and improves the functional activity of patients with debilitating arthritis of the hip. The success of the procedure depends on the surgeon's ability to provide an implant with immediate stability that restores the biomechanics of the hip (3,4,6,15). Attainment of these surgical goals is limited by the fact that no single prosthesis is suitable for all patients because of individual variations in bone quality, bone anatomy, activity level, and the postoperative expectations of the patient. However, with thorough preoperative planning, these goals are attainable and any unexpected problems during surgery can be avoided.

Preoperative planning is presented as a five-step process and begins with the surgeon's introduction to the patient. A thorough history and physical examination constitute the first step in this process. Secondly, radiographs that accurately assess the patient's anatomy with measurable dimensions of the bones are needed. The third step requires the selection of the implant along with the method of implant fixation to bone. Next, the selected implants are templated onto the radiographs and the appropriate sizes are selected. The final step of this process evaluates any special considerations, such as underlying metabolic diseases, that require medical treatment either before or after surgery, anatomic deformities requiring correction, and any significant leg-length discrepancy. The surgical approach is also selected at this point and is based both on the need for any anatomical correction and also on the patient's activities or occupation. Certain patient lifestyles or occupations may be better addressed with the use of the posterior approach. The objective of revision total hip arthroplasty is presented separately. The same five-step approach is used for planning. Owing to the complex nature of revision surgery, each step of the planning process requires many additional considerations, which makes careful preoperative planning even more important.

II. STEP I—HISTORY AND PHYSICAL EXAMINATION

The first step in preoperative planning for THA begins with a thorough history. The underlying cause of arthritis is defined in the specific patient. A large percentage of patients with arthritic hips have significant underlying abnormalities that predispose to the development of arthritis (9). These abnormalities may be either congenital or developmental, such as various epiphyseal dysplasias, developmental dysplasia of the hip, Legg-Calve-Perthes disease, or slipped capital femoral epiphysis. Other possibilities are the various types of inflammatory arthritis, posttraumatic arthritis, avascular necrosis, and Paget's disease. It is important to define the underlying etiology, because each specific abnormality may be associated with either specific anatomical or biological characteristics that may need to be addressed either surgically or medically. Another important part of the history is determination of the patient's preoperative pain and function. Established tools such as the Harris hip score form or the SF-36 may be used and are helpful in documenting the improvement following surgery as well as to report the results in studies.

In addition to a thorough history, careful physical examination is an essential part of preoperative planning. This examination begins with inspection of the skin to check for previous incisions and to identify accompanying rashes. Psoriatic arthritis may often have psoriatic lesions on the skin overlying the hip. The range of motion is then measured in both the affected and the unaffected hips and any contractures are also noted. Typically there may be a flexion, adduction, or abduction contracture. The clinical leg-length discrepancy (LLD) is also calculated as measured from the umbilicus to the medial malleolus or from the anterior superior iliac spine to the medial malleolus. Muscle strength, especially of the hip abductors, is assessed both through manual testing and the presence of the Trendelenburg sign. A neurological exam documenting the integrity of the sciatic nerve function along with the documentation of the peripheral vasculature is also essential. The best way to ensure that all parts of the physical examination are completed is through the use of a form with a checklist (Figure 1).

III. STEP II—RADIOGRAPHIC EVALUATION

Good-quality radiographs with magnification markers are essential for accurate preoperative planning. The typical views include an anteroposterior (AP) pelvic along with AP and Lowenstein lateral views of the affected hip. The AP pelvic and the AP views are obtained with the legs internally rotated by 15–20 degrees (Figure 2) and allow assessment of the neck shaft angle, the lateral offset, and comparison with the opposite unaffected hip. In case of severe contractures, the patient may be unable to rotate the hip internally. A posteroanterior (PA) view of the hip may then be obtained with the patient prone and rolled toward the affected side and the hip externally rotated (Figure 3). The Lowenstein lateral view allows assessment of the femoral neck anteversion and also the level and extent of bow in the shaft of the femur (Figure 4) (6,7).

IV. STEP III—IMPLANT SELECTION

Several factors are considered in selecting an appropriate implant. The patient's age and activity level are important. Generally, the younger, more active patients are considered to be those with the highest demand; for them, cementless implants and some of the newer bearing surfaces may be appropriate. For older, less active, or low-demand patients treatment with hybrid THA and the traditional bearing surfaces is usually indicated.

The quality of bone is another factor that influences the method of implant fixation. Canal configurations, as described by Noble et al. (16), are defined by calculating the ratio of canal width 20 mm proximal to the lesser trochanter in relation to the width of the canal at the femoral isthmus (Figure 5) (16). This ratio is known as the canal flair index (CFI). If the ratio is less than 3.0, the canal has a stovepipe configuration; if the ratio is greater than 4.7, the canal has a champagne flute configuration. A ratio of 3.0–4.7 is considered to be in the normal range. Generally, a femur with a stovepipe canal is more amenable to a cemented femoral component, while a champagne-flute canal will be better suited for a cementless femoral component.

Next, the extent of arthritic involvement in the joint can influence the type of implant selected. In the case of isolated femoral wear, as seen in the early stages of avascular necrosis, some surgeons prefer a resurfacing hemi-

NAME: _____ DATE: _____

HT: _____ WT: _____ M F D.O.B.: _____ SIDE: _____

NEW PATIENT HIP EXAM FORM

1. Pain Degree: None, SL, Mild, Moderate, Marked, Totally Disabled

   Location: Groin, Side, Ant. Thigh, Lat. Thigh, Butt, Knee

   Type: Start up, Walking, Rest, Night, Other: _____

   Particularly painful activities: _____

   _____

2. Limp — 0, SL,, Mod, Sev, Unable to Walk

3. Support — None, Cane long walks, Cane full time, One crutch, Two crutches or walker, Unable to walk

4. Distance Walks — Unlimited, 8 blks, 2-3 blks, 1 blk, Unable

5. Stairs — Normal, FOF w/hand rail, One at a time, Unable

6. Shoes — Easy, difficult, unable

7. Sit — Any 1 h, high 1/2 h, unable

8. Gait — Normal, antalgic, trendelenberg, short leg, other _____

9. Trendelenberg sign: +, −, Level, NT

10. ROM   Right   Left   ROM   Right   Left
    Ext.   _____ _____   AD   _____ _____
    Flex   _____ _____   ER   _____ _____
    AB   _____ _____   IR   _____ _____

11. Tender? Yes, No — If Yes, where?

12. Active SLR painful? Yes, No - If yes, where?

13. Abductor Strength (L) _____   (R) _____

14. Leg lengths: equal, (L) short _____ (R) short _____

15. Pelvic Obliquity: Yes   No

16. Neuro-Vascular:
    Sensation: Intact, decreased where _____
    other: _____ Other:
                    (R)   (L)   PULSES: (R)   (L)
    Motor: EHL's _____   _____   DP   _____ _____
    DTR's: KJ   _____   _____   PT   _____ _____
           AJ   _____   _____   FEM   _____ _____

17. Prior incisions?   Yes   No

18. Outside X-rays: Date   Comments:
                   _____   _____
                   _____   _____
                   _____   _____

Figure 1 Form utilized for documenting basic history and physical examination findings.

arthroplasty (Figure 6), where only the femoral head is resurfaced. In addition, the extent of anatomic distortion also influences the selection of implant. In cases of DDH, where the proximal femur is excessively anteverted, the surgeon may choose a modular or custom prosthesis that allows for derotation of the neck if cementless fixation is used (Figure 7). Furthermore, on the acetabular side, a protrusio configuration can be accommodated with a deeper profile acetabular component (Figure 8). Therefore, any anatomical distortion, whether on the femoral or acetabular side, must be well defined. Numerous implant options are currently available to accommodate specific

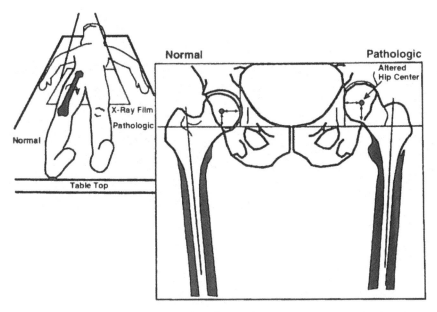

Figure 2 Anteroposterior view of the hip and proximal femur obtained with the leg internally rotated by 15–20 degrees. (From Ref. 6.)

situations, and in many cases specialized implants can minimize the need for either osteotomies or bone grafting procedures.

V.   STEP IV—RADIOGRAPHIC TEMPLATING

Once the specific implant and the type of implant fixation have been selected, the templates specific to that implant are used to determine the approximate sizes and the level of femoral neck resection. The first part of this process begins with the AP pelvic radiograph. A line connecting the base of the two ischial tuberosities is first drawn. If the tuberosities appear asymmetrical, alternatively the interteardrop line (connecting the base of the acetabular teardrops) can be drawn. The distance from either of these lines to a similar point on each lesser trochanter is drawn. The difference between these two distances is the radiographic LLD (Figure 9). The clinical LLD is then compared with the radiographic LLD. A significant difference exists between these two measurements, and it is usually due to pelvic obliquity or to anomalies in the level of the hip. If any pelvic obliquity is present, the desired leg-length correction may be determined by splitting the difference between the clinical and radiographic LLD. It is important to know whether

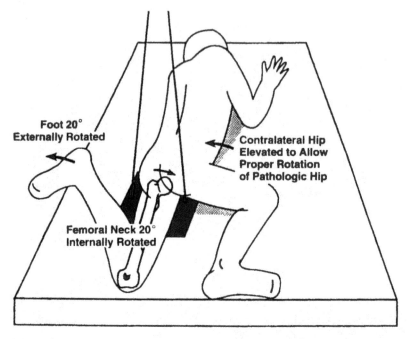

Figure 3 Posteroanterior view of the hip obtained with the patient prone. This is used in case of severe contractures when the patient is unable to internally rotate the leg. (From Ref. 10.)

the pelvic obliquity is fixed or not. In case of a fixed obliquity due to problems above the level of the hip joint—i.e., lumbosacral spine—correcting the measured clinical LLD is more important. Although these individuals may have a greater radiographic LLD, complete correction of this may lead to clinical overlengthening of the limb because of the pelvic obliquity. On the other hand, if the pelvic obliquity is fixed at the hip joint due to ipsilateral hip adduction or abduction contractures, correcting the radiographic LLD is more important, because the obliquity will self-correct through surgical release of the contractures. Therefore the combination of all these factors is essential in establishing the desired leg length gain on the operative hip.

Next, the planned center of the acetabular component is marked after placing the template at a 45 degree angle lateral to the teardrop and minimizing the resection of subchondral bone (3). Conventional implant templates are available generally with 20% magnification, which is typically encountered with most radiographs and confirmed with magnification markers. In the case of a severely deformed hip, the method of Ranawat, where

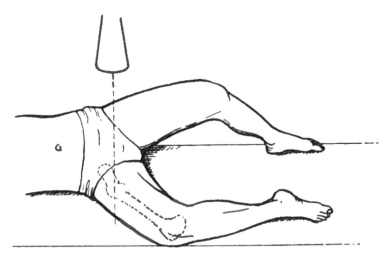

Figure 4 Lowenstein lateral view of the hip and proximal femur. The patient's hip, thigh, and knee are placed flat on the operating table, with the x-ray beam at 90 degrees to the hip. (From Ref. 7.)

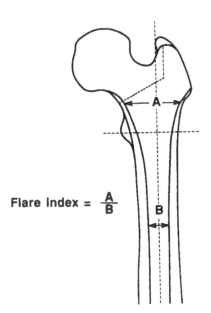

Flare Index = $\dfrac{A}{B}$

Figure 5 The canal flare index as defined by Noble—the ratio of the proximal and distal widths of the medullary canal in the anteroposterior view. (From Ref. 16.)

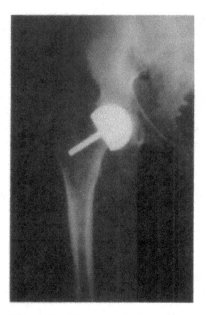

Figure 6 The case of a resurfacing hemiarthroplasty performed in a patient with isolated femoral involvement secondary to avascular necrosis of the hip.

the opposite hip is used as a reference, may serve to determine the center of rotation (Figure 10) (18). The lateral radiograph is then used to assess the level and the extent of bow of the femur. The presence of excessive anteversion of the femoral neck may also be suggested on the lateral radiograph. A computed tomography (CT) scan may be used to document the extent of the anteversion present. The method of correcting for the anteversion may then be selected (covered in Sec. VI, below). The femoral component is then templated on the AP radiograph. Fit and fill are maximized if a cylindrical cementless femoral component is planned and 2–3 mm of cement mantle are taken into account if a cemented component is planned. Conventional femoral component templates are used and the vertical and lateral offset are restored, accounting for the LLD. The planned level of neck resection is then marked on the radiograph, measuring either from the top of the femoral head or from the lesser trochanter (Figure 11) (3,4,6).

VI. SPECIAL CONSIDERATIONS

There are several instances where hip arthritis is secondary to underlying anatomical and biological abnormalities, which present unique problems and

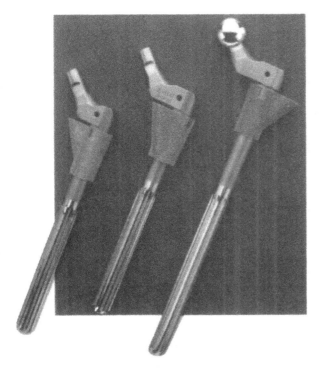

Figure 7 A modular femoral component which allows rotation of the neck and alteration of lateral offset to compensate for variability in anteversion and offset of the proximal femur. (Courtesy of Johnson and Johnson.)

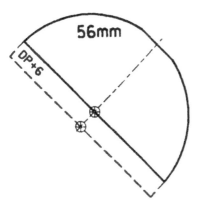

Figure 8 Template of a regular and deep profile acetabular component which allows an additional 6 mm buildout on the acetabulum in cases of protrusio. (Courtesy of Johnson and Johnson.)

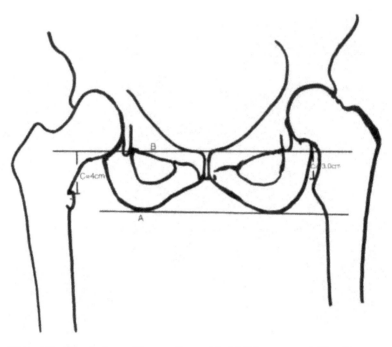

Figure 9 Illustrations of how radiographic LLD is measured. The distance (c) from B (interteardrop line) to the top of the lesser trochanter on each hip is measured. Alternatively, the distance from the transischial line to the top of the lesser trochanter can also be measured. The difference between C on the unaffected and the affected hip is the radiographic LLD.

require specific medical and surgical treatment. Some of the more commonly encountered problems are reviewed here.

The patient's lifestyle and ability to maintain certain positional restrictions after surgery are very important considerations for selecting the surgical approach. Typically, the posterior approach provides an easier and wider exposure of the hip joint, but it is accompanied by a higher dislocation rate. This is especially a problem in an individual who is unable to maintain the positional precautions either due to occupational risk factors or simple noncompliance. In these cases, an anterior or anterolateral surgical approach is preferred. On the other hand, if a significant LLD needs to be corrected, it may be helpful to check the intraoperative status of the sciatic nerve, which is easily done with the posterior approach to the hip joint.

Acetabular protrusio is an anatomical finding encountered in cases of rheumatoid arthritis, ankylosing spondylitis, Paget's disease, and even in

Measurement Method to Determine the
True Acetabular Region and
Approximate Femoral Head Center

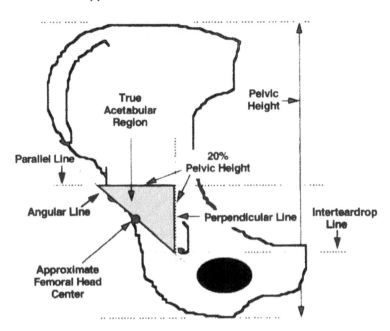

Figure 10   Illustration of how the center of rotation can be measured in the case
of a severely deformed hip by the method of Ranawat. The interteardrop line connecting the base of two acetabular teardrops is drawn. A vertical line is drawn just
lateral to the teardrop and a horizontal line at a vertical distance equaling 20 percent
of the total pelvic height from the interteardrop line is then drawn, and a triangle is
then formed. The approximate center of rotation is at the midpoint of the base of
the triangle. (From Refs. 18 and 20.)

some patients with severe osteoporosis. Radiographic assessment of protrusio is established by noting the extent of femoral head displacement medially
relative to Kohler's line (ilioischial line) or can be defined by a center edge
angle of Wiberg exceeding 35 degrees (Figure 12) (16). Protrusio can be
treated by restoring the center of acetabular rotation to the correct anatomic
position. During surgery, any medial reaming of the acetabulum should be
avoided. Acetabular component fixation is then obtained through good peripheral rim contact with the acetabular bone. Any medial defect can then
be filled with bone graft or by utilizing a deep profile acetabular component,
whose need should be anticipated preoperatively (Figure 13).

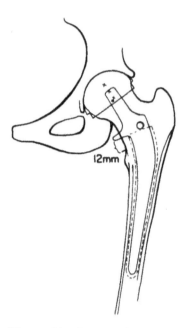

Figure 11   The acetabular component is templated and the center of rotation is marked. The femoral component is then templated and the level of neck resection is measured as the distance from the top of the lesser trochanter. (From Ref. 7.)

Coxa vara is an anatomical abnormality encountered at times. Generally, the surgical goal is to restore the anatomical center of rotation of the hip by the accurate placement of the acetabular component. The femoral component that best restores the host vertical and lateral offset is then selected. The majority of implant manufacturers now have implants with varying offsets and neck shaft angles readily available as off the shelf products for these types of cases (Figure 14).

DDH is a complex problem often encountered during hip replacement surgery. Numerous issues need to be addressed both in preoperative planning as well as during the surgical procedure. The major issues facing the surgeon include LLD, acetabular bone stock, location of acetabular component placement with potential need for structural bone grafting, the correction of excessive femoral anteversion, and the need for a femoral shortening osteotomy. The extent of acetabular dysplasia has been well documented in the Crowe classification (5). Based on the degree of dysplasia, which can range from a slightly shallow acetabulum to a complete dislocated hip, the surgical plan can be the placement of the acetabular component either at the true joint center or in the high hip center position. If a high hip center is used

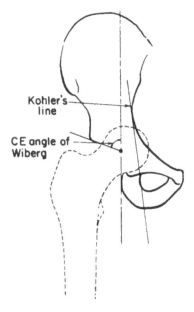

Figure 12 Measurement of protrusio. Acetabular protrusio is present if the femoral head migrates medial to Kohler's line or if the center edge angle is greater than 35 degrees. (From Ref. 7.)

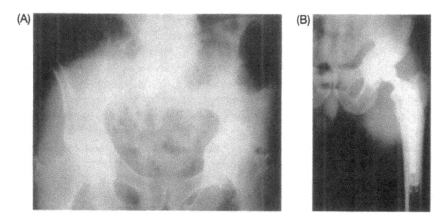

Figure 13 A and B. A patient with acetabular protrusio secondary to rheumatoid arthritis treated with hybrid total hip arthroplasty. A cementless deep profiled acetabular component with some medial bone grafting was used.

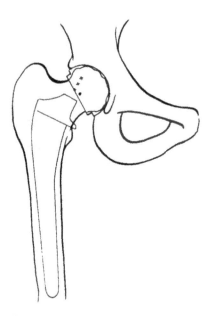

Figure 14 Coxa vara with increased lateral offset. Implants with regular and increased lateral offset are typically available to accommodate these cases. (From Ref. 7.)

(19), the acetabular component is often very small and may require a thin polyethylene liner and smaller femoral head or a very long-necked femoral component with higher risk of impingement and dislocation. In restoring the true hip joint center, the acetabular component is usually very small, or in some cases oblong-shaped and may require structural bone grafting. Other issues include correcting LLDs and the excessive anteversion that is typically present. Femoral osteotomy may be used for shortening and/or for derotation. Modular femoral components can eliminate the need for a derotation osteotomy. Some components have cutting flutes in the stem which can generally provide enough stability to eliminate the need for any additional fixation for stabilizing a shortening osteotomy. Furthermore, in planning for the femoral component, special order components may be required owing to a very small diameter of the femur (Figure 15A to C).

Paget's disease presents both biological and anatomical problems that require special consideration. There is a higher risk of postoperative heterotopic ossification, which can be minimized by pre- and postoperative treatment with bisphosphonates (13). Cemented components are favored to help decrease the amount of surgical blood loss, which is generally higher intra-

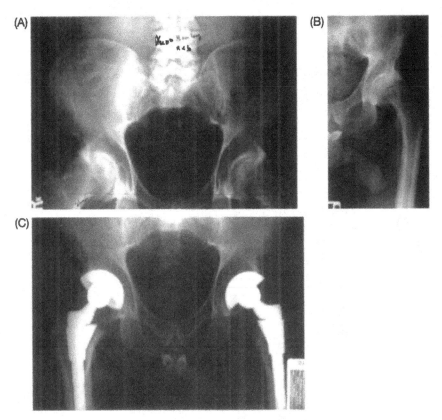

Figure 15 A to C. A patient with bilateral hip arthritis with high lateral offset treated with a modular implant to restore his offset.

operatively. Furthermore, femoral deformities may be present and osteotomies may be necessary to accommodate conventional implants. In some cases, smaller implants may be used to avoid an osteotomy (Figure 16A to C). Also, the bone is often hard and sclerotic, which can make reaming and broaching very difficult (Figure 17A to C).

A very convenient method for comprehensive preoperative planning is the use of a checklist form. A sample form is shown where the selected acetabular and femoral components are noted (Figure 18). Backup implants are also listed in case unexpected intraoperative problems are encountered with the original preoperative plan. The clinical and radiographic LLD is listed along with the desired correction. Any special surgical considerations are also noted. Additionally, specific surgical equipment—such as special drills, high-speed burrs, hardware for internal fixation, extraction devices for retained hardware

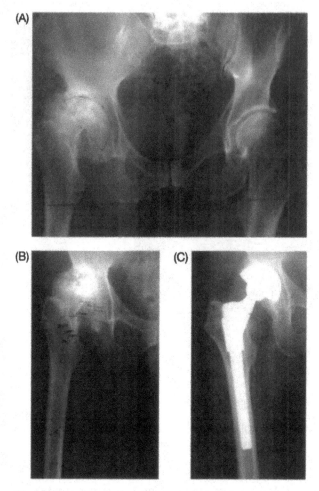

Figure 16 A to C. A patient with severe hip arthritis secondary to DDH. Treatment was undertaken with a modular femoral prosthesis to correct the anteversion and a deep profile acetabular component was used to restore the hip point center.

or a cell saver—are noted. It is also a helpful practice to draw the radiographic templating plan directly on the radiographs with a grease pencil.

VII.   REVISION TOTAL HIP ARTHROPLASTY

Revision hip arthroplasty is discussed separately, as it presents a spectrum of problems that make this one of the biggest challenges in orthopedic sur-

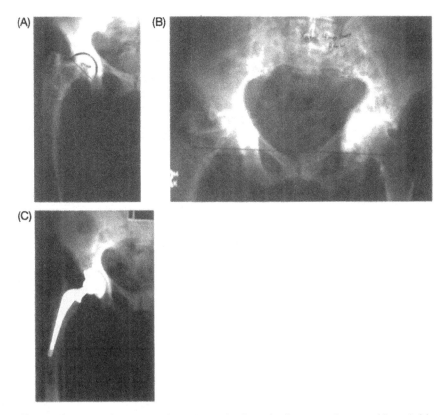

Figure 17 A to C. An elderly patient with Paget's disease and severe hip arthritis who had an angular deformity of the proximal femur. Treatment was undertaken with a hybrid technique and small diameter femoral component was used and osteotomy was avoided in this elderly patient.

gery. These problems include either acetabular or femoral bone loss, bone deformation, compromised soft tissues, and other problems, such as stem fracture and osteolysis, that are unique to revision hip surgery (2). Furthermore, removal of the failed implant either with or without cement also poses an additional challenge, and a variety of specialized techniques with specific tools must be available at the time of the surgical procedure. As a result, a comprehensive preoperative plan is even more important before proceeding with revision hip arthroplasty.

The goals of surgical reconstruction include restoring the hip joint center, establishing bone continuity, providing an implant that is well fixed to the host bone, and using bone graft with favorable biological and me-

HIP FORM

Complete:_____   Date:_____

DR. RAJIT SALUJA, M.D.

Name:_____Surgery Date:_____

TOTAL HIP TEMPLATING

Stem Plan   Manufacturer   Type   Call Rep ?
A.   _____

B/U 1.   _____

B/U 2.   _____

Cup Plan   Manufacturer   Type   Call Rep?
A.   _____

B/U 1.   _____

B/U 2.   _____

Pre-Op Planning Notes:_____

_____

XLLD=:_____CLLD=:_____

Target LL Change:_____

Bone Graft: Iliac Crest Graft_____
          Allograft: Femoral Head_____
          Other: Specify Size & Type_____

          _____

Special Instructions: Other Notes:

Midas Rex   _____

Moreland   _____

Fluoro   _____

Cell Saver   _____

Pelvic Recon plates/screws   _____

Synthese: Large Frag/Small Frag _____
Dall-Miles Cable/Trochanteric grip

Faxed/Called/Slot/Mailed   Date:_____By:_____

Figure 18 A preoperative planning worksheet is utilized which lists the templated implants and the respective backup prosthesis. Both the clinical and radiographic leg-length discrepancy are noted and the desired leg length gain is noted. The need for specialized equipment and bone graft is also noted.

chanical characteristics wherever necessary (2). To accomplish these goals, the five-step approach is again utilized in formulating the surgical plan. As part of the clinical history, it is helpful to obtain previous surgical records if possible. The type and the manufacturer of the existing implant can be identified and specific extraction tools may be available for removal of this implant. Additionally, if only a partial revision is undertaken, the corresponding femoral heads and liners can be ordered. As a part of the physical examination, previous incisions and surgical approaches are noted. Although prior incisions of the hip are less likely to pose any problems as compared with those of the knee, it is generally recommended to avoid crossing previous incisions and leaving any narrow skin bridges (3). Magnification markers are very important in the radiographic assessment. Both the femoral head sizes of the existing implant as well as the femoral canal diameter can be accurately measured. The femoral canal diameter can dictate the type of implant selected. For very large canals, either proximally fixed cementless implants or impaction grafting may be used. The bone defects either on the femoral or acetabular side may be identified on the radiographs. Additional views such as Judet views or CT scans may be done to better identify the defects. Based on the CT scan data, polyurethane models can also be obtained to get a 3D view of the defects (12). Implant selection is based on the goal of attaining maximum stability on host bone. Cementless implants are generally favored for revision surgery, although cement is used with impaction grafting on the femoral side and with reconstruction cages and large structural allografts on the acetabular side. Having various implants available for the revision surgery is generally necessary because unexpected situations are frequently encountered during surgery. Specialized implants such as long-stem femoral components, impaction grafting stems, acetabular reconstruction cages, and constrained acetabular liners can be ordered for the surgical procedure. Various types of bone grafts—such as allograft struts, femoral heads, distal femurs, morcellized bone, and bone graft substitutes —should also be available. Special considerations include appropriate management of underlying diseases and planning the method of removing the existing implants. Many specialized tools, such as mechanical chisels and gouges and ultrasonic cement removal instruments, may be used. In some cases, osteotomy of the femur may also be necessary in order to simplify cement removal, and the length of the osteotomy can be planned on the radiographs preoperatively. A typical revision total hip arthroplasty case is illustrated in Figure 19.

VIII. DISCUSSION

In summary, preoperative planning for THA is an integral part of the procedure and is essential for deciding the correct size and orientation of the components, for minimizing postoperative LLD, and for avoiding potential intraoperative complications. The five-step approach described here is a comprehensive method. A thorough history and physical examination is obtained, along with accurate radiographs with magnification markers. The

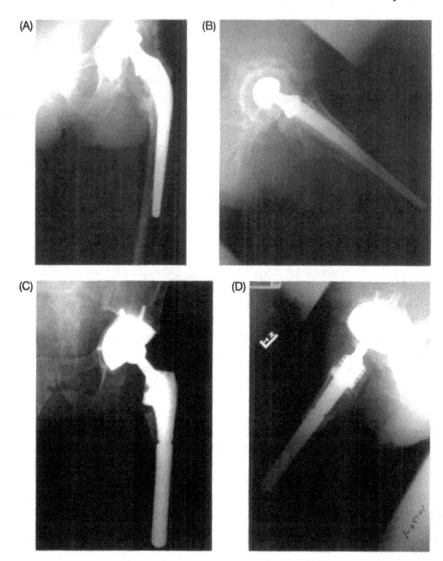

Figure 19 A to D. A typical revision case is shown when loose cemented femoral and acetabular components were revised with larger cementless implants.

implants and the method for implant fixation are then selected and conventional templates are used to template the patient's individual radiographs. Any special anatomical and biological considerations are taken into account and a checklist form is very helpful in organizing the surgical plan. Careful preoperative planning is even more important in revision hip surgery, and the same five steps can be followed. However, at each step, additional factors need to be considered owing to the complexity of the procedures and the need for specialized implants, operative tools, and the surgical approaches utilized.

The value of preoperative planning for THA is well documented (1,3, 4,6,8,11,14,17). In one review, electronically digitized and hand-sketched preoperative plans were compared with postoperative radiographs, and the correct type and size of the prosthesis was planned in greater than 90 percent of cases. The mean postoperative LLD was 0.3 cm clinically and 0.2 cm radiographically, and more than 80 percent of intraoperative difficulties were anticipated (8). A major limitation of preoperative planning is the inaccurate estimation of radiographic magnification, the inability of plain radiographs to fully assess rotational abnormalities in the limb, and inadequate assessment of bone quality from radiographic parameters, which can affect the selection of implant size and the method of fixation (14). Therefore, the development of measurable radiographic techniques, which are reproducible and also provide information on bone quality, is needed for accurate preoperative planning in the future.

REFERENCES

1. Abraham WD, Dimon JH III: Leg length discrepancy in total hip arthroplasty. Orthop Clin North Am 1992;23:201–209.
2. Bierbaum BE, Liebelt RA: Surgical considerations and planning for acetabular and femoral deficiencies in revision hip replacement. Bull Hosp Joint Dis Orthop Inst 1989;49:1–9.
3. Blackley HRL, Howell GED, Rorabeck CH: Planning and management of the difficult primary hip replacement: preoperative planning and technical considerations. Instr Course Lect 2000;49:3–10.
4. Capello WN: Preoperative planning of total hip arthroplasty. Instr Course Lect 1994;43:323–327.
5. Crowe JF, Mani VJ, Ranawat CS: Total hip replacement in congenital dislocation and dysplasia of the hip. J Bone Joint Surg 1979;61A:15–23.
6. D'Antonio JA: Preoperative templating and choosing the implant for primary THA in the young patient. Instr Course Lect 1994;43:339–346.
7. Dore DD, Rubash HE: Primary total hip arthroplasty in the older patient: optimizing the results. Instr Course Lect 1994;43:347–357.

8. Eggli S, Pisan M, Muller ME: The value of preoperative planning for total hip arthroplasty. J Bone Joint Surg 1998;80-B:382–389.
9. Harris WH: Etiology of osteoarthritis of the hip. Clin Orthop 1986;213:20.
10. Engh CA: Recent advances in cementless total hip arthroplasty using the AML prosthesis. Techniques Orthop 1991;6(3):59–72.
11. Jasty M, Webster W, Harris W: Management of limb length inequality during total hip replacement. Clin Orthop Rel Res 1996;333:165–171.
12. John JF, Talbert RE, Taylor JK, Bargar WL: Use of acetabular models in planning complex acetabular reconstructions. J Arthrop 1995;10:661–666.
13. Kaplan FS, Singer FR: Paget's disease of bone: pathophysiology, diagnosis, and management. J Am Acad Orthop Surg 1995;3:336–344.
14. Knight JL, Atwater RD: Preoperative planning for total hip arthroplasty: quantitating its utility and precision. J Arthrop 1992;7:403–409.
15. McCarthy JC, Bono JV, Lee J: The difficult femur. Instr Course Lect 2000;49:63–68.
16. Noble PC: Biomechanical advances in total hip replacement. Biomech Orthop 1992;46–75.
17. O'Toole RV III, Jaramaz B, DiGioia AM III, Visnic CD, Reid RH: Biomechanics for preoperative planning and surgical simulations in orthopaedics. Comput Biol Med 1995;25:183–191.
18. Ranawat CS, Dorr LD, Inglis AE: Total hip arthroplasty in protrusio acetabuli of rheumatoid arthritis. J Bone Joint Surg 62A:1059, 1980.
19. Russotti GM, Harris WH: Proximal placement of the acetabular component in total hip arthroplasty. J Bone Joint Surg 1991;73A:587–592.
20. Stans AA, Pagnano MW, Shaughnessy WJ, Hanssen AD: Results of total hip arthroplasty for Crowe type III developmental hip dysplasia. Clin Orthop Rel Res 1998;348:149–157.

Index